4th Edition

LECTURE NOTES ON
INFECTIOUS
DISEASES

+ INCLUDED

☑ Highlight
☑ General Review
☑ Review Test

Ken K. S. Wang

nfectious diseases stand as a persistent challenge in the realm of public health, necessitating a nuanced and comprehensive understanding for effective management. **"Lecture Notes on Infectious Diseases"** An Introduction emerges as an indispensable cornerstone for students and professionals navigating the intricate landscape of health science. This foundational textbook converges an integrated approach, elucidating the fundamental methodologies inherent in infectious disease epidemiology while concurrently unraveling the social and environmental determinants pivotal in comprehending disease propagation and its impact on population health.

The text unfolds in four discernible parts, accurately dissecting the origins, occurrences, spread, and management of infectious diseases. Delving into the intricacies of disease emergence, modes of transmission, and the multifaceted dimensions of social, behavioral, cultural, and environmental factors influencing communicable spread, this work offers a compelling synthesis of basic science and clinical practice. Each chapter follows a systematic structure, addressing essential components from infectious agent identification to methods of control, all encapsulated within an engaging narrative. This fourth edition, a testament to the commitment to currency and relevance, has been meticulously updated. A novel chapter has been introduced, casting light upon infections in special groups, while modern infectious diseases take center stage. Acknowledging the dynamic nature of the field, the introductory chapter now incorporates contemporary control measures and emerging infections, with additional global occurrence data interwoven into the epidemiological fabric.

The streamlined and improved structure of the text is tailored for facile accessibility, rendering it an invaluable resource for clinical attachments and comprehensive revision. The inclusion of information on fast-evolving topics, such as SARS, MERS, COVID-19, and influenza epidemic underscores the commitment to providing an up-to-date and informative guide. In essence, **Lecture Notes on Infectious Diseases** serves as a succinct yet all-encompassing compendium. Tailored to resonate with public health students, nursing professionals, junior doctors, and allied health practitioners, it beckons as an ideal companion for those seeking a brief introduction or a comprehensive revision of this critical subject.

Dr. Ken K. S. Wang Ph.D.
Department of Public Health
Chung Shan Medical University
July 2024

Ken K. S. Wang

▌ Educational qualifications

Doctor of Science, National Chung Hsing University

Master of Science, Kaohsiung Medical College

Bachelor of Science, Chung Shan Medical College

▌ Academic experiences

Associate Professor, Chung Shan Medical University

Assistant Professor, Chung Shan Medical University

Vector Control Technician (PCO)

Medical Examiner

▌ Current position

Professor, Department of Public Health, Chung Shan Medical University

CONTENTS

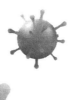

Lecture Notes on
Infectious Diseases

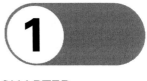

1

CHAPTER

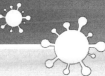

An Introduction to the Infectious Diseases

For Health: A state of complete physical, mental, and social well-being and not merely the absence of disease or infirmity. [The World Health Organization (WHO) defined health in its broader sense in 1946]

An infectious disease is an infection that is capable of spreading from person to person. Not all infections are communicable diseases. The term infectious means communicable. Infectious diseases may be transmitted by many routes: direct person-to-person transfer; respiratory transmission; parenteral inoculation; by way of fomites; sexual or mucosal contact; and by insect vectors. Infectious diseases occur as the result of interactions between pathogenic (disease- producing) microorganisms and the host (Fig. 1-1). All infectious disease begins at some surface of the host, whether it be the external surfaces such as the skin and conjunctiva or internal surfaces such as the mucous membranes of the respiratory tract, intestine, or urogenital tract.

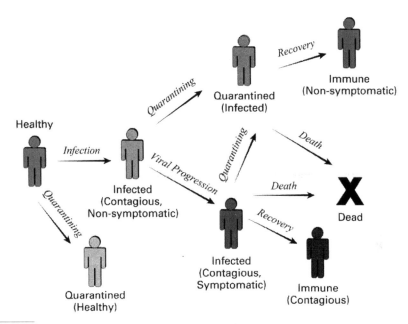

Figure 1-1   Individual infection progression (WHO, 2007)

Infectious disease:

Infectious diseases, also known as communicable diseases or transmissible diseases, are illnesses caused by pathogenic microorganisms such as bacteria, viruses, fungi, or parasites. These microorganisms can be spread from one person to another, from animals to humans, or through contaminated objects or environments. Infectious diseases can range from mild to severe and can affect various parts of the body.

Here are some key points to consider when discussing infectious diseases:

1. **Types of Microorganisms**: Infectious diseases can be caused by different types of microorganisms, including:

- Bacteria: These are single-celled organisms that can multiply rapidly. Most of bacterial infections include tuberculosis, strep throat, and urinary tract infections.

- Viruses: Viruses are much smaller than bacteria and require a host cell to reproduce. Common viral infections include the flu, HIV/AIDS, and COVID-19.

- Fungi: Fungal infections can affect the skin, nails, or internal organs. Fungus infection include athlete's foot and candidiasis (yeast infection).

- Parasites: Parasitic infections are caused by organisms that live in or on a host organism. Malaria, giardiasis, and tapeworm infections are examples of parasitic diseases.

2. **Transmission**: Infectious diseases can spread through various modes of transmission, including:

- Direct Contact: Through physical contact with an infected person, such as touching, kissing, or sexual activity.

- Indirect Contact: Via contaminated surfaces, objects, or food and water.

- Airborne Transmission: Some diseases can spread through respiratory droplets when an infected person coughs or sneezes. which include influenza and tuberculosis.

- Vector-Borne: Certain diseases are transmitted by vectors, such as mosquitoes (malaria, dengue fever) or ticks (Lyme disease).

- Infectious diseases often involve practicing good hygiene, vaccination, safe food and water practices, and avoiding contact with infected individuals or vectors.

3. **Symptoms**: The symptoms of infectious diseases can vary widely but may include fever, fatigue, cough, diarrhea, skin rashes, and more, depending on the specific disease.

4. **Treatment**: Treatment depends on the type and severity of the infection. It may involve antibiotics for bacterial infections, antiviral medications for viral infections, antifungal drugs for fungal infections, or anti-parasitic medications for parasitic diseases.

5. **Global Impact**: Infectious diseases have a significant impact on public health worldwide. Efforts to control and eradicate infectious diseases have led to the development of vaccines, antibiotics, and public health measures that have saved countless lives.

It's important to stay informed about infectious diseases, particularly during outbreaks or pandemics, and to follow guidance from healthcare authorities to prevent their spread. Proper hygiene, vaccination, and early medical intervention are crucial elements in managing and controlling infectious diseases. Understanding the basis of these differences in infectious agent, occurrence, reservoir, mode of transmission, incubation period, period of communicability, susceptibility, and methods of control et al., which are the fundamental goal of this book.

Transmission route:

1. The pathway of causative agents from a source to infection of a susceptible host is called "transmission route". Infectious diseases may be transmitted by many routes, detail as following: Direct Contact Transmission: This occurs when an infected person or animal comes into physical contact with a susceptible host. include:

- Skin-to-skin contact: Touching an infected person's skin or mucous membranes, which can transmit diseases like herpes and scabies.

- Sexual contact: Engaging in sexual activity with an infected person can lead to the transmission of sexually transmitted infections (STIs) such as HIV, syphilis, and gonorrhea.

- Droplet transmission: Respiratory droplets produced when an infected person coughs, sneezes, talks, or breathes can be inhaled by others nearby, leading to diseases like the flu and COVID-19.

2. **Indirect Contact Transmission**: Infectious agents can be transmitted indirectly through contaminated objects or surfaces. include:

- Fomite transmission: Touching contaminated surfaces or objects (e.g., doorknobs, toys, money) and then touching the face or mouth can lead to the transmission of diseases like the common cold and gastrointestinal infections.

- Vehicle-borne transmission: Consuming contaminated food, water, or drugs can result in diseases like food poisoning, cholera, and hepatitis A.

3. **Airborne Transmission**: Some infectious agents can remain suspended in the air for extended periods and be inhaled by individuals who are in close proximity. include:

- Airborne droplet nuclei: Tiny particles that contain infectious agents and can remain suspended in the air for prolonged periods. Tuberculosis is an example of a disease transmitted via airborne droplet nuclei.

- Aerosol transmission: Fine respiratory droplets produced during medical procedures (e.g., intubation, nebulization) can transmit diseases like COVID-19.

4. **Vector-borne Transmission**: Certain infectious agents are transmitted by vectors, which are organisms that can carry and transmit the disease. include:

- Mosquitoes: Mosquitoes can transmit diseases such as malaria, dengue fever, Zika virus, and West Nile virus.

- Cockroaches: Cockroaches are known to be potential vectors for several diseases because they can carry pathogens on their bodies and in their feces. Some of the diseases that cockroaches can transmit Salmonellosis, Dysentery, and Gastroenteritis.

- Ticks: Ticks can transmit Lyme disease and Rocky Mountain spotted fever.

- Fleas: Fleas can transmit the bacterium responsible for bubonic plague.

5. **Vertical Transmission**: Some infectious agents can be passed from a mother to her offspring during pregnancy, childbirth, or breastfeeding. include:

- Mother-to-child transmission (perinatal transmission): HIV, syphilis, and hepatitis B can be transmitted from a mother to her baby during childbirth or breastfeeding.

6. **Blood-borne Transmission**: Exposure to infected blood or blood products can result in the transmission of blood-borne pathogens such as HIV, hepatitis B, and hepatitis C. This can occur through needle stick injuries, transfusions, or sharing of contaminated needles.

Understanding these transmission routes is essential for implementing appropriate prevention measures, such as vaccination, hygiene practices, safe sex practices, and vector control, to reduce the spread of infectious diseases. Public health authorities and healthcare providers play a critical role in educating the public and implementing strategies to mitigate the transmission of infectious agents.

Infectious diseases occur:

Infectious diseases occur as the result of interactions between pathogenic, microorganisms and the host. All infectious disease begins at some surface of the host, whether it be; 1. External surfaces such as the skin and conjunctiva, and 2. Internal surfaces such as the mucous membranes of the respiratory tract, intestine, or urogenital tract.

Infectious diseases kill more than 14 million people each year, mainly in the developing world. In these countries, approximately 46% of all deaths are due to infectious diseases, and 90% of these deaths are attributed to acute diarrhea and respiratory infections of children, AIDS, tuberculosis, malaria, measles, and recent SARS. Other diseases, that rarely kill, maim millions. Large populations living in remote areas of the developing world are at risk of disabling diseases, such as poliomyelitis, leprosy, lymphatic filariasis, and onchocerciasis. For these diseases, the toll of suffering and permanent disability is compounded by a double economic burden (Fig. 1-2).

For all these reasons, concern about the impact of infectious diseases has increased, with some encouraging results. Lack of access to effective vaccines and drugs has been a long-standing problem in the developing world. Major new initiatives, including the Global Fund to Fight AIDS, Tuberculosis and Malaria, the Global Alliance for Vaccines and Immunization, and the Roll Back Malaria and Stop TB partnerships, have formed to attack the main infectious diseases that kill and are delivering badly needed drugs and vaccines. The concern of international community is also evident in time-limited drives to eradicate or eliminate polio, leprosy, lymphatic filariasis, onchocerciasis and other diseases that maim. While microbial agents will always deliver surprises, the shock of SARS has encouraged a number of countries to give infrastructures for protecting public health much higher priority. All health care will benefit.

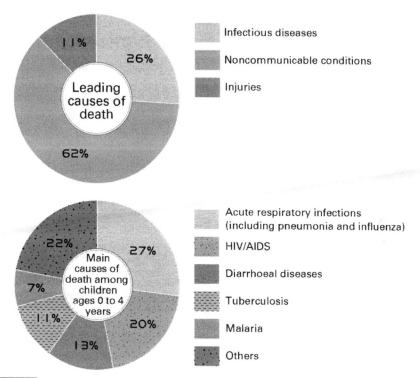

Figure 1-2   The trend of global infectious disease (JICA, 2004) (www.jica.jp/english/publications/report/network/archive_20 04/vol_24_3.html)

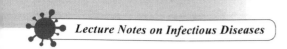

The impact of infectious diseases:

Lack of access to effective vaccines and drugs has been a long-standing problem in the developing world. The major new initiatives from non-government organism that including 1. The Global Fund to Fight AIDS, Tuberculosis and Malaria, 2. The Global Alliance for Vaccines and Immunization, and 3. The Roll Back Malaria and Stop TB partnerships, which have formed to attack the main infectious diseases that kill and are delivering badly needed drugs and vaccines.

Causes of infectious disease:

An infection is a disease caused by a pathogen. The human body is colonized on the skin and mucosal surfaces with numerous microorganisms that form the normal flora of the body. In order to cause infectious disease a pathogen must accomplish the following: It must enter the host, it must metabolize and multiply on or in the host tissue, it must resist host defenses, and it must damage the host. The simple illustration as follows:

Infectious dose of microbe → (Contact) → Portal of entry → (Invasion) → Host defense barrier → Body compartment → Target tissue → Portal of exit → Microbe spreads to other host.

An infection is a disease caused by a pathogen. The human body is colonized on the skin and mucosal surfaces with numerous microorganisms that form the normal flora of the body.

The medical terms of infection:

The medical terms used in discussion of infectious diseases are constantly changing to keep pace with changes in our knowledge and understanding. We will start by defining some of the common terms used in this book.

1. **Communicable disease:** an infection that is capable of spreading from person to person.

2. **Epidemiology:** the study of the distribution and determinants of diseases in population.

3. **Incubation period:** is the time interval between initial contact with the infectious organism and the first appearance of symptoms associated with the infection.

4. **Infection:** a disease caused by a pathogen.

5. **Infectious agent:** identifies the specific agent or agents causing the disease; classifies the agent; and may indicate its important characteristics.

6. **Infectiousness:** the ease with which a pathogen can spread in a population.

7. **Methods of control:** contain preventive measures and control of patient, contacts and the immediate environment.

8. **Mode of transmission:** describes the mechanisms by which the infectious agent is spread to humans.

9. **Occurrence:** provides information on where the disease is known to occur. Information on past and current outbreaks may also be included.

10. **Outbreak:** an occurrence of a disease clearly in excess of normal expectancy.

11. **Pathogen:** an organism that can invade the body and cause disease.

12. **Pathogenicity:** the ability to cause disease.

13. **Period of communicability:** is the time during which an infectious agent may be transferred directly or indirectly from an infected person

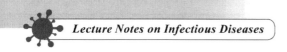

to another person; from an infected animal to humans; or from an infected person to animals, including arthropods.

14. **Quarantine**: Isolation or restriction of the movement of individuals who have been exposed to a contagious disease to prevent its spread.

15. **Reservoir:** indicates any person, animal, arthropod, plant, substance in which an infection agent normally lives and multiplies, on which it depends primarily for survival, and where it reproduces itself in such a manner that it can be transmitted to a susceptible host.

16. **Susceptibility:** provides information on human or animal populations at risk of infection, or that are resistant to either infection or disease. Information on subsequent immunity consecutive to infection is also given.

17. **Vaccination (Immunization)**: The process of administering a vaccine to stimulate the immune system's response to a specific pathogen, providing immunity against future infections.

18. **Vector:** a living creature that can transmit infection from one host to another.

19. **Virulence:** a pathogen's power to cause severe disease.

20. **Zoonosis:** an animal disease that can spread to humans.

Clinical aspects of infectious disease:

Fever, pain, and swelling are the universal signs of infection. Beyond this, the particular organs involved and the speed of the process dominate the signs and symptoms of disease. Cough, diarrhea, and mental confusion represent disruption of three different body systems. On the basis of clinical experience, physicians have become familiar with the range of behavior of the major pathogens. However, signs and symptoms overlap considerably. Skilled physicians use this knowledge to begin a deductive process leading to a list of suspected pathogens and strategy to make a specific diagnosis and provide patient care. Through the probability assessment, an understanding of how the diseases work is a distinct advantage in making the correct decisions.

🔖 Reporting of communicable diseases:

Reporting of some communicable diseases is required within countries and in some instances internationally to world health organization (WHO). Reporting can take the form of either a case report or an outbreak report.

- **Class I:** Case report required internationally to WHO by the international health regulations or as a disease under surveillance by WHO.

- **Class II:** Case report regularly required wherever the disease occurs.

- **Class III:** Selectively reportable in recognized endemic areas.

- **Class IV:** Obligatory report of outbreaks only – no case report required.

- **Class V:** Official report not ordinarily justifiable.

- **Case reports:** Case reporting provides diagnosis, age, sex and date of **onset** for each person with the disease. Sometimes it includes identifying information such as the name and address of the person with the disease. Additional information such as treatment provided, and its duration are required for certain case reports. If there is a requirement for international case reporting, national governments report to WHO.

- **Outbreak reports:** Outbreak reporting provides information about an increase above the expected number of persons with a communicable disease that may not be included in the list of diseases officially **reportable**, or it may be of unknown etiology if it is newly recognized or emerging. If there is a requirement for outbreak reporting, international national governments report to WHO (Tab. 1-1).

Infectious diseases remain as important and fascinating as ever. Where else do we find the emergence of new diseases, together with improved understanding of the old ones? At a time when the revolution in molecular biology and genetics has brought us to the threshold of new and novel means of infection control, the perpetrators of bioterrorism threaten us with diseases we have already conquered. Meeting this challenge requires a secure knowledge of the pathogenic organisms and how they produce disease, as well as an understanding of the clinical aspects of those diseases. In the collective judgment of the authors, this book presents the principles and facts required for students of Public Health to understand the most important infectious diseases.

Table 1-1   Current WHO phases of pandemic alert (WHO, 2007)

Phase	Definition	Level
Interpandemic phase New virus in animals, no human cases	Low risk of human cases	1
	Higher risk of human cases	2
Pandemic alert New virus causes human cases	No or very limited human-to- human transmission	3
	Evidence of increased human-to- human transmission	4
	Evidence of significant human-to- human transmission	5
Pandemic	Efficient and sustained human-to- human transmission	6

General review

1. Communicable disease:

2. Pathogenicity:

3. Virulence:

4. Zoonosis:

5. Fever:

6. Pain:

7. Swelling:

8. Cough:

9. Diarrhea:

10. Mental confusion:

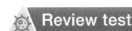 **Review test**

SCAN ME

Check Your Answers

I. Multiple-choice questions (four selected one):

1. ( ) Infectious diseases can be transmitted through various routes, including: (A) parenteral inoculation, (B) by way of fomites, (C) sexual or mucosal contact, (D) all of the above

2. ( ) In many developing countries, approximately what percentage of all deaths are attributed to infectious diseases? (A) 15%, (B) 25%, (C) 36%, (D) 46%

3. ( ) The study of the distribution and determinants of diseases in a population is known as: (A) communicable disease, (B) epidemiology, (C) infection, (D) mode of transmission

4. ( ) The ability of a pathogen to cause severe disease is often referred to as its: (A) communicable disease, (B) epidemiology, (C) virulence, (D) susceptibility

5. (　) A case report must be submitted to the WHO either in accordance with the International Health Regulations or as part of a disease under surveillance by WHO, depending on its classification: (A) class I, (B) class II, (C) class III, (D) class V

6. (　) Among the thousands of species of viruses, bacteria, fungi, and parasites, only a small fraction are associated with any form of disease. What are these referred to as? (A) antigen, (B) pathogen, (C) virulence, (D) infectious disease

7. (　) What is the term for the route taken by causative agents from their source to the infection of a susceptible host? (A) infecting, (B) infectious disease, (C) transmission route, (D) occurrence

8. (　) Which of the following provides information on human or animal populations susceptible to infection, or those that exhibit resistance to either infection or disease? (A) susceptibility, (B) occurrence, (C) medical news, (D) outbreak

9. (　) What term is used to describe the practice of isolating or restricting the movement of individuals who have been exposed to a contagious disease in order to prevent its spread? (A) Infectiousness, (B) Quarantine, (C) Prevention, (D) Isolation

10. (　) Which of the following terms describes the mucous membranes of the respiratory tract, intestine, or urogenital tract? (A) external surfaces, (B) external skin, (C) Internal membrane, (D) Internal surfaces

II. Simple answer:

1. To cause an infectious disease, a pathogen must have accomplished which 4 steps?

2. Would you please tell me the clinical aspects of infectious disease?

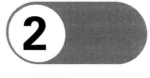

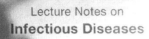

Lecture Notes on
Infectious Diseases

The Infectious Disease Process

INTRODUCTION

The infectious disease process provides a scientific explanation for the factors that determine the relationships among humans, the many microorganisms that are in the environment, and normal flora. There are many variables that determine the relationship between microorganisms and human host. This interaction has illustrated in various ways, including the epidemiologic chain; **Host** ←→ **Agent** ←→ **Environment**. The chain portrays the three key elements in infection – agent, host, and environment – and their dynamic interaction. This model demonstrates this interaction for other types of disease as well. In this chapter, we discuss specific characteristics or changes in any one of the three elements that can lead to the development of an infectious disease. In order to cause infectious disease a pathogen must accomplish the following: 1) It must enter the host, 2) It must metabolize and multiply on or in the host tissue, 3) It must resist host defenses, 4) It must damage the host.

The infectious disease process commences when an individual encounters a disease-causing pathogen. This pathogen gains entry into the body, metabolites and multiplies within host tissues, and often triggers the host's immune system, leading to the emergence of symptoms such as fever, pain, swelling, fatigue, and inflammation. The course of the infection can vary, with some individuals recovering due to the effective elimination of the pathogen by their immune systems, while others may experience a progression of the disease marked by more severe symptoms and potential complications. Some infectious diseases are contagious, allowing transmission to others through various means. Successful recovery frequently results in immunity against the same pathogen, providing protection against future infections.

In conclusion, the infectious disease process is a multifaceted sequence triggered by pathogen exposure. It encompasses invasion, immune response, symptom development, and diverse outcomes. It highlights the significance of vaccination, hygiene, and public health in disease prevention and management.

2-1 Types of Infection

The term infection refers to the presence and multiplication of microorganisms in the tissue of a host. The host's response to this invasion and replication varies. When there are signs and symptoms caused by this invasion, such as fever, swelling, pain, and inflammation, we recognize these as characteristics of infection. Some infectious diseases are evident and produce acute signs and symptoms. Infectious diseases occur as the result of interactions between pathogenic (disease-producing) microorganisms and the host. All infectious disease begins at some surface of the host, whether it be the external surfaces such as the skin and conjunctiva or internal surfaces such as the mucous membranes of the respiratory tract, intestine, or urogenital tract. The types of infection content as follows:

1. **Infection:** It can result in little or no illness.

2. **Acute infection:** Has a short and relatively severe course. For example, Streptococcal pharyngitis (Sore throat caused by *Streptococcus pyogenes*).

3. **Chronic infection:** Has a long duration. For example, Tuberculosis is caused by *Mycobacterium tuberculosis*.

4. **Fulminating infection:** Occurs suddenly and with severe intensity. For example, Cerebrospinal meningitis is caused by *Neisseria meningitidis*.

5. **Localized infection:** Restricted to a limited area of the body. For example, Urinary tract infection is caused by *Escherichia coli*.

6. **Generalized infection:** Affects many or all parts of the body. For example, Blood infections, such as typhoid fever is caused by *Salmonella typhi*.

7. **Mixed, or polymicrobial infection:** More than one kind of microorganism contributes to the infection. For example, Gaseous gangrene, in which a combination of *Clostridium* species may occur.

8. **Primary infection:** An initial localized infection that decreases resistance and thus paves the way for further invasion by the same microorganisms. For example, Viral influenza.

9. **Secondary infection:** Infection that is established after a primary infection has caused a decreased resistance. For example, Pneumococcal pneumonia is following viral influenza.

10. **Inapparent infection:** It is termed subclinical, and the individual is sometimes referred to as a carrier.

11. **Carrier:** It can be asymptomatics, but infectious to others.

12. **Horizontal transmission:** It is direct or indirect infection from person-to-person.

13. **Vertical transmission:** It is direct infection, which occur from transplacentally, during birth, or through breast milk.

14. **Zoonotic transmission:** It is direct or indirect infection from animals to humans.

15. **Opportunistic Infections:** These occur in individuals with weakened immune systems, often seen in people with HIV/AIDS or undergoing immunosuppressive treatments.

16. **Hospital-Acquired Infections (Nosocomial Infections):** Infections acquired in healthcare settings, such as surgical site infections and bloodstream infections.

17. **Latent Infections:** In some cases, pathogens can remain dormant in the body for an extended period before becoming active, as seen in latent tuberculosis infection.

2-2   Chain of Infection

The interaction among the agent, the host, and the environment leading to infection has been described in a model called the chain of infection (Fig. 2-1).

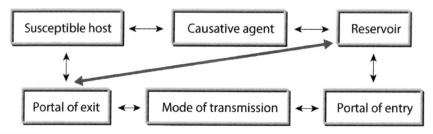

Figure 2-1   The chain of infection

The "Chain of Infection" is a model used in healthcare and epidemiology to understand and break down the various elements necessary for an infection to occur and spread. It consists of a series of interconnected links, each of which represents a crucial step in the transmission of infectious diseases. By identifying and disrupting these links, healthcare professionals can implement strategies to prevent infections. Specific conditions and characteristics affecting each element in the chain and element's interaction with the other elements determine whether an infection will result.

The traditional Chain of Infection consists of six links:

1. **Causative agent:** This is the first link in the chain and represents the pathogen (e.g., bacteria, virus, fungus, parasite) responsible for causing the infection. Understanding the nature of the infectious agent helps in developing targeted interventions.

2. **Reservoir:** The reservoir is the second link and refers to the source of the infectious agent. This can be a person, animal, or environment where the pathogen resides and multiplies. For example, humans can be

reservoirs for diseases like COVID-19, while animals like bats can be reservoirs for diseases like Ebola.

3. **Portal of exit:** This link describes how the pathogen leaves the reservoir. Common portals of exit include respiratory secretions (e.g., coughing, sneezing), bodily fluids (e.g., blood, saliva), and feces. Identifying these routes helps in infection control.

4. **Mode of transmission:** The fourth link outlines how the pathogen is transmitted from the reservoir to a susceptible host. Transmission can occur through various means, including direct contact, droplets, airborne particles, contaminated surfaces (fomites), or vectors (e.g., mosquitoes carrying malaria). Preventing transmission is a key focus in infection control.

5. **Portal of entry:** Once the pathogen is transmitted, it needs a way to enter a susceptible host. This is represented by the fifth link. Common portals of entry include the mouth, nose, eyes, and broken skin. Understanding these entry points helps in designing protective measures.

6. **Susceptible host:** The final link in the chain is the person or organism that is at risk of becoming infected. Factors influencing susceptibility include the individual's overall health, immunization status, and genetic factors. Reducing susceptibility through vaccination and maintaining good health is a key strategy in infection prevention.

2-3 Mode of Transmission

The mechanism by which an organism moves from the portal of exit or environmental reservoir through a susceptible host's portal of entry is referred to as the mode of transmission.

Table 2-1   The common routes of transmission

Route of exit	Route of transmission	Example
Respiratory	Aerosol droplet inhalation	Influenza virus
Salivary	Direct salivary transfer; animal bite	Oral-labial herpes Rabies
Gastrointestinal	Stool-hand-mouth Stool-object-mouth	Enterovirus infection; hepatitis A
Skin	Skin discharge-air-respiratory tract; skin to skin	Human papilloma virus; syphilis
Blood	Transfusion or needle prick; Insect bite	Hepatitis B; AIDS; malaria; relapsing fever
Genital secretions	Urethral or cervical secretions; semen	Gonorrhea; herpes simplex; CMV
Urine	Urine-hand-catheter	Hospital-acquired urinary tract infection
Eye	Conjunctival	Adenovirus
Zoonotic	Animal bite; contact with carcasses; arthropod	Rabies; tularemia; plague; Lyme disease

1. **Respiratory spread:** Many infections are transmitted by the respiratory route, often by aerosolization of respiratory secretions with subsequent inhalation by others. Droplet particle in diameter: 100 um: requires only seconds to fall the height of a room. 10 um: remains airborne for about 20 minutes. 0.6-5.0 um: attach to mucous sites at various levels along the URT or LRT.

2. **Salivary spread:** Transmission of infectious secretions, are by direct contact with the nasal mucosa or conjunctiva. Above often accounts for the rapid dissemination of agents such as respiratory syncytial virus (RSV) and adenovirus.

3. **Fecal-Oral spread:** Fecal-oral spread involves direct or finger-to-mouth spread, the use of human feces as a fertilizer, or fecal contamination of food or water. Reduced gastric hydrochloric acid can facilitate enteric infections.

4. **Skin-to-Skin transfer:** Skin is the portal of entry, such as: Syphilis, caused by *Treponema pallidum*, Impetigo, caused by strains of gr. A Streptococci, Ringworm and athlete's foot that caused by dermatophyte fungi.

5. **Blood-borne transmission:** Blood-borne transmission may caused by Insect vector, human blood transfusions, illicit drugs by intravenous or subcutaneous route, and using shared non-sterile equipment. Hepatitis B and C viruses as well as HIV were frequently transmitted in this way prior to the institution of blood screening tests.

6. **Genital transmission:** Spread can occur between sexual partners or from or from the mother to the infant at birth. A major factor in these infections has been the persistence, high rates of asymptomatic carriage, such as *Chlamydia trachomatis*, cytomegalovirus (CMV), herpes simplex virus (HSV), and *Neisseria gonorrhoeae*.

7. **Eye-to-Eye transmission:** Infections of the conjunctiva may occur in epidemic or endemic form. Epidemics of adenovirus and *Haemophilus* conjunctivitis may occur and highly contagious. The major endemic disease is trachoma, caused by *Chlamydia*.

Understanding the mode of transmission is essential for developing appropriate preventive measures, including vaccination, hand hygiene, respiratory etiquette, and the use of personal protective equipment (PPE). Public health interventions also play a crucial role in controlling the spread of infectious diseases, especially during outbreaks and pandemics.

General review

1. Acute infection:

2. Chronic infection:

3. Fulminating infection:

4. Localized infection:

5. Generalized infection:

6. Polymicrobial infection:

7. Inapparent infection:

8. Horizontal transmission:

9. Vertical transmission:

10. Blood-borne transmission:

11. Opportunistic Infections:

12. Nosocomial Infections:

Review test

SCAN ME

Check Your Answers

I. Multiple-choice questions (four selected one):

1. (   ) What is the first step in the infectious disease process? (A) Metabolization and multiplication, (B) Damage to the host, (C) Entry into the host, (D) Resistance to host defenses

2. (   ) What symptoms are commonly associated with the host's immune response during an infectious disease? (A) Headache and dizziness, (B) Fever, pain, swelling, and fatigue, (C) Loss of appetite and insomnia, (D) Skin discoloration and joint stiffness

3. (　) Why is successful recovery from an infectious disease often associated with immunity against the same pathogen? (A) The pathogen becomes weaker after an infection, (B) The immune system adapts and becomes stronger, (C) The host develops tolerance to the pathogen, (D) The pathogen is eliminated by antibiotics

4. (　) What distinguishes chronic infections from acute infections? (A) Severity of symptoms, (B) Duration of illness, (C) Generalized nature, (D) Sudden onset

5. (　) Which infectious disease has a sudden onset and severe intensity? (A) Tuberculosis, (B) Streptococcal pharyngitis, (C) Urinary tract infection, (D) Cerebrospinal meningitis

6. (　) What characterizes a localized infection? (A) Affects many parts of the body, (B) Has a short and severe course, (C) Is restricted to a limited area of the body, (D) Results in little or no illness

7. (　) What characterizes a mixed or polymicrobial infection? (A) Infection caused by a single microorganism, (B) More than one kind of microorganism contributing to the infection, (C) Infection that occurs horizontally, (D) Infection acquired in healthcare settings

8. (　) Which type of infection serves as an initial localized infection that paves the way for further invasion by the same microorganisms? (A) Secondary infection, (B) Inapparent infection, (C) Opportunistic infection, (D) Primary infection

9. ( ) What is the term for an individual who is asymptomatic but can infect others? (A) Carrier, (B) Latent carrier, (C) Inapparent carrier, (D) Symptomatic carrier

10. ( ) How is horizontal transmission of infection defined? (A) Infection from animals to humans, (B) Infection that occurs during birth, (C) Direct or indirect infection from person to person, (D) Direct infection from transplacentally

11. ( ) What characterizes opportunistic infections? (A) They are caused by a single microorganism, (B) They occur in individuals with weakened immune systems, (C) They are acquired in healthcare settings, (D) They result from vertical transmission

12. ( ) Which link in the Chain of Infection involves understanding the nature of the infectious agent to develop targeted interventions? (A) Reservoir, (B) Portal of exit, (C) Causative agent, (D) Mode of transmission

13. ( ) What is the reservoir in the context of the Chain of Infection? (A) The person or organism at risk of becoming infected, (B) The source of the infectious agent, (C) The route through which the pathogen leaves the reservoir, (D) The portal of entry for the pathogen

14. ( ) How is the mode of transmission defined in the Chain of Infection? (A) The person or organism at risk of becoming infected, (B) The route through which the pathogen leaves the reservoir, (C) How the pathogen is transmitted from the reservoir to a susceptible host, (D) The nature of the infectious agent

15. (   ) Which size range of droplet particles, when aerosolized, remains airborne for about 20 minutes? (A) 100 um, (B) 10 um, (C) 5.0 um, (D) 0.6 um

16. (   ) What is the primary mode of transmission for infections such as respiratory syncytial virus (RSV) and adenovirus? (A) Respiratory spread, (B) Salivary spread, (C) Fecal-oral spread, (D) Blood-borne transmission

17. (   ) How does fecal-oral spread typically occur? (A) Skin-to-Skin transfer, (B) Respiratory spread, (C) Direct contact with nasal mucosa, (D) Direct or finger-to-mouth spread

18. (   ) Which infection is primarily transmitted through skin-to-skin contact as the portal of entry? (A) Hepatitis B, (B) Impetigo, (C) Respiratory syncytial virus (RSV), (D) Ringworm

19. (   ) What is a common factor contributing to blood-borne transmission of infections? (A) Insect vector, (B) Direct contact with nasal mucosa, (C) Use of human feces as fertilizer, (D) Shared non-sterile equipment

20. (   ) Which infection can be transmitted between sexual partners or from the mother to the infant at birth? (A) Trachoma, (B) Hepatitis B, (C) Cytomegalovirus (CMV), (D) Ringworm

II. Simple answer:

1. Please provide an example of a generalized infection and the microorganism responsible for it.

2. Please provide an example of a latent infection and explain its characteristics.

3. Please explain the significance of identifying the portal of exit in the Chain of Infection and provide an example of a common portal of exit.

4. Please explain the significance of reduced gastric hydrochloric acid in facilitating enteric infections through fecal-oral spread.

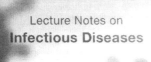

Lecture Notes on
Infectious Diseases

3

CHAPTER

Gastrointestinal Tract Infectious Diseases

The alimentary tract is the passageway from the mouse to the anus. It is a major route for pathogens to enter the body. The system is composed of the mouth and saliva producing glands, esophagus, stomach, small intestine, liver, pancreas, and large intestine (Fig. 3-1). The gastrointestinal (GI) tract is a complex and vital system responsible for the ingestion, digestion, absorption, and elimination of food and waste products in the human body. It is a long, continuous tube that starts at the mouth and ends at the anus. This system plays a central role in nourishing the body by breaking down food into nutrients that can be absorbed and utilized for energy and other physiological functions. In intestine, the normal fasting stomach is devoid of microorganisms, which make up about one-third of the weight feces.

Gastrointestinal infections (infectious intestinal disease) can be acquired directly, through the ingestion of contaminated food or water, or may be spread from person to person through contact with infected body fluid such as feces or vomit. Poor personal hygiene or food-handling practices in the kitchens of a hospital or nursing home can cause outbreaks of infection affecting large numbers of patients and stuff. Measures to prevent cross-infection are also particularly important as contact with body fluids and the movement of staff and equipment between patients may greatly facilitate the transmission of gastrointestinal infections.

Gastrointestinal infections, often referred to as GI infections or stomach infections, are a group of diseases that affect the digestive system, primarily the stomach and intestines. These infections can be caused by various microorganisms such as bacteria, viruses, parasites, and sometimes fungi. They are a common global health concern, leading to a significant burden of illness and healthcare costs.

The familiar G.I. tract infectious diseases in Taiwan contain cholera, poliomyelitis, typhoid fever, paratyphoid fever, Shigellosis, amoebiasis, EHEC, and enteroviruses groups. G.I. tract infectious diseases can be caused by viruses, bacteria, protozoans, parasites and other diseases and inevitably cause diarrhea.

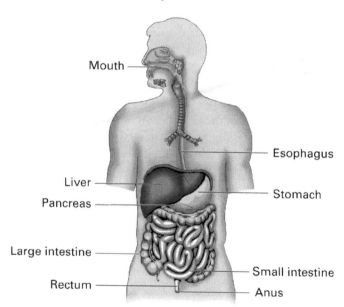

Figure 3-1　The alimentary tract is the passageway from the mouth to the anus. It is a major route for pathogens to enter the body.

This chapter focuses on microorganisms that cause food-borne infection and how the principles of food hygiene, and environmental hygiene should be used to prevent infection. It also considers other gastrointestinal pathogens associated with outbreaks of infection in communities and the infection control precautions required to prevent their transmission. Practicing good hygiene and safe food handling, along with early diagnosis and appropriate treatment, are key strategies for controlling these infections.

3-1 Cholera (ICD-9 001; ICD-10 A00)

 Highlight

1. *Vibrio cholerae*, cholera toxin, enterotoxin
2. Acute bacterial enteric disease, profuse watery stools
3. Rapid dehydration, acidosis, circulatory collapse
4. Fatality rate may exceed 50%

Cholera is a highly contagious and potentially life-threatening bacterial infection caused by the bacterium *Vibrio cholerae*. It is primarily characterized by severe diarrhea and dehydration and can lead to rapid and severe illness if left untreated.

Vibrio cholerae is a Gram-negative bacterium that produces cholera toxin, an enterotoxin, whose action on the mucosal epithelium lining of the small intestine is responsible for the characteristic massive diarrhea of the disease. In its most severe forms, cholera is one of the most rapidly fatal illnesses known, and a healthy person may become hypotensive within an hour of the onset of symptoms; infected patients may die within three hours if treatment is not provided. In a common scenario, the disease progresses from the first liquid stool to shock in 4 to 12 hours, with death following in 18 hours to several days without rehydration treatment.

In spite of its rarity in developed countries, cholera is still an important infection worldwide. It may occur as part of an epidemic or arise sporadically in the developing world, particularly in parts of Africa, Asia, and the Caribbean. It can lead to large-scale epidemics with substantial morbidity and mortality. It is occasionally found in travelers returning from endemic countries. Cholera is an acute bacterial enteric disease with sudden onset, profuse watery stools, occasional vomiting, rapid dehydration, acidosis and circulatory collapse. Asymptomatic infection is much more frequent than clinical illness (O139), especially with organisms of the El Tor biotype.

Identification to the Cholera:

Mild cases with only diarrhea are common, particularly among children. In severe untreated cases, death may occur within a few hours and the case fatality rate may exceed 50%; with proper treatment, the rate is below 1%. In epidemics, once laboratory confirmation and antibiotic sensitivity have been established, it becomes unnecessary to confirm all subsequent cases. Shift should be made to using primarily the clinical case definition proposed by WHO as follows: 1) Disease unknown in area: severe dehydration or death from acute watery diarrhea in a patient aged 5 or more. 2) Endemic cholera: acute watery diarrhea with or without vomiting in a patient aged 5 or more. 3) Epidemic cholera: acute watery diarrhea with or without vomiting in any patient. However, monitoring an epidemic should include laboratory confirmation and antimicrobial sensitivity testing of a small proportion of cases on a regular basis.

The clinical symptoms of choler:

1. **Profuse diarrhea**: Cholera is characterized by sudden and severe watery diarrhea, often described as "rice water" stools. The diarrhea is odorless, grayish-white, and may contain mucus.

2. **Dehydration**: Rapid fluid loss from diarrhea and vomiting can lead to dehydration. Signs of dehydration include dry mouth, sunken eyes, reduced skin elasticity, and extreme thirst.

3. **Vomiting**: Cholera-infected individuals may also experience vomiting, which can contribute to fluid loss and dehydration.

4. **Muscle cramps**: Dehydration and electrolyte imbalances can lead to muscle cramps.

5. **Rapid heart rate**: An increased heart rate (tachycardia) may be present due to the body's attempt to compensate for fluid loss.

6. **Low blood pressure**: In severe cases, cholera can cause low blood pressure and shock, leading to organ failure and death if not treated promptly.

Infectious agent:

Only *Vibrio cholerae* serogroups O1 and O139 are associated with the epidemiological characteristics and clinical picture of cholera. *Vibrio cholera* serogroup O1, which includes the serologically indistinguishable classical and El Tor biotypes and either Inaba or Ogawa serotypes. These organisms elaborate the same enterotoxin so that the clinical pictures are similar. Presently the El Tor biotype is predominant in Taiwan. The infectious dose of *Vibrio cholreae* O1 is 10^6-10^8 organisms, which varies with vehicle of transmission and gastric acidity.

Occurrence:

During the 19th century pandemic cholera repeatedly spread from India to most of the world. Since 1992 serotype O139 organisms sporadic imported cases have continued to occur among travelers returning Asia. *V. cholerae* O139 almost completely replaced *V. cholerae* O1 strains in hospitalized cholera patient and in samples of surface water. The epidemic continued to spread through 1994, with cases of O139 cholera reported from 11 countries in Asia. This new strain was soon introduced into other countries by infected travelers, but secondary spread outside of Asia has not been reported and *V. cholerae* O139 remains confined to the southeastern areas of the Asian continent. According to the report from WHO, overall cholera cases, 54% of cases were reported from Africa, 13% from Asia and 32% from Hispaniola (Fig. 3-2) (WHO, 2017).

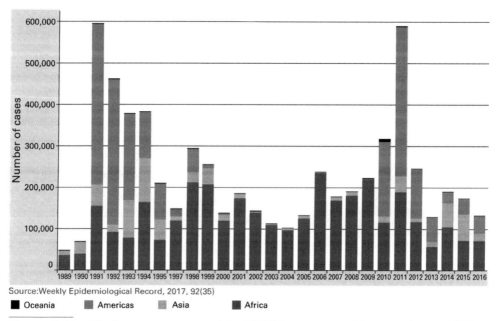

Source:Weekly Epidemiological Record, 2017, 92(35)

■ Oceania ■ Americas ■ Asia ■ Africa

Figure 3-2 Cholera cases report to WHO by year and by continent 1989-2016 (WHO, 2017).

▶ Reservoir:

Man (environments). Recent observations in the USA, Australia and Taiwan suggest presence of environmental reservoirs. The author believes that the natural reservoir of cholera is aquatic environments, especially brackish and coastal waters.

Mode of transmission:

Cholera is acquired through ingestion of an infective dose of contaminated food or water and can be transmitted through many mechanisms. The transmission ways include: Ingestion of water contaminated with feces, vomits of patients, feces of carries, and ingestion of food which had been contaminated by dirty water, feces, soiled, hand, or flies. Study report been indicated El Tor organisms can persist in water for long periods and multiply in moist leftover food. Raw or uncooked sea foods from polluted eaters caused outbreaks or epidemics in Asia. Cases have been reported Ping-ton epidemic was traced to eating at home-prepared bullfrogs taken from pond and estuary water contaminated with *V. cholerae*, serotype Inaba in Taiwan. Clinical cholera in endemic areas is usually confined to the lowest socioeconomic groups.

Incubation period:

It is from a few hours to 5 days, usually 2-3 days.

Period of communicability:

It is presumably for the duration of the stool-positive stage, usually only a few days after recovery. The carrier state may persist for several months. Effective antibiotics, e.g., tetracycline, shorten the period of communicability. Chronic biliary infection, lasting for years, has been observed in adults, associated with intermittent shedding of vibrios in the stool.

Susceptibility and Resistance:

Variable, the achlorhydria increases risk of disease. Clinical cholera usually is confined to the lowest socioeconomic group. Infection results in a rise in agglutinating, vibriocidal and antitoxic antibodies and increased resistance to reinfection which lasts longer against the homologous serotype. In endemic area, most persons acquire antibodies by early adulthood.

Methods of control:

Oral cholera vaccines (OCVs), such as Vaxchora, Dukoral, ShanChol, and Euvichol-Plus, have become available on the international market, offering a crucial means of combating cholera. These vaccines are characterized by their safety and effectiveness in providing significant protection against cholera, particularly for several months, especially when caused by O1 strains (Tab. 3-1). While OCVs are increasingly utilized in various contexts, they are notably favored by travelers from more developed nations who seek to safeguard themselves against cholera exposure during trips to high-risk areas. Additionally, OCVs are strategically deployed in outbreak settings and among high-risk populations, playing a pivotal role in curbing the spread of cholera during outbreaks and contributing to the overall prevention and control of this infectious disease.

Isolation and Quarantine measures play a pivotal role in managing cholera cases effectively. When dealing with cholera patients, it is imperative to promptly isolate them while ensuring access to crucial medical care and rehydration therapy. Oral rehydration solutions (ORS) or intravenous fluids are vital for replenishing lost fluids and electrolytes, addressing dehydration. In severe cases, the administration of antibiotics is recommended to expedite recovery and reduce the severity of the illness. Hospitalization of severely ill patients, with appropriate enteric precautions, is advisable, although strict isolation is typically not necessary. Instituting quarantine measures for close contacts of cholera patients is a proactive step in containing potential outbreaks. Additionally, reporting cholera cases to the local health authorities is universally required under the International Health Regulations, specifically classified as Class 1, to facilitate timely response and comprehensive public health management.

Table 3-1   Characteristics of oral cholera vaccines

Vaccine name (Manufacturer)	How given	Number of doses recommended	Age range	How long vaccination is effective	Available in the US?
Vaxchora (Emergent BioSolutions)	By mouth	1 dose	2-64 years	At least 3-6 months	Yes
Dukoral (SBL Vaccines)	By mouth	2 doses, given1-6 weeks apart (Children aged 2-5 years need 3 doses, given 1 to 6 weeks apart)	2 years and older	2 years	No
ShanChol* (Sanofi Healthcare India Private Limited)	By mouth	2 doses, given at least 2 weeks apart	1 year and older	At least 3 years for 2 doses; short-term protection for 1 dose	No
Euvichol-Plus (EuBiologics)	By mouth	2 doses, given at least 2 weeks apart	1 year and older	At least 3 years for 2 doses; short-term protection for 1 dose	No

* Shanchol and Euvichol-Plus use the same vaccine formula but are produced by different makers. These vaccines are currently available for mass vaccination campaigns.

Source: Centers for Disease Control and Prevention, National Center for Emerging and Zoonotic Infectious Diseases (NCEZID), Division of Foodborne, Waterborne, and Environmental Diseases (DFWED), August 7, 2023

The most useful measure in preventing the spread of cholera is provision of safe drinking water and sanitary disposal of human feces. Food likely to be contaminated, especially fish and shellfish, should be thoroughly cooked before eating. Travel and trade restrictions between countries are not effective.

General review

1. Cholera

2. *Vibrio cholerae*

3. enterotoxin

4. Profuse watery stools

5. Rapid dehydration

6. Acidosis

7. Circulatory collapse

8. Asymptomatic infection

9. Chronic biliary infection

10. Achlorhydria (Gastric anacidity)

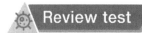 Review test

SCAN ME

Check Your Answers

I. Multiple-choice questions (four selected one):

   1. ( ) *Vibrio cholerae* can produce enterotoxin, which acts on which part of the small intestine? (A) mucus membrane, (B) mucosal squamous lining, (C) mucosal columnar lining, (D) mucosal epithelium lining

2. (　) How long is it possible for a person infected with cholera to survive without treatment? (A) 3 hours, (B) 6 hours, (C) 12 hours, (D) 48 hours

3. (　) In a common scenario, how long does it take for cholera to progress from the first liquid feces to shock? (A) 3 hours, (B) 4-12 hours, (C) 24 hours, (D) 24-48 hours

4. (　) What is the infectious dose of Vibrio cholerae O1? (A) 10^3-10^5, (B) 10^6-10^8, (C) 10^{10}-10^{12}, (D) 10^{12}-10^{16} organisms

5. (　) To which group among the following is clinical cholera usually confined? (A) the lowest socioeconomic group, (B) traveller group, (C) aged under 5 group, (D) aged over 65 group

6. (　) Cholera is one of the most rapidly fatal illnesses known, and how long does it take for a healthy person to become hypotensive after the onset of symptoms? (A) 1 hour, (B) 2 hours, (C) 4 hours, (D) 8 hours

7. (　) Cholera is an acute bacterial enteric disease with what kinds of symptoms? (A) sudden onset, (B) profuse watery stools, (C) acidosis and circulatory collapse, (D) all of the above.

8. (　) The case fatality rate of cholera may exceed how much? (A) 15%, (B) 30%, (C) 50%, (D) 80%

9. (　) Which of the following is the transmission route of cholera? (A) vomits of patients, feces of carriers, (B) ingestion of food contaminated by dirty water, (C) flies spread, (D) all of the above

10. (　) How long is the usual incubation period for cholera infection? (A) 4 hours, (B) 12 hours, (C) 2-3 days, (D) 4-5 hours

II. Simple answer:

1. Could you please provide me with clinical publications about a cholera-infected patient?

2. Could you please provide me with the transmission mode of cholera?

3. What are the most useful measures in preventing the spread of cholera?

3-2   Poliomyelitis (ICD-9 045; ICD-10 A80)

 Highlight

1. Poliomyelitis
2. Polioviral fever, infantile paralysis
3. Aseptic meningitis
4. Fecal-oral transmission; FOT
5. Vaccination: OPV; Sabin, IPV; Salk

Poliomyelitis, often called polio or infantile paralysis, is an acute viral infectious disease spread from person to person, primarily via the fecal-oral route. The term derives from the Greek polio (πολιός), meaning "grey", myelon (μυελός), referring to the "spinal cord", and -itis, which denotes inflammation. Although around 90% of polio infections have no symptoms at all, affected individuals can exhibit a range of symptoms if the virus enters the blood stream. In fewer than 1% of cases the virus enters the central nervous system, preferentially infecting and destroying motor neurons, leading to muscle weakness and acute flaccid paralysis. Different types of paralysis may occur, depending on the nerves involved. Spinal polio is the most common form, characterized by asymmetric paralysis that most often involves the legs. Bulbar polio leads to weakness of muscles innervated by cranial nerves. Bulbospinal polio is a combination of bulbar and spinal paralysis.

Polio has been known to humanity for thousands of years, with historical records describing outbreaks of a polio-like illness dating back to ancient civilizations. Major polio epidemics occurred in the late 19th and early 20th centuries, leading to significant disability and death among affected populations. Until recently (2007), polio was the commonest worldwide cause of paralysis and limb-wasting in young age groups. By 1958, the Taiwan Provincial Department of Health finally imported the Salk vaccine and started a free Salk vaccination program in large counties and cities. In 1965, Taiwan Provincial Department of Health promoted the full implementation of the oral Sabin vaccine (OPV) until now, and the disease in Taiwan was eradicated in the year of 2000. As of my last knowledge update in September 2023, polio cases had been reduced dramatically worldwide, with only a handful of countries reporting endemic cases. Continued vaccination efforts and surveillance are crucial to achieving complete global eradication.

Identification to the poliomyelitis:

Poliovirus infection occurs in the GI tract with spread to the regional lymph nodes and, in a minority of cases, to the central nervous system. Flaccid paralysis occurs in less than 1% of poliovirus infections; over 90% of infections are either inapparent or result in a nonspecific fever. Aseptic meningitis occurs in about 1% of infections. Poliomyelitis is acute viral infection with severity ranging from inapparent infection to a nonparalytic febrile illness, to an aseptic meningitis, to paralytic disease and possible death. Polio symptoms can vary widely, and many cases are asymptomatic.

In cases where symptoms do appear, they may include Fever, Fatigue, Headache, Stiff neck and pain in the limbs, Muscle weakness or paralysis (usually asymmetric, affecting one limb more than the other), Loss of muscle reflexes, Muscle pain and spasms.

Polio must now be distinguished from other paralytic conditions by isolation of virus from stool. Other enteroviruses (notably types 70 and 71), echoviruses and coxackieviruses can illness simulating paralytic poliomyelitis. The most frequent cause of acute flaccid paralysis (AFP) that must be distinguished from poliomyelitis and Guillain-Barre syndrome (GBS) (Tab. 3-2). Paralysis in GBS is typically symmetrical and may progress for periods as long as 10 days. The fever, headache, nausea, vomiting and pleocytosis characteristic of poliomyelitis are usually absent in GBS; high protein and low cell counts in the CSF and sensory changes are seen in the majority of GBS cases. Acute motor axonal neuropathy (China paralytic syndrome) is an important cause of AFP in northern China and is probably present elsewhere; it is seasonally epidemic and closely resembles poliomyelitis.

Table 3-2   Differences between Polio and Guillain-Barre syndrome

Neurological Conditions	Polio (poliomyelitis)	GBS (Guillain-Barré syndrome)
Cause	caused by infection with the poliovirus, which is a type of enterovirus	an autoimmune disorder. It often occurs following an infection, such as a RT or GI infection
Onset	symptoms typically develop rapidly after infection. A sudden onset of muscle weakness or paralysis	usually has a relatively sudden onset, with symptoms progressing over a period of days or weeks

Neurological Conditions	Polio (poliomyelitis)	GBS (Guillain-Barré syndrome)
Muscle Involvement	Polio primarily affects motor neurons in the spinal cord, leading to muscle weakness and, in severe cases, paralysis	GBS affects peripheral nerves outside the spinal cord and brain, leads to a symmetrical muscle weakness in the legs
Sensory Symptoms	Polio primarily affects motor function and may not involve significant sensory symptoms	GBS can involve sensory symptoms such as tingling, numbness, and pain in addition to muscle weakness
Recovery	some individuals with polio may experience partial or complete recovery over time, but others may have permanent paralysis	many people with GBS experience significant recovery with appropriate medical treatment and rehabilitation
Vaccination	can be prevented through vaccination	GBS is not preventable through vaccination

🔵 Infectious agent:

The poliovirus belongs to the Enterovirus genus, which is part of the Picornaviridae family. Polio is a highly contagious virus that primarily affects the nervous system, specifically the spinal cord, leading to symptoms that can range from mild or asymptomatic to severe paralysis. Poliovirus types I, II and III; all types cause paralysis. Type I is the most paralytogenic, that most frequently causes epidemics. Type III is less frequently, and type II uncommonly. Most vaccine-associated cases are due to type II or III.

▣ Occurrence:

Poliomyelitis occurred worldwide. Before large-scale immunization programs were carried out, the highest incidence of clinically recognized disease was in temperate zones and in the more developed countries, occurring as sporadic cases and in small epidemics. The diseases are more common during summer and early autumn in temperate climates.

Poliomyelitis remains primarily a disease of infants and young children. In the few remaining endemic countries, 80-90% of cases are under 3 and virtually all cases under 5. Clusters of susceptible persons, including groups that refuse immunization, minority populations, migrants and other unregistered children, nomads, refugees and urban poor are at high risk. While wild poliovirus cases decreased, there were occasional outbreaks of vaccine-derived poliovirus (VDPV) in various parts of the world. VDPV cases occurred when the live, attenuated virus in the oral polio vaccine mutated and caused paralysis. These cases required a public health response to stop the spread.

▣ Reservoir:

Man only, most frequently persons with inapparent infections, especially children. Long-term carriers have not been found. Fly may play as a mechanical carrier.

▣ Mode of transmission:

Poliovirus is primarily person-to-person spread, principally through the fecal-oral route; direct contact through close association. In rare instances milk, foodstuffs and other fecally contaminated materials have been incriminated as vehicles. During epidemics, pharyngeal spread and throat secretions are become relatively more important. It's important to note that not everyone who is infected with the poliovirus develops symptoms or becomes paralyzed. Many individuals who contract the virus remain asymptomatic or experience mild, flu-like symptoms. However, they can still excrete the virus and potentially spread it to others.

🔋 Incubation period:

It is commonly 7-14 days for paralytic cases, with a range of 3 to possibly 35 days.

🔋 Period of communicability:

It is not precisely defined, but transmission is possible as long as the virus is excreted. Poliovirus is demonstrable in throat secretions as early as 36 hours and in the feces 72 hours after exposure to infection in both clinical and inapparent cases. The virus persists in the throat for approximately 1 week and in the feces for 3-6 weeks or longer. Cases are probably most infectious during the first few days before and after onset of symptoms.

🔋 Susceptibility and resistance:

Susceptibility to polio refers to an individual's vulnerability to contracting the poliovirus and developing the disease. Individuals who have not been vaccinated against polio or have not received the recommended number of vaccine doses are more susceptible to the virus. Polio primarily affects young children, with the highest susceptibility occurring in infants and toddlers. Older individuals are generally less susceptible because they may have acquired immunity through vaccination or previous exposure to the virus.

Type-specific resistance of lifelong duration follows both clinically recognizable and inapparent infection. Second attacks are rare and result from infection with poliovirus of a different type. Infants born of immune mothers have transient passive immunity to paralysis. An increased susceptibility to paralytic poliomyelitis is associated with pregnancy.

Resistance to polio involves the ability of an individual or a population to prevent infection or minimize the severity of the disease. Key factors contributing to resistance include vaccination, herd immunity, improved sanitation and hygiene.

❶ Methods of control:

Vaccination: Advantages of oral poliovaccine (OPV; Sabin), which can be administered orally, confers mucosal as well as systemic immunity, and the vaccine could infects and immunizes close contacts. Disadvantages of poliovaccine (IPV; Salk), which must be kept refrigerated, three doses are needed, there is a small risk of mutation to virulence, and paralytic disease, and the vaccine is infectious within the family and the community (Tab. 3-3).

Table 3-3   Inactivated *v.s.* attenuated vaccines

	Inactivated IPV (Formalin treated)	Live attenuated OPV
Cost	Higher (Greater mass required)	Lower (Agent replicates in the body)
Administration	Parenteral	Oral
Adjuvant	Need	Not needed
Stability	Good	Poor
Reversion	Absent	Possible
Immunity	Mucosal immunity absent	Mucosal immunity present
	Antibody-mediated	Antibody-mediated and cytotoxic T cells
	Short-lasting	Long-lasting

Although polio remains endemic in many Asian countries, it has been virtually eradicated in most developing countries, notably in the Americas, Europe, and Taiwan. The WHO aims to eliminate polio globally by the year 2000. Polio is a notifiable disease. Case should be isolated in hospital. In an outbreak, extensive virus circulation usually precedes the first case; a single case of indigenously acquired polio requires vaccination of a wide network of contacts. Global annual reported cases of Poliomyelitis and immunization coverage (3rd dose); number of reported cases is less than 10,000, and immunization coverage rate are close to 90% (Fig. 3-3).

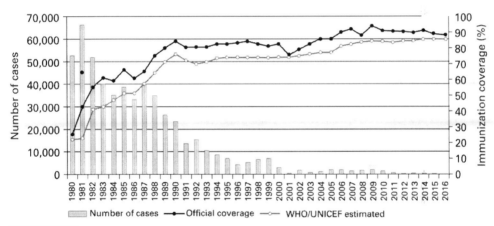

Figure 3-3   Global annual reported cases of Poliomyelitis and immunization coverage (3rd dose) between 1980-2016 (WHO, 2017).
(www.who.int/immunization/monitoring_surveillance/burden/diphtheria/en/index.html)

⚕ General review

1. Poliomyelitis

2. Infantile paralysis

3. Enteroviral infection

4. Aseptic meningitis

5. Flaccid paralysis

6. Anterior horn region

7. OPV

8. IPV

⚕ Review test

SCAN ME

Check Your Answers

I. Multiple-choice questions (four selected one):

1. ( ) In which year was poliomyelitis eradicated in Taiwan and reported to the WHO? (A) 1990, (B) 1995, (C) 2000, (D) 2005.

2. ( ) Among the three types of poliovirus, which type is the most paralytogenic? (A) type I, (B) type II, (C) type III, (D) both type I and type II.

3. ( ) Which types of poliovirus are responsible for most polio vaccine-associated cases? (A) type I, (B) type II, (C) type III, (D) type II or type III

4. ( ) In temperate climates, during which season is the prevalence of poliomyelitis more common? (A) spring, (B) summer, (C) autumn, (D) summer and early autumn

5. ( ) During which stage of the following are poliomyelitis cases most likely to be infectious? (A) the first few days after infection, (B) before onset of symptoms, (C) after onset of symptoms, (D) B and C

6. ( ) What percentage of people infected with polio are approximately asymptomatic? (A) >90%, (B) 70%, (C) 35%, (D) <1%

7. ( ) How many cases of poliomyelitis involve the poliovirus entering the CNS, preferentially infecting and destroying motor neurons? (A) 90%, (B) 70%, (C) 35%, (D) <1%.

8. ( ) In both clinical and inapparent cases, for how long can poliovirus be confirmed to persist in throat secretions? (A) 12 hours, (B) 24 hours, (C) 36 hours, (D) 72 hours

9. ( ) In both clinical and inapparent cases, how long can poliovirus be confirmed to persist in feces? (A) 12 hours, (B) 24 hours, (C) 36 hours, (D) 72 hours

10. ( ) Which of the following is associated with an increased susceptibility to paralytic poliomyelitis? (A) inactivated polio vaccine, (B) live attenuated polio vaccine, (C) pregnancy, (D) all of the above.

II. Simple answer:

1. According to a report from the Ministry of Health and Welfare, in which year was polio eradicated in Taiwan?

2. Could you please provide me with the time frame of poliomyelitis occurrence in Taiwan?

3. Could you please explain the transmission mode of poliomyelitis?

4. Please provide a detailed comparison of the advantages and disadvantages of the Sabin and Salk vaccines.

3-3

Typhoid Fever (ICD-002.0; ICD-10 A01.0)
Paratyphoid Fever (ICD-9 002.1-002.9; ICD-10 A01.1-A01.4)

 Highlight

1. Typhoid fever (enteric fever, bilious fever or Yellow Jack)
2. Enteric fevers are mainly associated with travel
3. Water borne disease
4. Typhoid fever is a systemic bacterial disease
5. Constipation more commonly than diarrhea
6. Fecal carriers are more common than urinary carriers
7. Immunization programmes; Vi vaccine, WCK vaccine

Typhoid fever, also known as enteric fever, bilious fever or Yellow Jack, is an illness caused by the bacterium *Salmonella enterica* serovar Typhi. Common worldwide, it is transmitted by the ingestion of food or water contaminated with feces from an infected person. The bacteria then multiply in the blood stream of the infected person and are absorbed into the digestive tract and eliminated with the waste. The organism is a Gram-negative short bacillus that is motile due to its peritrichous flagella. The bacteria grow best at 37°C (human body temperature).

Salmonella infections are important to appreciate the difference between salmonella food poisoning, and typhoid and paratyphoid fevers caused by specific enteric fever salmonellae. The food-poisoning organisms infect both human and animals, and are biochemically and clinically distinct from "enteric" salmonellae which are exclusively human pathogens. This disease is characterized by a range of symptoms, including high fever, abdominal pain, and gastrointestinal disturbances. Typhoid fever has been a significant public health concern throughout history and continues to be a health issue in many parts of the world, particularly in regions with poor sanitation and limited access to clean drinking water.

▶ Identification to the typhoid fever:

Typhoid fever is also known as enteric fever or typhus abdominalis. Enteric fevers are mainly associated with travel. It is a systemic bacterial disease with insidious onset of sustained high fever (103-104°F (39-40°C)), marked headache, abdominal pain (the lower right quadrant is common), gastrointestinal symptoms (include diarrhea or constipation, nausea, vomiting, and loss of appetite), malaise, anorexia, relative bradycardia, splenomegaly, nonproductive cough in the early stage of the illness, rash (rose spots on their chest or abdomen), and involvement of the lymphoid tissues. Patients often experience extreme weakness and fatigue. Inapparent or mild illnesses occur, especially in endemic area; 60-90% of patients with typhoid fever do not receive medical attention or are treated as outpatients. Mild cases show no systemic involvement; the clinical picture is that of gastroenteritis.

Paratyphoid fever, also known as paratyphoid, is an infectious disease caused by the bacterium Salmonella enterica. This bacterium consists of several serotypes, and two of these, *Salmonella* Paratyphi A and *Salmonella*

Paratyphi B, are responsible for causing paratyphoid fever. This illness is similar in many ways to typhoid fever, but it is generally less severe. The ratio of disease caused by *Salmonella* enterica subsp. *enterica serova* Typhi, (commonly the latter not italicized) to that caused by *S*. Paratyphi A and B is about 10:1. Relapses occur in approximately 3-4% of cases.

Infectious agents:

Salmonella typhi, the typhoid bacillus. Presently 106 types can be distinguished by phage typing, of value in epidemiological studies. In the recently proposed nomenclature for *Salmonella* the agent formerly known as *S. typhi* is called *S. enterica* subsp. *enterica* serovar Typhi (commonly *S.* Typhi). For paratyphoid fever, mainly *S.* Paratyphi A and Paratyphi B.

Occurrence:

The occurrence of typhoid fever varies widely across the world, and it is influenced by factors such as sanitation practices, access to clean water, healthcare infrastructure, and vaccination coverage. Typhoid fever is most common in regions with poor sanitation and limited access to clean drinking water. It tends to be endemic in parts of South Asia, Southeast Asia, sub-Saharan Africa, and some parts of South America. In these areas, the disease can be relatively common and may occur throughout the year. Travelers who visit regions where typhoid fever is endemic or where outbreaks are occurring may contract the disease. Travel-related cases can occur in individuals from countries with better sanitation and healthcare systems when they are exposed to contaminated food or water while abroad.

In Taiwan the number of sporadic cases has remained relatively constant for several years and, with development of sanitary facilities and detection and treatment of cases and carriers, has been virtually eliminated from many areas. Most cases now represent importation from endemic areas. At present, most of typhoid and paratyphoid confirmed cases belong to imported cases in Taiwan, especially foreign workers and those returning to Southeast Asia, but there are still sporadic cases occur annually domestic (Centers for Disease Control, R.O.C., Taiwan) (Fig. 3-4, 3-5).

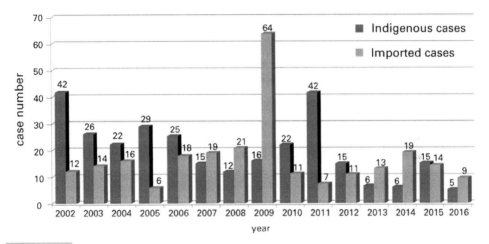

Figure 3-4   Typhoid Fever Confirmed Cases in Taiwan, 2002-2016.

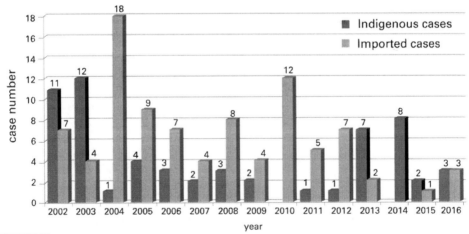

Figure 3-5   Paratyphoid Fever Confirmed Cases in Taiwan, 2002-2016.
(http://www.cdc.gov.tw/english/info.aspx?treeid=e79c7a9e1e
9b1cdf&nowtreeid=e02c24f0dacdd729&tid=58E17AB0E98687
80)

Paratyphoid fever is most commonly reported in regions with limited access to clean water and poor sanitation, similar to typhoid fever. It tends to occur in the same endemic regions as typhoid fever, particularly in parts of: South Asia, Southeast Asia, Sub-Saharan Africa, and South America. Of the 3 serotypes, paratyphoid B is most common, A less frequent and C caused by *S.* Paratyphi C extremely rare. In China and Pakistan more cases have been reported as caused by *S.* Paratyphi than *S.* Typhi.

▶ Reservoir:

Man, both patients and especially carriers. Family contacts may be transient carriers. In most parts of the world fecal carriers are more common than urinary carriers.

A carrier state may follow acute illness or mild or even subclinical infections. In most parts of the world short-term fecal carriers are more common than urinary carriers. The chronic carrier state is most common (2-5%) among persons infected during middle age, especially women; carriers frequently have biliary tract abnormalities including gallstones, with *S.* Typhi located in the gallbladder.

Mary Mallon (1870-1938) was nicknamed "Typhoid Mary". Mary Mallon was an Irish-born woman who immigrated to the United States in the late 19th century. She worked as a cook and became known as a skilled and sought-after cook in the New York City area. She was a carrier of Salmonella Typhi, the bacterium responsible for typhoid fever. Although she never showed any symptoms of the disease herself, she shed the bacteria in her feces and, possibly, her urine. Mary Mallon worked in various households as a cook, and wherever she went, outbreaks of typhoid fever tended to follow. Multiple people in the households where she worked fell ill with the disease, and some died. In 1907, health authorities in New York

City began to investigate the source of the typhoid outbreaks. After extensive testing, Mary Mallon was identified as an asymptomatic carrier of the bacteria. She was placed in quarantine to prevent further transmission. She was forcibly quarantined as a carrier of typhoid fever in 1907 for three years and then again from 1915 until her death in 1938 (Fig. 3-6).

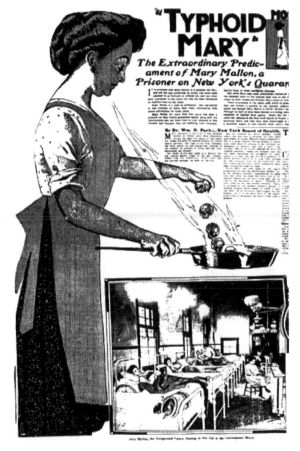

Figure 3-6   Mary Mallon (1870-1938) was nicknamed "Typhoid Mary".
(Typhoid Mary: An Urban Historical publisher=Anthony
Bourdain Hardcover. New York. 2001:148. ISBN 1582341338)

⬧ Mode of transmission:

It is ingestion of food and water contaminated by feces and urine of patients or carriers. Shellfish taken from sewage-contaminated beds and raw fruits, vegetables, milk and milk products contaminated usually by hands of carriers or missed cases are important vehicles in some part of the world. Flies can infect foods in which the organisms may multiply to achieve an infective dose.

Epidemiological data suggest that, while waterborne transmission of *S.* Typhi usually involves small inocula, foodborne transmission is associated with large inocula and high attack rates over short periods.

⬧ Incubation period:

Depends on size of infecting dose and host factors; usual range 8-14 days. The incubation period for paratyphoid is 1-10 days.

⬧ Period of communicability:

It is as long as typhoid bacilli appear in excreta; usually from the 1st week throughout convalescence. About 10% of untreated patients will discharge bacilli for 3 months after onset of symptoms. About 2-5% untreated patients become permanent carriers. Fewer persons infected with paratyphoid organisms may become permanent gallbladder carriers.

⬧ Susceptibility and resistance:

Susceptibility is general; it is increased in individuals with gastric achlohydria. Relative specific resistance follows recovery from clinical disease. In endemic areas attack rates usually decline with age.

🔹 Methods of control:

Prevention is based on access to safe water and proper sanitation as well as adhesion to safe food handling practices. Patient isolation, enteric precaution while ill; hospital care is desirable during acute illness. Inoculation with typhoid vaccine is advised for international travelers to endemic areas. The choice of antibiotic for enteric fevers lies between ciprofloxacin, high dose amoxicillin, co-trimoxazole and chloramphenicol.

Typhoid Vaccines: The use of typhoid vaccines is a primary method of preventing typhoid fever. There are two types of typhoid vaccines available:

1. **Inactivated Typhoid Vaccines**: These are administered as a shot. The Vi capsular polysaccharide vaccine (Typhim Vi or Typherix) and the Vi-conjugate vaccine (TCV) are examples of inactivated vaccines. Vi-polysaccharide vaccine, given in a single 0.5 ml dose, provide protection equivalent to whole-cell vaccine. A booster is recommended after 3 years. They provide protection against *Salmonella* Typhi, the bacterium that causes typhoid fever.

2. **Oral Typhoid Vaccines**: The live attenuated Ty21a vaccine (Vivotif) is administered orally in multiple doses. It offers protection against both *Salmonella* Typhi and *Salmonella* Paratyphi A. Oral Ty21a live vaccine, given in three doses of one capsule each on alternative days. Booster doses are recommended at yearly intervals.

👍 General review

1. Enteric fever, Typhus abdominalis

2. Bradycardia

3. Splenomegaly

4. Constipation

5. *Salmonella typhi*

6. Fecal carriers, urinary carriers

7. F.O.T.

8. Vi typhoid vaccine

9. WCK typhoid vaccine

10. Paratyphoid fever: Mild and asymptomatic infections.

11. *Salmonella paratyphi* A. B. C.

12. Serotype paratyphoid B is most common

13. Gastroenteritis

SCAN ME

Check Your Answers

Review test

I. Multiple-choice questions (four selected one):

1. (　) The characterized and clinical publication of typhoid fever are? (A) fever and headache, (B) general malaise and anorexia, (C) rose spots on trunk and nonproductive cough, (D) all of the above.

2. (　) The reservoirs of typhoid fever transmission are? (A) patients, (B) family contacts, (C) fecal carriers, (D) all of the above.

3. (　) In the USA, Canada, and Taiwan, paratyphoid fever is infrequently identified. Among the three varieties, which serotype is the most common? (A) paratyphoid A, (B) paratyphoid B, (C) paratyphoid C, (D) paratyphoid A and B

4. (　) What percentage of untreated typhoid patients will become permanent carriers? (A) 1%, (B) 2-5%, (C) 10%, (D) 25%

5. (　) In Taiwan, which serotype of paratyphoid fever is most common in frequently identified? (A) paratyphoid A, (B) paratyphoid B, (C) paratyphoid C, (D) paratyphoid D.

6. (　) For the Vi-polysaccharide vaccine (Typhim Vi or Typherix), when is the recommended booster shot after the initial vaccination? (A) yearly, (B) 2 years, (C) 3 years, (D) no need

7. (　) For the Oral Ty21a live vaccine (Vivotif), when are the recommended booster doses and at what intervals? (A) yearly, (B) 2 years, (C) 3 years, (D) no need.

8. (　) What are the potential consequences for a small number of people who are infected with Paratyphoid bacteria? (A) become permanent gallbladder carriers, (B) become asymptomatic carriers, (C) become healthy carriers, (D) all of the above.

9. (　) For how long after the onset of symptoms will approximately 10% of untreated typhoid fever patients continue to discharge bacilli? (A) 4 weeks, (B) 2 months, (C) 3 months, (D) all year round.

II. Simple answer:

1. What are the alternative names for typhoid fever?

2. With whom are enteric fevers mainly associated?

3. Could you please tell me the transmission mode of typhoid fever?

4. Could you please tell me what types of immunization vaccines can prevent typhoid fever?

5. Could you please tell me the infectious agents responsible for paratyphoid fever?

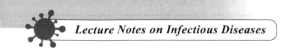

6. Which serotype of paratyphoid is the most commonly occurring in Taiwan?

 | **3-4** | **Shigellosis** (ICD-9 004; ICD-10 A03) |

⊙ Highlight

1. Shigellosis (bacillary dysentery)
2. An important worldwide disease
3. An acute bacterial disease (diarrhea, fever, nausea, toxemia, vomiting, cramps and tenesmus)
4. Watery diarrhea (enterotoxin)
5. Direct or indirect fecal-oral transmission

Shigellosis, also known as bacillary dysentery, is a highly contagious bacterial infection primarily caused by a group of bacteria known as Shigella. This illness primarily affects the gastrointestinal tract, leading to symptoms such as diarrhea, abdominal cramps, fever, and sometimes bloody stools. Shigellosis can range in severity from mild to severe, and in some cases, it can be life-threatening, especially in vulnerable populations. It accounts for less than 10% of the reported outbreaks of foodborne illness in the Taiwan. In Western countries the endemic *Shigella* spp. causes self-limiting illnesses which are generally mild. Tropical shigellosis tends to be both more severe and persistent, causing serious morbidity, especially in children. Shigellosis rarely occurs in animals other than humans and other primates like monkeys and chimpanzees. The causative organism is frequently found in water polluted with human feces, and is transmitted via the fecal-oral route. The usual mode of transmission is directly person-to-person hand-to-mouth, in the setting of poor hygiene among children.

Bacillary dysentery is an important worldwide disease. If left untreated or in severe cases, bacillary dysentery can lead to complications such as dehydration, kidney problems, and in rare instances, seizures or death. Infants, young children, the elderly, and individuals with weakened immune systems are at higher risk of severe complications. Preventing bacillary dysentery relies on maintaining good hygiene practices, including frequent handwashing with soap and clean water, safe food handling and preparation, and access to clean drinking water. Vaccines for Shigella are in development but are not yet widely available.

Identification to the Shigellosis:

Shigellosis is an acute bacterial disease involving the large and small intestine, characterized by diarrhea accompanied by fever, nausea and sometimes toxemia, vomiting, cramps and tenesmus. In typical cases the stools contain blood, mucus and pus resulting from the confluent microabscesses caused by the invasive organisms; watery diarrhea with vomiting may also occur, attributable to an enterotoxin elaborated by the organisms. Convulsions may be an important complication in young children. Bacteraemia is uncommon. Mild and asymptomatic infections occur; illness is usually self-limited, lasting on average 4-7 days. *S. sonnei* incidence is annually in Taiwan. After promoting series of surveillance and management plans, such as building access to safe drinking water and leading health education programs, the indigenous cases decreasing significantly (Centers for Disease Control, R.O.C., Taiwan) (Fig. 3-7).

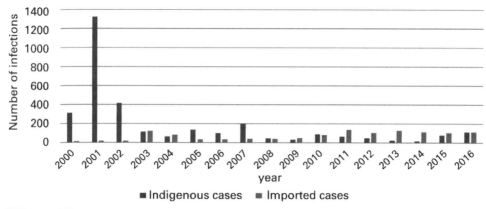

Figure 3-7   Number of *Shigella* Infections by Year– Taiwan, 2000-2016.
(http://www.cdc.gov.tw/English/info.aspx?treeid=E79C7A9E1
E9B1CDF&nowtreeid=E02C24F0DACDD729&tid=6E3416131D
149BD5)

It's important to note that the identification of Shigellosis should be done by a healthcare professional. Self-diagnosis or self-treatment with antibiotics is not recommended, as it can lead to inappropriate antibiotic use and potentially worsen antibiotic resistance. Once Shigellosis is confirmed, treatment can include antibiotics, rehydration therapy to address fluid and electrolyte loss, and in severe cases, hospitalization. Additionally, measures to prevent further spread of the infection should be implemented, including isolating infected individuals, practicing good hygiene and sanitation, and notifying close contacts to seek medical evaluation if they develop symptoms. Public health authorities may also conduct investigations to identify the source of the outbreak and implement control measures.

Infectious agents:

There are several species and subtypes of Shigella that can cause shigellosis, with some being more common in certain regions. The primary infectious agents of shigellosis are as follows:

- Group A: *Shigella dysenteriae* is less common but has been associated with more severe and potentially life-threatening cases of shigellosis. It is known for producing a potent toxin called Shiga toxin, which can lead to complications.

- Group B: *Shigella flexneri* is another common species that can cause shigellosis worldwide. It is known to cause more severe cases of the illness, particularly in children.

- Group C: *Shigella boydii* is relatively rare and is responsible for a smaller proportion of shigellosis cases compared to the other species. It can cause both mild and severe infections.

- Group D: *Shigella sonnei* is the most common species of Shigella responsible for causing shigellosis in many developed countries, including the United States. It tends to cause milder cases of the disease.

The genus *Shigella* contain a specific plasmid has been associated with virulence. The infectious dose for humans is low; 10-100 bacteria have caused disease in volunteers (Fig. 3-8).

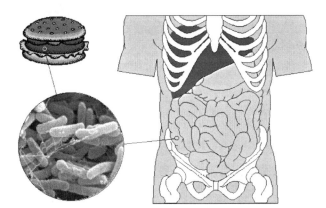

Figure 3-8   *Shigella* infection may occur after the ingestion of very few (10-100) organisms.
(www.doctortipster.com)

Occurrence:

Shigellosis is a common bacterial infection globally, particularly in developing countries with inadequate sanitation and hygiene practices. It is estimated that there are millions of cases of shigellosis each year worldwide. The prevalence of shigellosis varies by region. It is more common in areas with poor sanitation and overcrowding. Regions with limited access to clean water and proper sewage disposal systems are at higher risk. In some regions, shigellosis may exhibit seasonal patterns, with increased cases during the warmer months. This can be attributed to factors such as contaminated water sources and food handling practices in hot weather.

In Taiwan *S. sonnei* infection is most common. Two-thirds of the cases, and most of the deaths, are in children under 10 years. Secondary attack rates in households are high, range from 10-40%. Outbreaks commonly occur under conditions of crowding and poor sanitation, such in jails, camps, mental hospitals and aboard ships. More than one serotype is commonly present in a community; mixed infections with other intestinal pathogens also occur. Travelers to regions with poor sanitation may contract shigellosis if they consume contaminated food or water. This is sometimes referred to as "traveler's diarrhea."

Reservoir:

Man is the only significant reservoir. However, outbreaks have occurred in primate colonies.

Mode of transmission:

It is mainly by direct or indirect fecal-oral transmission from a patient or carrier. Infection may occur after the ingestion of very few (10-100) organisms. Shigella can be highly contagious, and several modes of transmission can lead to the spread of the disease: Person-to-person contact, contaminated food, contaminated water, contaminated surfaces, food handlers, daycare centers and institutions, sexual transmission, and travel-related transmission. Individuals primarily responsible for transmission include those who fail to clean hands and under fingernails thoroughly after defecation. Water, milk, cockroach and fly-borne transmission may occur as the result of direct fecal contamination.

Incubation period:

Incubation period is usually 1-3 days, but may range from 12 to 96 hours; up to one week for *S. dysenteriae*.

Period of communicability:

During acute infection and until the infectious agent is no longer present in feces, usually within 4 weeks after illness. Asymptomatic carriers may transmit infection. The carrier state may persist for months, or longer. Appropriate antimicrobial treatment usually reduces duration of carriage to a few days.

Susceptibility and resistance:

Susceptibility is general with infection following ingestion of a small number of organisms; individuals of all ages can be susceptible to shigellosis if they are exposed to Shigella bacteria. Young children, the elderly, and those with weakened immune systems may be at higher risk of severe illness. The disease is more severe than in adults, among whom many infections may be asymptomatic.

Natural immunity to Shigella bacteria is generally not long-lasting. A person who recovers from shigellosis can become reinfected with a different

Shigella strain in the future. Breast feeding is protective for infants and young children. Studies with experimental serotype-specific live oral vaccines and parenteral polysaccharide conjugate vaccines show protection of short duration against infection with the homologous serotype.

🔋 Methods of control:

Local health authorities must be prepared to evaluate the local situation and take appropriate steps to prevent the spread of infection. In contrast, an infection with *S. sonnei* in a private home would not merit such an approach. The most difficult epidemics to control are those involving young children, the mentally defective, and situations where there is an inadequate supply of water. Concurrent disinfection is necessary, of feces and contaminated articles. In communities with an adequate sewage disposal system, feces can be discharged directly into sewers without preliminary disinfection. Patients should avoid handling food until their feces are normal.

Isolate individuals with shigellosis, especially in institutional settings, during the acute phase of the illness to prevent further spread. This may involve staying home from school or work until they are no longer contagious. In certain situations, close contacts of individuals with shigellosis may be quarantined to prevent secondary cases. Antibiotics are typically reserved for individuals with moderate to severe shigellosis, as well as for those at higher risk of complications. Antibiotics are also recommended for individuals in outbreak situations and institutional settings. The choice of antibiotics should be guided by susceptibility testing whenever possible to ensure that the selected antibiotic is effective against the specific Shigella strain causing the infection. Commonly used antibiotics include Ciprofloxacin, Ceftriaxone, and Azithromycin.

General review

1. Shigellosis

2. Bacillary dysentery

3. An acute bacterial disease

4. Cramps and tenesmus

5. Microabscesses

6. Group A, *S. dysenteriae*

7. Group B, *S. flexneri*

8. Group C, *S. boydii*

9. Group D, *S. sonnei*

Review test

SCAN ME

Check Your Answers

I. Multiple-choice questions (four selected one):

1. ( ) In Taiwan, which subgenus of Shigella causes the most common infections? (A) group A, (B) group B, (C) group C, (D) group D

2. ( ) Two-thirds of the Shigellosis cases, and most of the deaths, are in children under what age? (A) 1 year, (B) 3 years, (C) 5 years, (D) 10 years

3. ( ) What are the secondary attack rates of Shigellosis in households, as a percentage? (A) 3%, (B) 5%, (C) 10-40%, (D) 50%

4. ( ) Among the following modes of transmission, which one may occur as a result of direct fecal contamination? (A) water, (B) milk, (C) cockroach, (D) all of the above.

5. ( ) During an acute infection with shigellosis, how long does it usually take until the infectious agent is no longer present in the stool? (A) 1 week, (B) 2 weeks, (C) 3 weeks, (D) 4 weeks

6. ( ) What is the infectious dose of Shigella? (A) 10-100, (B) 10^3-10^5, (C) 10^8-10^{12}, (D) 10^{16}-10^{18}

7. ( ) According to statistics, what proportion of Shigella cases accounts for the foodborne outbreaks reported annually in Taiwan? (A) <10%, (B) 10-12.5%, (C) 15-20%, (D) 25-40%.

8. ( ) Which subgenus of Shigella is less common but has been associated with more severe and potentially life-threatening cases of shigellosis? (A) group A, (B) group B, (C) group C, (D) group D

9. ( ) Which subgenus of Shigella is known to cause more severe cases of the illness, particularly in children? (A) group A, (B) group B, (C) group C, (D) group D

II. Simple answer:

1. Could you please tell me which species of bacterial dysentery infection is the most common in Taiwan?

2. Could you please provide detailed information on the transmission mode of Shigellosis?

3-5 Amoebiasis (ICD-9 006; ICD-10 A06)

 Highlight

1. Amoebiasis
2. Protozoan parasite
3. Acute amoebic dysentery
4. Extra-intestinal abscesses
5. *Entamoeba histolytica*
6. Transmission mode: Epidemic outbreaks, Endemic spread, Sexually transmitted

Amoebiasis, also known as amoebic dysentery or amoebic colitis, is a common parasitic infection caused by a microscopic single-celled organism called Entamoeba histolytica. This infection primarily affects the human intestine and can lead to a range of gastrointestinal symptoms, varying from mild to severe. Amoebiasis is a significant global health concern, particularly in regions with poor sanitation and limited access to clean water. It is usually contracted by ingesting water or food contaminated with amoebic cysts. Amoebiasis is an intestinal infection that may or may not be symptomatic. When symptoms are present it is generally known as invasive amoebiasis.

Amoebiasis is mainly spread via contaminated food, especially raw vegetables, and water. Infection is common in areas of poor sanitation and personal hygiene. The disease occurs principally in adults and is rare in children below 5 years of age. Up to 1000 cases are reported annually in Taiwan. Half of these are known to be acquired overseas, principally in the foreign labors. The disease is in many parts of the world where sanitation is poor. The effects of infection range from asymptomatic excretion of cysts to chronic intestinal infection, sometimes with granuloma formation, to acute amoebic dysentery. Extraintestinal abscesses may also occur and can threaten life if untreated.

Identification to the Amoebiasis:

Amoebiasis is an infection with a protozoan parasite that exists in two forms: The effects of infection range from asymptomatic excretion of cysts to chronic intestinal infection, sometimes with granuloma formation, to acute amoebic dysentery. Most infections are asymptomatic but may become clinically important under certain circumstances. Intestinal disease varies from acute or fulminating dysentery with fever, chills and bloody or mucoid diarrhea (amoebic dysentery), to mild abdominal discomfort with diarrhea containing blood or mucus, alternating with periods of constipation or remission. Amoebic granulomata (amoeboma), sometimes mistaken for carcinoma, may occur in the wall of the large intestine in patients with intermittent dysentery or colitis of long duration. Extra-intestinal abscesses may also occur and can threaten life if untreated.

Amebiasis is one of the Category 2 communicable diseases in Taiwan, and all cases should be reported to health departments. In a decade ago, many outbreaks took place in long-term care facilities. After leading health education programs to facility staff and residents screening plan before admission to a long-term care facility, the outbreaks decreased significantly. However, *E. histolytica* is much more prevalent among male homosexuals in Taiwan. On the other hand, importing foreign workers from Southeast Asia has led to an increase in imported cases in Taiwan (Centers for Disease Control, R.O.C., Taiwan) (Fig. 3-9).

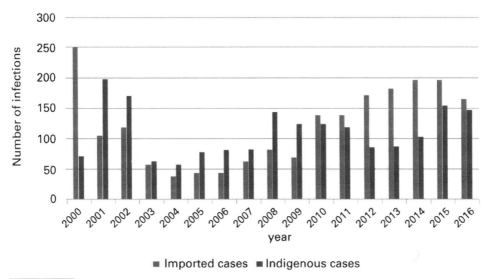

Figure 3-9   Number of Amebiasis by Year– Taiwan, 2000-2016.
(http://www.cdc.gov.tw/English/info.aspx?treeid=E79C7A9E1
E9B1CDF&nowtreeid=E02C24F0DACDD729&tid=75272F1629
A55481)

🔹 Infectious agent:

Entamoeba histolytica, a parasitic organism not to be confused with *E. hartmanni*, *E. coli*, or other intestinal protozoa. Most asymptomatic cyst passers carry strains of *E. dispar*. The life cycle of Entamoeba histolytica, the parasitic amoeba responsible for amoebiasis in humans, is relatively straight forward. It involves two main stages: the trophozoite stage and the cyst stage (Fig. 3-10).

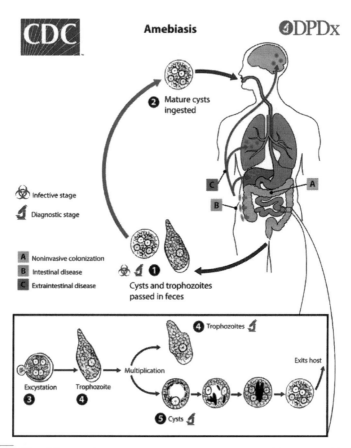

Figure 3-10 The life cycle of *Entamoeba histolytica* (Source: CDC, US.) (http://www.dpd.cdc.gov/dpdx)

Occurrence:

Worldwide, amoebiasis is a significant public health concern, particularly in regions with poor sanitation and limited access to clean water. It is estimated to affect millions of people worldwide, with a substantial burden of disease in developing countries. Published prevalence rates vary widely from place to place. In general, rates are higher in young adult man, and in areas with poor sanitation such as parts of the tropics, in mental institutions and among sexually promiscuous male homosexuals (probably *E. dispar*). Travelers, foreign labors may play as a carrier. In areas with good sanitation, amoebic infections tend to cluster in households and institutions.

Reservoir:

Man, man is usually a chronically ill or asymptomatic cyst passer. Contaminated Environments, in settings with poor sanitation, such as overcrowded or unsanitary living conditions, the environment itself can become contaminated with feces containing cysts. This increases the risk of exposure and infection for individuals living in such environments.

Mode of transmission:

It is mainly through ingestion of fecally contaminated food or water containing amoebic cysts, which are relatively chlorine resistant. Epidemic outbreaks result mainly from ingestion of fecally contaminated water containing amoebic cysts. Endemic spread is by hand-to-mouth transfer of feces, by contaminated raw vegetables, by flies, possibly by soiled hands of food-handlers. Sexually transmitted is by oral-anal contact.

Incubation period:

Incubation period is variable, from a few days to several months or years. The commonly are 2-4 weeks.

Period of communicability:

During the period of cysts are passed, which may continue for years. *E. histolytica* infection makes up approximately 10% of those cases with cysts present in the stool.

Susceptibility and resistance:

Although susceptibility to infection is general, most persons harboring the organism do not develop disease. Children and infants may be more susceptible to amoebiasis due to their immature immune systems and the likelihood of engaging in behaviors that expose them to contaminated environments. Malnourished individuals may have compromised immune function, making them more susceptible to amoebiasis. Individuals with weakened or compromised immune systems, such as those with HIV/AIDS or malnutrition, are at higher risk of severe amoebiasis. A person's immune system plays a crucial role in resisting and controlling amoebiasis. Prior exposure to *Entamoeba histolytica* may confer some degree of immunity or resistance.

Methods of control:

The disease can be prevented by providing water that has been treated by filtration, and adequate disposal of human feces. Travelers to tropical countries should avoid drinking water that is not known to have been properly treated and unpeeled fruit and raw vegetables. Known carriers should be given instruction in thorough hand-washing after defecation.

Protect public water supplies from fecal contamination. Educate the general public in personal hygiene. Control flies. Cysts are killed by desiccation and temperatures above 50°C. Medical treatment with specific antibiotics, such as Metronidazole or Tinidazole, is effective in treating symptomatic cases and preventing complications. Medical care should be sought promptly if symptoms arise.

📖 Supplementary information:

Acanthamoeba keratitis:

Acanthamoeba keratitis is a rare but serious eye infection caused by the microscopic amoeba called Acanthamoeba. This condition primarily affects the cornea, which is the clear, front surface of the eye responsible for focusing light onto the retina. Acanthamoeba keratitis can result in painful and potentially vision-threatening complications.

The infection typically occurs when Acanthamoeba comes into contact with the cornea, often through the use of contaminated contact lenses, lens solutions, or exposure to contaminated water, such as while swimming or using hot tubs. Individuals who wear contact lenses, particularly those who do not follow proper lens hygiene and cleaning practices, are at a higher risk of developing Acanthamoeba keratitis.

Acanthamoeba keratitis can cause a range of symptoms, including severe eye pain, redness, blurred vision, sensitivity to light (photophobia), excessive tearing, and a feeling of a foreign body in the eye. Symptoms may develop gradually and can be mistaken for other eye conditions, such as a corneal abrasion or bacterial or viral conjunctivitis.

🖎 General review

1. Amoebiasis

2. Acute amoebic dysentery

3. Granuloma formation

4. Extra-intestinal abscesses

5. Extra-intestinal amoebiasis

6. *Entamoeba histolytica*

7. Asymptomatic cyst passer

8. Acanthamoeba keratitis

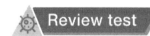 **Review test**

SCAN ME

Check Your Answers

I. **Multiple-choice questions (five selected one):**

1. ( ) According to statistics from Taiwan Centers for Disease Control, how many cases of amoebiasis are reported in Taiwan annually? (A) 10, (B) 100, (C) 500, (C) 1000 cases

2. ( ) Which type of infection almost exclusively occurs in contact lens wearers? (A) *Entamoeba histolytica*, (B) *Entamoeba hartmanni*, (C) *Entamoeba keratitis*, (D) Acanthamoeba keratitis

3. ( ) At what temperature can Entamoeba cysts be killed by desiccation? (A) 50°C, (B) 60°C, (C) 70°C, (D) all of the above

4. ( ) In which age group does amoebiasis primarily occur? (A) under 5 years of age, (B) teenagers, (C) young adults, (D) adults

5. ( ) What percentage of patients with Entamoeba infection present with cysts in their feces? (A) 10%, (B) 25%, (C) 33%, (D) over 50%.

6. ( ) In Taiwan, which of the following groups exhibits a higher prevalence of Entamoeba histolytica? (A) teenagers, (B) travelers, (C) foreign labors, (D) male homosexuals.

7. ( ) What is the approximate proportion of asymptomatic and self-limited cases among all cases of amoebiasis? (A)< 1%, (B) 10%, (C) 35-50%, (D) 90%

II. Simple answer:

1. Could you please explain the transmission mode of amoebiasis?

2. Could you please tell me the major risk factors for Acanthamoeba keratitis infection?

3-6 \ Diarrhea Caused by Enterohemo-rrhagic Strains (ICD-9 008.0; ICD-10 A04.3)

 Highlight

1. Diarrhea caused by Enterohemorrhagic strains

2. Enteropathogenic

3. Zoonotic infectious disease

4. HUS (hemolytic uremic syndrome)

5. TTP (thrombotic thrombocytopenic purpura)

6. *Escherichia coli* (O157: H7)

7. Toxin-mediated traveler's diarrhea

8. Haemorrhagic colitis

9. Uncooked beef and row milk.

Escherichia is named after German bacteriologist Theodore Escherich (1857-1911), who first described them in 1885. They are Gram-negative non-sporeforming, rod-shaped bacteria, often motile and possessing a facultative metabolism. However, some strains of *E. coli* are enteropathogenic strains that can cause intestinal disease. These diarrheagenic *E. coli* strains are further subdivided on the basis of the symptomology of infections, aka virotype. Pathogenesis among *E. coli* is associated with the possession of virulence factors, often encoded by plasmids, bacteriophage, or 'islands' integrated into the chromosome. It is likely that these factors, not all of which have been identified, are traded and reassorted among *E. coli* and the other Enterobacteriaceae via lateral, or horizontal, gene transfer.

Enterohemorrhagic *Escherichia coli* (EHEC) is a specific strain of the bacterium *Escherichia coli* (*E. coli*) that is known to cause a type of diarrhea often associated with severe complications. This strain of *E. coli* is particularly notorious for its ability to produce toxins that can lead to bloody diarrhea and potentially life-threatening conditions. The diarrheagenic *E. coli* are transmitted via the fecal-oral route, either from person-to-person or from contaminated food or water sources. Domestic, agricultural, and wild animals, as well as humans, can be sources of contamination. Some strains, including many enterohemorrhagic *E. coli* (EHEC) isolates, are resistant to stomach acid and have infectious doses as low as 10 organisms.

Diarrhea caused by enterohemorrhagic strains contain: diarrhea caused by enterohemorrhagic *E. coli* (EHEC), Shiga toxin producing *E. coli* (STEC), verocytotoxic *E. coli* (VTEC), enteropathogenic *E. coli* (EPEC), enteroaggregative *E .coli* (EAEC), and enterotoxigenic *E. coli* (ETEC). Most gastrointestinal illness produced by *E. coli* is non-specific and must be suspected on epidemiological evidence. Outbreaks of traveler's diarrhea or HUS (hemolytic uremic syndrome) will alert clinicians and public health specialist.

🔹 Identification to the EHEC:

EHEC is typically transmitted to humans through the consumption of contaminated food or water. Undercooked ground beef, unpasteurized milk, and fresh produce contaminated with EHEC are common sources of infection. Person-to-person transmission can also occur, especially in close-contact settings such as households and daycare centers. In the 1982's certain serotype of *Escherichia coli* (O157: H7) caused large epidemics of gastroenteritis in infants of U.S. The important *E. coli* disease now include: Toxin-mediated traveler's diarrhea and haemorrhagic colitis that associated with certain serotypes of verocytotoxin-producing organisms.

In EHEC, 5-10% of the patients may got the disease of HUS and TTP. HUS (hemolytic uremic syndrome) is mainly a disease of children but can also affect adults. The pathogenesis of HUS is based on mucosal damage and microangiopathic anemia, together with renal vascular damage. TTP is the adult form overlaps clinically with the syndrome of thrombotic thrombocytopenic purpura. Hemolytic uremic syndrome (HUS) and thrombotic thrombocytopenic purpura (TTP) are microangiopathic disorders. They are characterized by abnormalities (chiefly blood clots) that occur within the small blood vessels of the body. Both HUS and TTP are distinguished by blood clots within the capillaries and arterioles of many organs. Such clotting is associated with hemolytic anemia (low red blood cell count due to cell rupture) and low numbers of platelets (cell-like bodies responsible for blood coagulation). The clinical publications of HUS and TTP are anemia (pale complexion), weakness, chronic fatigue, confusion (not thinking right or clearly, memory loss), low grade fever (99.5°F or 37.8°C in orally, or greater), bleeding (without clotting), bruising (easily) (Fig. 3-11).

The case report standard on CDC, Taiwan: Suspected case: diarrhea with HUS or TTP. Probable case: isolated *E. coli* O157 from clinical specimen. Confirmed case: isolated *E. coli* O157: H7 from clinical specimen or detect out Shiga-like toxin of *E. coli* O157 (NM) from clinical specimen.

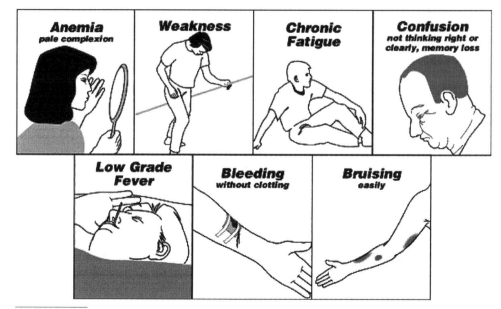

Figure 3-11 Clinical publications of HUS and TTP.
(www.healthylive world.com)

🔘 Infectious agent:

E. coli O157 : H7 or *E. coli* O157 (NM), *E. coli* O26: H11, *E. coli* O111: H8, *E. coli* O104: H21.

The main EHEC serotype in North America is *E. coli* O157: H7; this serotype is thought to cause over 90% of cases of diarrhea-associated HUS. The other most common serogroups in the United States are O26, O111, O103, O45, and O121.

🔘 Occurrence:

The routes of transmission and epidemiological features of *E. coli* vary considerably between different pathogenic types and in different geographical locations (ex. North America, Europe, South Africa, Japan, and South America). *E. coli* O157:H7 has ever been recognized from cattle feces in Taiwan. So far, there has no case report in Taiwan (D.O.H., 2005). As of my last knowledge update in September 2023, I do not have access to real-time or the most current information regarding specific infectious agents or outbreaks in Taiwan or any other region. The infectious agents responsible for outbreaks can change over time, and new outbreaks can occur.

Reservoir:

Cattle are the most important reservoir of EHEC; humans may also serve as a reservoir for person-to-person transmission. Other animals, including deer, may also carry EHEC.

Mode of transmission:

It is mainly through ingestion of food contaminated with ruminant feces. EHEC are usually spread from person-to-person by the fecal-oral route, although transmission via contaminated baby food also occurs. In general, *E. coli* O157:H7 is transmitted to humans primarily through consumption of contaminated foods, such as raw or undercooked ground meat products and raw milk. Fecal contamination of water and other foods, as well as cross-contamination during food preparation (with beef and other meat products, contaminated surfaces and kitchen utensils), will also lead to infection. Examples of foods implicated in outbreaks of *E. coli* O157:H7 include undercooked hamburgers, dried cured salami, unpasteurized fresh-pressed apple cider, yogurt, and cheese made from raw milk.

Incubation period:

Incubation period is relative long, 3-8 days, usually 3-4 days.

🔬 Period of communicability:

The duration of excretion of the pathogen is typically 1 week or less in adults. 1/3 of children could be communicable for 3 weeks.

🔬 Susceptibility and resistance:

The infective dose of EHEC is very low, probably between 10 and 100 organisms. In child and old man are high-risk populations. The hypochlorhydria patient may be a risk factor. Under 5-year-old child is HUS high-risk population.

🔬 Methods of control:

Prevention of *E. coli* gastroenteritis is by adequate sanitary and hand-washing facilities. Scrupulous attention to hygiene is important, particularly in nurseries, where infection is common. Hamburger meat should be cooked (75°C, 15 sec) (ground beef preferably to an internal temperature of 68°C) thoroughly before eating. Travelers to tropical countries should avoid drinking untreated water and eating high risk foods such as raw vegetables, salad, peeled fruit and undercooked meat. Here are several methods of control:

1. **Proper Food Handling and Preparation**: Cooking meat thoroughly, avoid cross-contamination, and avoid raw or unpasteurized dairy products.

2. **Safe Food Storage**: Store perishable foods in the refrigerator at or below 40°F (4°C) and use them promptly.

3. **Hand Hygiene**: Wash hands thoroughly with soap and water for at least 20 seconds before handling food, after using the restroom, and after contact with animals or their environments.

4. **Avoiding Contaminated Water**: Be cautious when consuming untreated or unfiltered water, especially while traveling in regions with uncertain water quality.

 General review

1. Diarrheagenic *E. coli*

2. EHEC: Diarrhea Caused by Enterohemorrhagic *E. coli*

3. Enteropathogenic

4. Diarrheagenic *E. coli*

5. *Escherichia coli*

6. HUS: hemolytic uremic syndrome

7. Microangiopathic anemia

8. Haemorrhagic colitis

9. TTP: thrombotic thrombocytopenic purpura

Review test

SCAN ME

Check Your Answers

I. Multiple-choice questions (four selected one):

1. (   ) In the case of EHEC, how likely is it for patients to develop HUS and TTP? (A) 5-10 %, (B) 10-15 %, (C) 20-25 %, (D) more than 50 %

2. (   ) Among the following, which population is at a higher risk of developing hemolytic uremic syndrome? (A) under 5-year-old child, (B) 10-15 year-old juvenile, (C) 18-25 year-old young man, (D) over 65-year old man

3. (   ) Which of the following is the primary reservoir for EHEC? (A) wild animals, (B) cattle, (C) pigs, (D) all of the above.

4. (   ) Enterohemorrhagic *E. coli* (O157:H7) typically spreads from person to person via the fecal-oral route. Which of the following methods can also result in infection? (A) undercooked hamburgers, (B) dried cured salami, (C) unpasteurized fresh-pressed apple cider, (D) all of the above.

5. (   ) From a clinical perspective, what is the infectious dose that causes enterohemorrhagic *E. coli* infection? (A) 10-100, (B) 10^3, (C) 10^4, (D) 10^8-10^{12} organisms

6. (   ) Which of the following is a clinical finding in a patient with HUS? (A) Anemia, (B) Weakness, (C) Low grade fever, (D) all of the above

7. (   ) Which of the following is a clinical finding in a patient with HUS? (A) Bruising, (B) Weakness, (C) Low grade fever, (D) all of the above

II. Simple answer:

1. *Escherichia coli* (O157:H7) causes an epidemic of gastroenteritis in infants. What are the two important current symptoms of enterohemorrhagic *E. coli*?

2. In the case of EHEC, 5-10% of patients may experience what kinds of complications?

3. Could you please provide detailed information on the transmission mode of EHEC?

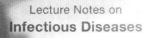

Lecture Notes on
Infectious Diseases

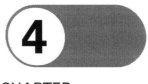

4

CHAPTER

Enteroviruses Groups Infectious Diseases

More than 70 serotypes of enterovirus have been isolated from human sources. Enteroviruses are a diverse group of viruses that belong to the Picornaviridae family. These viruses are responsible for a wide range of infectious diseases in humans, with symptoms ranging from mild to severe. Enteroviruses are highly contagious and are primarily transmitted through the fecal-oral route, respiratory secretions, and direct contact with infected individuals. They are often associated with outbreaks, particularly in crowded settings like schools and daycare centers. Enteroviruses can be categorized into several groups, with the most prominent ones being:

Group 1; Polioviruses: Polioviruses are perhaps the most well-known enteroviruses and are the causative agents of polio (poliomyelitis). Polio is a highly contagious disease that can lead to paralysis or even death in severe cases.

Group 2; Coxsackieviruses: Coxsackieviruses are responsible for a variety of diseases, including hand, foot, and mouth disease (HFMD), which primarily affects infants and young children. HFMD is characterized by fever, sores in the mouth, and a rash on the hands and feet.

Group 3; Echoviruses: Echoviruses can cause a range of illnesses, from mild respiratory infections to more severe diseases involving the central nervous system. They are often associated with aseptic meningitis, a condition characterized by inflammation of the brain and spinal cord.

Group 4; Enteroviruses: This group includes a diverse set of enteroviruses that can cause a wide range of illnesses, including respiratory infections, gastrointestinal problems, and viral myocarditis.

Enterovirus infections are generally more common during the summer and fall months. They can affect individuals of all ages but are often more severe in infants, young children, and individuals with weakened immune systems. Enteroviruses enter the body through the pharynx and the alimentary tract. The virus multiplies locally in the tonsils, Peyer's patches and other bowel-assiciated lymphoid tissue. A viraemic phase often occurs, and this may be followed by disease in different organs, for example meninges, myocytes, brain or skin. Diagnosis typically involves laboratory tests on samples of bodily fluids, such as throat swabs, stool samples, or cerebrospinal fluid.

Enteroviruses are most easily recovered from feces, but throat swabs and cerebrospinal fluid should also be examined in cases of meningitis. Culture of an enterovirus from a sterile site is diagnostic, whereas isolation from feces is less certainly so. Enteroviruses grow well in cultures of human embryonic lung fibroblasts. The infected cells become rounded and refractile before separating from the monolayer. Isolates are typed by neutralization using pooled antisera. The spectrum of enteroviral infections includes lymphocytic meningitis, myositis, pericarditis and acute myocarditis. Patients with significant meningism, precordial pain, dysrhythmias or heart failure require further investigation.

In Taiwan, Enteroviruses group's infections are incidence from March to October. According to survey data gathered over a period of several years by Taiwan CDC and the National Health Insurance (NHI) Administration, the number of weekly outpatient and emergency visits, as shown by the data transferred from the database of NHI, increases in late March and peaks around mid-June. It decreases after mid-June. There is usually another smaller outbreak when schools reopen in September (Fig.4-1). Those survey data also indicate that children under the age of 5 are more prone to critical complications and death. In Taiwan, the case-fatality rate of enterovirus infection with severe complications (EVSC) are ranged from 1.3% to 33.3%. The major symptoms of enterovirus infection are herpangina and hand-foot-and-mouth disease (HFMD). EVA71 is the most commonly seen serotype of cases of EVSC in Taiwan (Fig.4-1, 4-2).

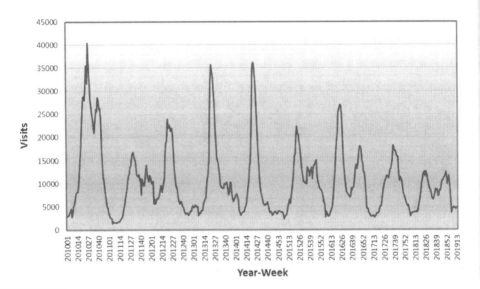

Figure 4-1　The number of weekly outpatient and emergency visits for enterovirus infection in Taiwan, 2010-2018.
(https://www.cdc.gov.tw/En/Category/ListContent/bg0g_VU_Ysrgkes_KRUDgQ?uaid=zRqpJ3zn3ll6Tc0LgD0Clw)

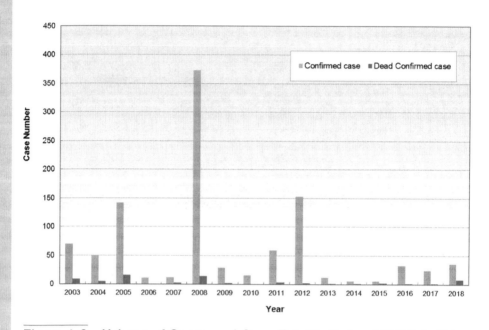

Figure 4-2　Volume of Cases and Case Fatality Rate of EVSC in Taiwan, 2003-2018.
(https://www.cdc.gov.tw/En/Category/ListContent/bg0g_VU
_Ysrgkes_KRUDgQ?uaid=zRqpJ3zn3II6Tc0LgD0CIw)

4-1 Enteroviral Vesicular Pharyngitis
(ICD-9 074.0; ICD-10 B08.5)

Highlight

1. Pharyngitis: a painful inflammation of the pharynx, as a sore throat
2. Tonsillitis and laryngitis may occur simultaneously
3. Enteroviral vesicular pharyngitis is also known as herpangina or aphthous pharyngitis
4. EVP is an acute, self-limited, viral disease
5. Herpangina: occur on the anterior pillars of the tonsillar fauces, soft palate, uvula and tonsils
6. Coxsackievirus, group A
7. It is direct contact with nose and throat discharges and feces of infected people and by aerosol droplet spread.

Pharyngitis is in most cases, a painful inflammation of the pharynx, and is colloquially referred to as a sore throat (Fig. 4-3). Infection of the tonsils (tonsillitis) and/or larynx (laryngitis) may occur simultaneously. About 90% of cases are caused by viral infection, with the remainder caused by bacterial infection and, in rare cases, oral thrush (fungal candidiasis e.g. in babies). Some cases of pharyngitis are caused by irritation from elements such as pollutants or chemical substances.

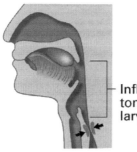

Inflammation of the
tonsils, pharynx and
larynx

Figure 4-3 Enteroviral vesicular pharyngitis cases are painful
inflammation of the pharynx, and is colloquially referred to
as a sore throat.

Identification to the vesicular pharyngitis:

Pharyngitis due to enterovirus infections is common. Enteroviral
vescular pharyngitis is also known as herpangina or aphthous pharyngitis,
which is an acute, self-limited, viral disease characterized by sudden onset,
fever, sore throat and small (1-2 mm), discrete, grayish papulovesicular
pharyngeal lesionson an erythematous base, gradually progressing to
slightly larger ulcers. These lesions usually occur on the anterior pillars of
the tonsillar fauces, soft palate, uvula and tonsils, and may persist 4-6 days
after the onset of illness. No fatalities have been reported. In one series,
febrile convulsions occurred in 5% of cases.

Individuals with enteroviral vesicular pharyngitis typically experience
symptoms such as:

1. **Sore throat**: Pharyngitis causes a painful, scratchy, or irritated throat.

2. **Vesicles in the throat**: Small, fluid-filled blisters or ulcers can develop
   in the throat, which can be seen during a medical examination.

3. **Fever**: Many enterovirus infections are accompanied by a fever.

4. **Difficulty swallowing**: The presence of vesicles in the throat can make swallowing uncomfortable.

5. **Respiratory symptoms**: Some individuals may also have symptoms like cough, runny nose, or sneezing.

Infectious agents:

Coxsackievirus, group A, types 1-10, 16 and 22.

Occurrence:

Probably worldwide, sporadically and in epidemics; maximal incidence in summer and early autumn; mainly in children under 10, but adult cases (especially young adults) are not unusual. The disease frequently occurs in outbreaks among groups of children (e.g. in nursery schools, childcare center).

Reservoir:

Human are the only known reservoir of infection.

Mode of transmission:

Enteroviral vesicular pharyngitis is highly contagious, and individuals infected with the virus should take precautions to prevent its spread. It is direct contact with nose and throat discharges and feces of infected people (who may be asymptomatics) and by aerosol droplet spread; no reliable evidence of spread by insects, water, food or sewage.

Incubation period:

Incubation period is usually 3-5 days.

Period of communicability:

It is during the acute stage of illness and perhaps longer, since viruses persist in stool for several weeks.

Susceptibility and resistance:

Susceptibility to infection is universal. Immunity to the specific virus is probably acquired through clinical or inapparent infection; duration unknown. Second attacks may occur with group A coxsackievirus of a different serological type.

General review

1. Herpangina are characterized by sudden onset, fever, sore throat and small, discrete, grayish papulovesicular pharyngeal lesionson, slightly larger ulcers.

2. No fatalities have been reported.

3. Coxsackievirus, group A, types 1-10, 16 and 22.

4. Maximal incidence in summer and early autumn; mainly in children under 10.

5. During the acute stage of illnes, viruses can persist in stool for several weeks.

4-2 Enteroviral Vesicular Stomatitis with Exanthema (ICD-9 074.3; ICD-10 B08.4)

 Highlight

1. Stomatitis

2. Exanthema

3. Poor oral hygiene

4. Hand-Foot-Mouth Disease

5. Blisters on the palmer

6. Purpura rash on the buttocks

7. Papulovesicular lesions

8. Maculopapular lesions

9. Coxsackievirus, group A, B

10. Enterovirus type71

Stomatitis is an inflammation of the mucous lining of any of the structures in the mouth, which may involve the cheeks, gums, tongue, lips, throat, and roof or floor of the mouth. The inflammation can be caused by conditions in the mouth itself, such as poor oral hygiene, poorly fitted dentures, or from mouth burns from hot food or drinks, or by conditions that affect the entire body, such as medications, allergic reactions, radiation therapy, or infections.

Enteroviral vesicular stomatitis with exanthema is a viral infection characterized by the presence of vesicles (small fluid-filled blisters) in the mouth (stomatitis) and a skin rash (exanthema). This condition is typically caused by certain enteroviruses, such as Coxsackievirus or Enterovirus 71.

🔟 Identification to the vesicular stomatitis with exanthema:

Vesicular stomatitis with exanthema (hand-foot-and-mouth disease; HFMD) differ from vesicular pharyngitis in that oral lesions are more diffuse and may occur on the buccal surfaces of the cheeks and gums and on the sides of the tongue. Papulovesicular lesions, which may from 7 to 10 days, also occur commonly as an exanthema, especially on the palms, fingers and soles; maculopapular lesions occasionally appear on the buttocks. Although the disease is usually self-limited, rare cases have been fatal in infants. Hand-foot-and-mouth disease of baby cause similar lesions in the mouth, accompanies by blisters on the palmer aspects of the hands and feet, and a purpura rash on the buttocks.

Individuals with enteroviral vesicular stomatitis with exanthema may experience the following symptoms:

1. **Vesicular stomatitis**: This refers to the presence of small blisters or vesicles in the mouth, on the tongue, and inside the cheeks. These vesicles can be painful and make eating and drinking uncomfortable.

2. **Skin rash (exanthema)**: A rash may develop on the skin, which can vary in appearance but often consists of small, red spots that may become raised or develop into small blisters.

3. **Fever**: Many enterovirus infections are accompanied by fever.

4. **Irritability**: Infants and young children with this condition may be irritable due to the discomfort caused by mouth sores.

Infectious agents:

Coxsackievirus, group A, type A16 predominantly and types 4, 5, 9 and 10; group B, types 2 and 5; and enterovirus 71.

Occurrence:

Probably worldwide, sporadically and in epidemics; maximal incidence in summer and early autumn; mainly in children under 10, but adult cases (especially young adults) are not unusual. The disease frequently occurs in outbreaks among groups of children (e.g. in nursery schools, childcare center).

Reservoir:

Human are the only known reservoir of infection.

Mode of transmission:

It is direct contact with nose and throat discharges and feces of infected people (who may be asymptomatics) and by aerosol droplet spread; no reliable evidence of spread by insects, water, food or sewage.

Incubation period:

Incubation period is usually 3-5 days.

Period of communicability:

It is during the acute stage of illness and perhaps longer, since viruses persist in stool for several weeks.

🔳 Susceptibility and resistance:

Susceptibility to infection is universal. Immunity to the specific virus is probably acquired through clinical or inapparent infection; duration unknown. Second attacks may occur with group A coxsackievirus of a different serological type.

⌀ General review

1. Vesicular stomatitis with exanthema (hand-foot-and-mouth disease).

2. Exanthema, especially on the palms, fingers and soles; maculopapular lesions occasionally appear on the buttocks.

3. The disease is usually self-limited.

4. Coxsackievirus, group A, type A16 predominantly.

5. The disease frequently occurs in outbreaks among groups of children under 10.

4-3 Enteroviral Lymphonodular Pharyngitis (ICD-9 074.8; ICD-10 B08.8)

🔬 Highlight

1. Acute lymphonodular pharyngitis
2. Tonsillitis
3. Laryngitis
4. Coxsackievirus, group A, type 10

Pharyngitis is in most cases, a painful inflammation of the pharynx, and is colloquially referred to as a sore throat. Infection of the tonsils (tonsillitis) and/or larynx (laryngitis) may occur simultaneously. About 90% of cases are caused by viral infection, with the remainder caused by bacterial infection and, in rare cases, oral thrush (fungal candidiasis e.g. in babies).

Enteroviral lymphonodular pharyngitis is a medical condition characterized by inflammation of the pharynx (the back of the throat) and the presence of lymphonodular (lymphoid) tissue in the throat. This condition is primarily caused by enteroviruses, which are a group of Coxsackieviruses known to infect the gastrointestinal and respiratory systems.

⬤ Identification to the lymphonodular pharyngitis:

Acute lymphonodular pharyngitis also differs from vesicular pharyngitis in that the lesions are firm, raised, discrete, and whitish to yellowish nodules, surrounded by a 3-6 mm zone of erythema. They occur predominantly on the uvula, anterior tonsillar pillars and posterior pharynx, with no exanthema. The publications are fever, headache, and sore throat, the pale lesions could be found on the uvula and post pharyngitic wall.

Individuals with enteroviral lymphonodular pharyngitis typically experience the following symptoms:

1. **Sore throat**: Pharyngitis causes a painful, scratchy, or irritated throat.

2. **Lymphonodular pharyngitis**: This condition is characterized by the presence of small, raised, yellow or white nodules or lumps in the back of the throat, which are actually clusters of lymphoid tissue.

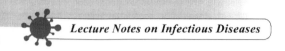

3. **Fever**: Many enterovirus infections are accompanied by a fever.

4. **Difficulty swallowing**: The presence of lymphonodular tissue and sore throat can make swallowing uncomfortable.

Infectious agents:

Coxsackievirus, group A, type 10.

Occurrence:

Probably worldwide, sporadically and in epidemics; maximal incidence in summer and early autumn; mainly in children under 10, but adult cases (especially young adults) are not unusual. The disease frequently occurs in outbreaks among groups of children (e.g. in nursery schools, childcare center).

Reservoir:

Human are the only known reservoir of infection.

Mode of transmission:

It is direct contact with nose and throat discharges and feces of infected people (who may be asymptomatics) and by aerosol droplet spread; no reliable evidence of spread by insects, water, food or sewage.

Incubation period:

Incubation period is usually 5 days.

Period of communicability:

It is during the acute stage of illness and perhaps longer, since viruses persist in stool for several weeks.

Susceptibility and resistance:

Susceptibility to infection is universal. Immunity to the specific virus is probably acquired through clinical or inapparent infection; duration unknown. Second attacks may occur with group A coxsackievirus of a different serological type.

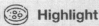
General review

1. Acute lymphonodular pharyngitis

2. Fever, headache, and sore throat, the pale lesions could be found on the uvula and post pharyngitic wall.

3. Coxsackievirus, group A

4-4 Coxsackievirus Carditis
(ICD-9 074.2; ICD-10 B33.2)

Highlight

1. Myocarditis (neonates)

2. Pericarditis (young adults)

3. Heart failure with pallor, cyanosis, dyspnea, tachycardia

4. Coxsackievirus Gr. A, B

5. Coxsackievirus carditis

6. Fecal-oral or respiratory droplet spread

Coxsackievirus carditis refers to inflammation of the heart muscle (myocardium) caused by Coxsackieviruses, which belong to the Enterovirus genus. These viruses are responsible for various infections, and they can sometimes affect the heart, leading to a condition known as viral myocarditis. Myocarditis is a serious condition because it can weaken the heart and interfere with its ability to pump blood effectively.

Identification to the coxsackievirus carditis:

Coxsackievirus carditis is also known as viral carditis, enteroviral carditis. It is an acute or subacute viral myocarditis or pericarditis occurring as a manifestation or infection with enteroviruses, especially group B coxsackievirus. The myocardium is affected, particularly in neonates, in whom fever and lethargy may be followed rapidly by heart failure with pallor, cyanosis, dyspnea, tachycardia and enlargement of heart and liver. Heart failure may be progressive and fatal, or recovery may take place over a few weeks. In young adults, pericarditis is the more common manifestation, with acute chest pain, disturbance of heart rate, and often dyspnea. The disease may be associated with aseptic meningitis, hepatitis, orchitis, pancreatitis, pneumonia, hand-foot-and-mouth disease, rash or epidemic myiagia.

Symptoms of Coxsackievirus carditis can vary and may include:

1. Chest pain or discomfort.

2. Shortness of breath.

3. Fatigue.

4. Rapid or irregular heartbeat (arrhythmia).

5. Swelling in the legs, ankles, or feet (edema).

6. Fluid retention (puffiness and swelling).

7. Signs of heart failure, such as difficulty breathing when lying down.

Infectious agents:

Group B coxsackievirus (types 1-5); occasionally group A coxsackievirus (types 1, 4, 9, 16, 23) and other enteroviruses.

Occurrence:

Coxsackievirus carditis is an uncommon disease, mainly sporadic, but increased during epidemics of group B coxsackievirus infection. Institutional outbreaks, with high case-fatality rates in newborns, have been described in maternity units.

Reservoir:

Human are the only known reservoir of infection.

Mode of transmission:

It is directly by fecal-oral or respiratory droplet contact with an infected person, or indirectly by contact with articles freshly soiled with feces or throat discharges of an infected person who may or may not have symptoms.

Group B coxsackievirus have been found in sewage and flies, though the relationship to transmission of human infection is not clear.

Incubation period:

Incubation period is usually 3-5 days.

Period of communicability:

Apparently during the acute stage of disease; stools may contain virus for several weeks.

Susceptibility and resistance:

Susceptibility to infection is probably general; type-specific immunity presumably results from infection.

General review

1. Coxsackievirus carditis is also known as viral carditis, enteroviral carditis.

2. It is an acute or subacute viral myocarditis or pericarditis.

3. Heart failure with pallor, cyanosis, dyspnea, tachycardia

4. Coxsackievirus Gr. A, B

5. In young adults, pericarditis is the more common manifestation, with acute chest pain.

6. With high case-fatality rates in newborns

7. Fecal-oral or respiratory droplet spread

4-5 ECHO Acute Febrile Respiratory Disease (ICD-9 461-466; 480; ICD-10 j01-06; j12)

 Highlight

1. Acute febrile respiratory disease

2. Enteric Cytopathic Human Orphan virus

3. Aseptic meningitis

4. High infant mortality rates

5. Transmitted person-to-person; fecal-oral route

The first isolation of echoviruses occurred from the feces of asymptomatic children early in the 1950s, just after cell culturing had been developed. The *echo–* part of the name was originally an acronym for "enteric cytopathic human orphan" virus: *Orphan virus* means a virus that is not associated with any known disease. Even though Echoviruses have since been identified with various diseases, the original name is still used.

An echovirus is a type of RNA virus that belongs to the genus *Enterovirus* of the *Picornaviridae* family. Echoviruses are found in the gastrointestinal tract (hence it being part of the enterovirus genus) and exposure to the virus causes other opportunistic infections and diseases.

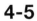 Identification to the acute febrile respiratory disease:

Echovirus is highly infectious, and its primary target is children. The echovirus is among the leading causes of acute febrile illness in infants and young children, and is the most common cause of aseptic meningitis. Infection of an infant with this virus following birth may cause severe systemic diseases, and is associated with high infant mortality rates.

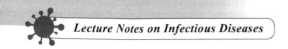

Most infections are subclinical; clinical manifestations vary from mild to lethal and acute to chronic; associated with aseptic meningitis (mostly serotypes 2, 5, 6, 7 and 9), muscle weakness and paralysis, exanthems and enanthems, pericarditis, myocarditis, common cold, conjunctivitis and infantile diarrhea, acute febrile respiratory illnesses.

Infectious agents:

Echovirus serotypes 1-9, 11-27, and 29-30. Naked, icosahedral virion, particle size is probably 20-30 nm in diameter; linear, positive-sense, single-stranded RNA; Picornaviridae.

Occurrence:

Worldwide; peak incidence in summer and fall; outbreaks common in daycare centers.

Reservoir:

Human are the only known reservoir of infection.

Mode of transmission:

Causes of echovirus infections can be placed in several categories. Main causes of infection are from overcrowded conditions such as the poor districts of a city and poor hygiene. Echoviruses are transmitted person-to-person; the fecal-oral route is the predominant mode, although transmission sometimes occurs via respiration of oral secretions such as saliva. Indirect transmission occurs through numerous routes, including via contaminated water, food, and fomites (inanimate objects). Contaminated swimming and wading pools can also transmit the virus. Also, there are well-documented reports of transmission via the contaminated hands of hospital personnel. Many ECHO virus infections are asymptomatic, meaning that individuals may carry the virus and shed it in their feces or respiratory secretions without experiencing noticeable symptoms.

🔋 Incubation period:

Incubation period is usually 2-14 days.

🔋 Period of communicability:

During the acute phase of the disease; excreted in feces for weeks after symptoms have subsided; person-to-person spread is common.

🔋 Susceptibility and resistance:

Susceptibility to infection is probably general; type-specific immunity presumably results from infection.

🔋 General review

1. Echovirus: enteric cytopathic human orphan virus

2. *Orphan virus* means a virus that is not associated with any known disease.

3. Echovirus is highly infectious, and its primary target is children.

4. Echovirus causes of acute febrile illness in infants and young children, and is the most common cause of aseptic meningitis.

5. High infant mortality rates

6. Echoviruses are transmitted person-to-person; the fecal-oral route is the predominant mode.

4-6 The Conclusions of Enteroviruses Groups Infectious Diseases

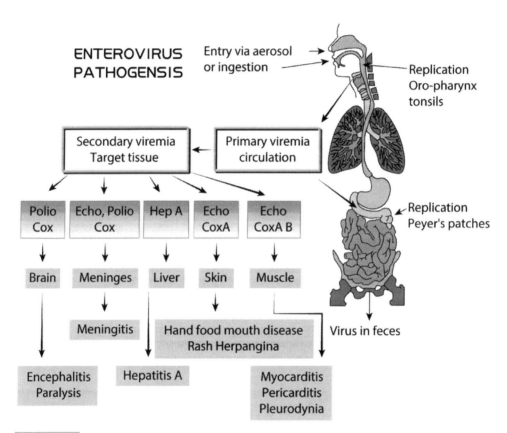

Figure 4-4   Enterovirus pathogensis

(www.pathmicro.med.sc.edu/virol/picorna.htm)

Most enterovirus infections are subclinical, especially in young children, but when they do cause clinically apparent disease, they can cause a wide range of clinical syndromes and can involve many of the body systems. Non-polio enteroviruses most commonly cause rashes, upper respiratory tract infections (URTIs) and summer colds. They can also cause neurological disease and are the most common cause of meningitis. In general, Coxsackievirus infections tend to cause more severe complications than echovirus infections resulting in: carditis, pleurodynia, herpangina, hand-foot-and-mouth disease, and occasionally paralysis, all of which are rarely seen in echovirus infection.

Recently there have been outbreaks of Enterovirus 71, which have caused fatal cases of hand-foot-and-mouth disease in Taiwan.

Human enteroviruses are found worldwide, and humans are the only natural hosts. Enteroviruses are transmitted primarily by the fecal-oral route, but respiratory spread is possible with some of the Coxsackieviruses, which can cause URTIs. Young children are most at risk for infection, which is usually inapparent, while older children and adults are more at risk for complications. In less developed areas of the world, most children become infected early in infancy, while in the developed world, first infection often does not occur until adolescence. Boys are more susceptible for the development of clinically apparent diseases than are girls. The virus may be shed from the stool for may weeks. Enteroviruses have been found in water, soil, vegetable, and shellfish. Thus, they may also be transmitted by contact with contaminated food or water. Enteroviruses are associated with seasonal infections, with epidemics peaking in late summer/early autumn in temperate climates, and epidemics occurring year-round in tropical climates.

Currently there are no vaccines available for the non-polio enteroviruses. Prevention includes improved sanitation and general hygiene, in addition to quarantine and possible closing of schools in the case of recognized epidemics. In addition to having no vaccines, there are no specific antiviral agents currently available for clinical use. Treatment is symptomatic and focuses on complications associated with infection. Administration of immune globulin may be useful in preventing severe disease in immunocompromised individuals or in those with life-threatening disease.

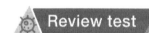 Review test

SCAN ME

Check Your Answers

I.   Multiple-choice questions (four selected one):

1. (   ) In Taiwan, during which seasons do Enterovirus group infections occur? (A) summer, (B) autumn, (C) summer and autumn, (D) winter and spring

2. (   ) What routes are used for the transmission of Enterovirus? (A) fecal-oral transmission, (B) air-droplets transmission, (C) contact transmission, (D) all of the above

3. (   ) Which disease publications frequently associate Coxsackie type A and Enterovirus type 71? (A) Herpangina, (B) Hand-Foot-Mouth Disease, (C) Infant Acute Myocarditis, (D) Epidemic pleurodynia

4. (   ) Which age group is more susceptible to enteroviral lymphonodular pharyngitis? (A) children under 10, (B) young adult, (C) old people, (D) all of the above

5. (   ) To which disease publications are Coxsackie types B and A frequently linked? (A) Herpangina, (B) Viral myocarditis or pericarditis, (C) Acute lymphonodular pharyngitis, (D) all of the above.

6. (   ) During epidemics of Group B Coxsackievirus infection, which of the following diseases could result in high case-fatality rates in newborns? (A) Viral myocarditis or pericarditis, (B) Hand-Foot-Mouth Disease, (C) Acute lymphonodular pharyngitis, (D) all of the above.

7. (   ) Which of the following methods could manage or prevent enteroviral infection? (A) Aspirin, (B) Erythromycin, (C) Pleconaril, (D) all of the above.

8. (   ) What is the target tissue that Hepatitis A virus invades in humans? (A) Brain, (B) Meninges, (C) Liver, (D) Muscle.

9. (   ) What is the target tissue that Echo virus, Polio virus, and Coxsackie virus invade in humans? (A) Brain, (B) Meninges, (C) Liver, (D) Muscle.

10. (   ) What is the target tissue that Echo virus and Coxsackievirus group A and B viruses invade in humans? (A) Brain, (B) Meninges, (C) Liver, (D) Skin

11. (   ) In Taiwan, during which season does the maximal incidence of Coxsackie type A10 epidemics occur? (A) spring, (B) summer and early autumn, (C) winter and spring, (D) all of the above

12. (   ) To which disease publications are Coxsackie type A and B infections frequently linked? (A) Herpangina, (B) Hand-Foot-Mouth Disease, (C) Acute lymphonodular pharyngitis, (D) Viral myocarditis or pericarditis

13. ( ) To which disease publications are Enterovirus type 71 and Coxsackie type A infections frequently linked? (A) Hand-Foot-Mouth Disease, (B) Infant Acute Myocarditis, (C) Epidemic pleurodynia, (D) Acute lymphonodular pharyngitis.

14. ( ) During epidemics of group B coxsackievirus infection, which disease of the following could induce high case-fatality rates in newborns? (A) Viral myocarditis or pericarditis, (B) Hand-Foot-Mouth Disease, (C) Acute lymphonodular pharyngitis, (D) all of the above.

15. ( ) In Taiwan, during which season does the peak incidence of ECHO acute febrile respiratory disease epidemics occur? (A) spring, (B) summer and fall, (C) winter and spring, (D) all of the above

16. ( ) What is the primary mode of transmission for enteroviruses? (A) Vector-borne transmission, (B) Airborne transmission, (C) Fomite transmission, (D) Fecal-oral route

17. ( ) Which enterovirus group is associated with diseases such as hand, foot, and mouth disease (HFMD)? (A) Group 1; Polioviruses, (B) Group 2; Coxsackieviruses, (C) Group 3; Echoviruses, (D) Group 4; Enteroviruses

18. ( ) What is a common symptom of infections caused by Coxsackieviruses? (A) Paralysis, (B) Skin rash, (C) Respiratory distress, (D) Encephalitis

19. ( ) Which group of enteroviruses is often associated with aseptic meningitis, a condition characterized by inflammation of the brain and spinal cord? (A) Group 1; Polioviruses, (B) Group 2; Coxsackieviruses, (C) Group 3; Echoviruses, (D) Group 4; Enteroviruses

20. ( ) What is a potential outcome of infections caused by enteroviruses from Group 4? (A) Paralysis, (B) Respiratory infections, (C) Hand, foot, and mouth disease, (D) Viral myocarditis

21. ( ) During which months are enterovirus infections more commonly observed? (A) Winter and spring, (B) Summer and fall, (C) Spring and summer, (D) Fall and winter

22. ( ) What is the most commonly observed serotype causing severe complications of enterovirus infections in Taiwan? (A) Coxsackievirus, (B) Echovirus, (C) Poliovirus, (D) Enterovirus A71 (EVA71)

23. ( ) Which term is used to describe enteroviral vesicular pharyngitis characterized by small, discrete, grayish papulovesicular lesions on an erythematous base? (A) Laryngitis, (B) Aphthous pharyngitis, (C) Herpangina, (D) Tonsillitis

24. ( ) In individuals with enteroviral vesicular pharyngitis, where do the lesions typically occur? (A) Nasal passages, (B) Anterior pillars of the tonsillar fauces, soft palate, uvula, and tonsils, (C) Lungs, (D) Esophagus

25. ( ) Which of the following is a symptom commonly experienced by individuals with enteroviral vesicular stomatitis with exanthema? (A) Respiratory distress, (B) Joint pain, (C) Irritability, (D) Vision problems

26. ( ) What is a characteristic feature of the skin rash in hand-foot-and-mouth disease (HFMD)? (A) Large, purple spots, (B) Raised blisters, (C) Itching and burning, (D) Yellow discoloration

27. ( ) How do the lesions in acute lymphonodular pharyngitis differ from those in vesicular pharyngitis? (A) Lesions are flat and red, (B) Lesions are firm, raised, discrete, and whitish to yellowish nodules, (C) Lesions occur predominantly on the palms and soles, (D) Lesions are itchy and may spread to other areas of the body

28. ( ) Where do the lesions occur predominantly in acute lymphonodular pharyngitis? (A) Palms and soles, (B) Uvula, anterior tonsillar pillars, and posterior pharynx, (C) Nasal passages, (D) Buttocks

29. ( ) Which group of Coxsackieviruses is particularly associated with myocarditis, especially in neonates? (A) Group A Coxsackieviruses, (B) Group B Coxsackieviruses, (C) Group C Coxsackieviruses, (D) Group D Coxsackieviruses

30. ( ) What is a common manifestation of Coxsackievirus carditis in young adults? (A) Hepatitis, (B) Aseptic meningitis, (C) Pericarditis, (D) Orchitis

31. ( ) What does the term "echo" in echovirus originally stand for? (A) Energetic cytopathic human orphan, (B) Enteric cytopathic human orphan, (C) Epidemic cytopathic human organism, (D) Echoic cytopathic human original

32. ( ) Which of the following diseases is echovirus most commonly associated with? (A) Pericarditis, (B) Myocarditis, (C) Aseptic meningitis, (D) Pharyngitis

33. ( ) What is the primary target demographic for echovirus infections? (A) Elderly population, (B) Adolescents, (C) Adults, (D) Children

34. (   ) What is the predominant mode of transmission for echovirus infections? (A) Blood transfusion, (B) Airborne particles, (C) Fecal-oral route, (D) Sexual contact

35. (   ) Apart from the fecal-oral route, what other mode of transmission is mentioned for echoviruses? (A) Vector-borne transmission, (B) Transmission through blood, (C) Respiration of oral secretions, (D) Skin-to-skin contact

36. (   ) Which of the following is mentioned as a complication more commonly associated with Coxsackievirus infections compared to echovirus infections? (A) Meningitis, (B) Pleurodynia, (C) Upper respiratory tract infections (URTIs), (D) Asymptomatic cases

II. Simple answer:

1. Could you please tell me that the enteroviruses can be differentiated into which main groups?

2. Could you please tell me during which seasons Enterovirus infections predominate in Taiwan?

3. Could you please tell me the transmission mode of enteroviruses infections?

4. Could you please tell me the predominant infectious agents of Hand-Foot-Mouth disease?

5. Fill in the blank

Enteroviruses groups' disease	Infectious agents
Enteroviral vesicular pharyngitis	
Enteroviral vesicular stomatitis with exanthema	
Enteroviral lymphonodular pharyngitis	
Coxsackievirus carditis	
ECHO acute febrile respiratory disease	

6. Fill in the blank (Enterovirus pathogenesis)

Pathogens	Target tissue	Pathogenesis
Polio, Cox		
Echo, Polio, Cox		
Hep A		
Echo, Cox A		
Echo, Cox A, B		

5

CHAPTER

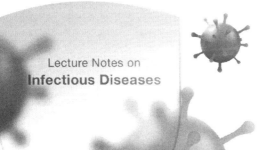

Lecture Notes on
Infectious Diseases

Respiratory Tract Infectious Diseases

The respiratory tract is divided into 3 segments: 1) Upper respiratory tract: nose and nasal passages, paranasal sinuses, and throat or pharynx. 2) Respiratory airways: voice box or larynx, trachea, bronchi, and bronchioles. 3) Lungs: respiratory bronchioles, alveolar ducts, alveolar sacs, and alveoli (Fig. 5-1). The respiratory tract is a common site for infections. Upper respiratory tract infections are probably the most common infections in the world. Most of the respiratory tract exists merely as a piping system for air to travel in the lungs; alveoli are the only part of the lung that exchanges oxygen and carbon dioxide with the blood.

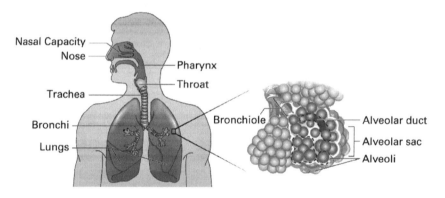

Nasal Capacity
Nose
Pharynx
Throat
Trachea
Bronchi
Bronchiole
Alveolar duct
Alveolar sac
Lungs
Alveoli

Figure 5-1   Respiratory tract is divided into 3 segments: upper respiratory, respiratory airways and Lungs.

Respiratory disease is an umbrella term for diseases of the lung, bronchial tubes, trachea and pharynx. These diseases range from mild and self-limiting (coryza/common cold) to life-threatening (e.g., bacterial pneumonia, pulmonary embolism etc.). Infectious respiratory diseases are, as the name suggests, typically caused by one of many infectious agents able to infect the mammalian respiratory system (for example the bacterium *Streptococcus pneumoniae*). The clinical features and treatment options vary greatly between infectious lung disease sub-types as each type may be caused by a different infectious agent, with different pathogenesis and virulence. Features also vary between: Upper respiratory tract infection, including strep throat and the common cold; and Lower respiratory tract infection, including pneumonia and pulmonary tuberculosis. About 20% of all deaths in children fewer than 5 years are duo to Acute Lower Respiratory Infections (ALRIs - pneumonia, bronchiolitis and bronchitis); 90% of these deaths are due to pneumonia. Early recognition and prompt treatment of pneumonia is lifesaving. Causative organisms may be bacterial (most commonly *Streptococcus pneumoniae* and *Haemophilus influenzae*) or viral. However, it is not possible to differentiate between bacterial and viral ALRIs based on clinical signs or radiology. Low birth weight malnourished and non-breastfed children and those living in overcrowded conditions are at higher risk of getting pneumonia. These children are also at a higher risk of death from pneumonia (WHO, 2008).

The familiar respiratory tract infectious diseases in Taiwan contains diphtheria, meningococcal meningitis, measles, pertussis, scarlet fever, rubella & CRS, mumps, chickenpox, tuberculosis, legionellosis, influenza, SARS, MERS, and COVID-19.

5-1 Diphtheria (ICD-9 032; ICD-10 A36)

Highlight

1. Diphtheria
2. Cutaneous diphtheria
3. Necrotic debris
4. Pseudomembrane
5. *Corynebacterium diphtheriae*
6. MLD: median lethal dose (LD50)
7. DPT: a triple antigen with diphtheria toxoid, tetanus toxoid and pertussis vaccine

Diphtheria was once a major public health concern, particularly in the late 19th and early 20th centuries. The development of effective vaccines has greatly reduced its incidence, but it remains a concern in some parts of the world. Diphtheria (Greek διφθερα (*diphthera*); "pair of leather scrolls"), is an upper respiratory tract illness characterized by sore throat, low fever, and an adherent membrane (a *pseudomembrane*) on the tonsils, pharynx, and/or nasal cavity. A milder form of diphtheria can be restricted to the skin. It is caused by *Corynebacterium diphtheriae*, an aerobic organism Gram-positive bacterium. Diphtheria is a contagious disease spread by direct physical contact or breathing the aerosolized secretions of infected individuals. Once quite common, diphtheria has largely been eradicated in developed nations through widespread vaccination. In Taiwan the DPT (*Diphtheria – Pertussis - Tetanus*) vaccine is given to all school children. Boosters of the vaccine are recommended for adults since the benefits of the vaccine decrease with age without constant re-exposure; they are particularly recommended for those traveling to areas where the disease has not been eradicated.

Diphtheria is a rare infection of the respiratory mucosa, and sometimes of broken skin. Although controlled in most communities by childhood immunization, elderly unvaccinated travelers. Vaccine- induced immunity declines in adult life. Tourists may unwittingly pass through endemic areas and be unexpectedly infected. Travelers who visit regions where diphtheria is more common can be at risk if they are not vaccinated. It's important for travelers to check their vaccination status and, if necessary, get vaccinated before traveling to areas where diphtheria is a concern. Diphtheria can still cause outbreaks in areas with suboptimal vaccination coverage. These outbreaks can occur in both developing and developed countries. Factors contributing to outbreaks may include vaccine hesitancy, challenges in vaccine distribution, and population mobility.

Identification to the Diphtheria:

It is an acute bacterial disease of tonsils, pharynx, larynx, nose, occasionally of other mucous membranes or skin and sometimes the conjunctiva or genitalia. The characteristic lesion, caused by liberation of a specific cytotoxin, is marked by patch or patches of an adherent grayish membrane with surrounding inflammation. Late effects of adsorption of toxin, appearing after 2-6 wks, include cranial and peripheral motor and sensory nerve palsies and myocarditis, and are often severe. The consequences of infection with *C. diphtheriae* are twofold: 1) the effects of the potent exotoxin. 2) obstruction of the airway by necrotic debris, which forms a tough pseudomembrane on infected respiratory mucosa.

A second type of diphtheria can affect the skin, causing the typical pain, redness and swelling associated with other bacterial skin infections. Ulcers covered by a gray membrane also may develop in cutaneous diphtheria. Although it's more common in tropical climates, cutaneous diphtheria also occurs in the Southeast Asia, particularly among people with poor hygiene who live in crowded conditions.

Infectious agent:

Corynebacterium diphtheriae of gravis, mitis, or intermedius biotype. Toxin production results when the bacteria are infected by corynebacteriophage containing the gene *tox*; toxigenic strains cause severe and fatal disease.

Occurrence:

Diphtheria is now most found in parts of the world with lower vaccination rates and limited access to healthcare. Countries in Africa, Asia, and the former Soviet Union have reported cases in recent years. Diphtheria is a disease of colder months in temperate zones, involving primarily unimmunized children less than 15 years of age. The case often found among adults in population groups whose immunization was neglected. In Taiwan the affected persons were from 6 months to 2-5 years of age. Endemics season are autumn (Oct., Nov., Dec.).

Reservoir:

Man.

Mode of transmission:

There are air droplets transmission, contact with patient or carrier, more rarely with articles solid with discharges from lesions of infected persons, and raw milk has served as a vehicle.

🔖 Incubation period:

Incubation period is usually 2-5 days, occasionally longer.

🔖 Period of communicability:

Variable, usually 2 weeks or less and seldom more than 4 weeks. The rare chronic carrier may shed organisms for 6 months or more.

🔖 Susceptibility and resistance:

People with weakened immune systems due to conditions like HIV/AIDS, cancer, or immunosuppressive medications may be more susceptible to diphtheria. Therefore, people who have not been vaccinated against diphtheria are highly susceptible to the disease. Infants born of immune mothers are relatively immune; protection is passive and usually lost before the 6th month. Recovery from clinical attack is not always followed by lasting immunity. Immunity is often acquired through inapparent infection. Prolonged active immunity can be induced by toxoid.

The diphtheria vaccine, which is often administered as part of the DTaP or Tdap vaccine series, stimulates the immune system to produce antibodies against the diphtheria toxin. These antibodies provide protection if the person is exposed to the bacterium. Immunity acquired from vaccination may decrease over time. To maintain resistance, individuals are often recommended to receive booster shots, such as the Tdap vaccine for adolescents and adults. Boosters help reinforce immunity.

The Schick test is a test used to determine whether a person is susceptible to diphtheria. The test is a simple procedure. A small amount (0.1 ml) of diluted (1/50 MLD) diphtheria toxin is injected intradermally into one arm of the person and a heat inactivated toxin on the other as a control. If a person does not have enough antibodies to fight it off, the skin around the injection will become red and swollen, indicating a positive result. This swelling disappears after a few days. If the person has an immunity, then little or no swelling and redness will occur, indicating a negative result. Results can be interpreted as:

1. **Positive**: when the test results in a wheal of 5-10 mm diameter, reaching its peak in 4-7 days. The control arm shows no reaction. This indicates that the subject lacks antibodies against the toxin and hence is susceptible to the disease.

2. **Pseudo-positive**: when there is only a red colored inflammation (erythema) and it disappears within 4 days. This happens on both the arms since the subject is immune but hypersensitive to the toxin.

3. **Negative reaction**: Indicates that the person is immune.

4. **Combined reaction**: Initial picture is like that of the pseudo-reaction, but the erythema fades off after 4 days only in the control arm. It progresses on the test arm to a typical positive. The subject is interpreted to be both susceptible and hypersensitive.

Methods of control:

Diphtheria is a medical emergency, and prompt treatment with antitoxin and antibiotics is essential to stop the infection and prevent complications. Patients with severe diphtheria may require hospitalization and supportive care. The only effective control is by a community program of active immunization with diphtheria toxoid, including an adequate program to maintain immunity. It is generally administered as a triple antigen with diphtheria toxoid combined with tetanus toxoid containing an aluminum adjuvant and pertussis vaccine (DPT). Vaccination is highly effective in preventing diphtheria. The diphtheria vaccine is typically given in combination with other vaccines, such as the tetanus (See Appendix: Introduction to Tetanus) and pertussis vaccines, as part of the DTaP or Tdap vaccine series for children and adults, respectively. Diphtheria toxoid was introduced to Taiwan in 1948. Until now, there was no more confirmed case after 1981 (Fig. 5-2).

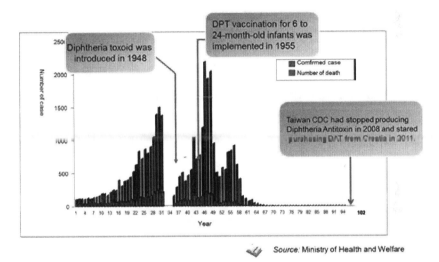

Source: Ministry of Health and Welfare

Figure 5-2   Diphtheria case in Taiwan, 1911-1981 (CDC, Taiwan).
(https://www.cdc.gov.tw/Category/ListContent/bg0g_VU_Ysr
gkes_KRUDgQ?uaid=9GTISWUmUE40xA_W9ZTWmA)

General review

1. Diphtheria

2. Cutaneous diphtheria

3. Necrotic debris

4. Pseudomembrane

5. *Corynebacterium diphtheriae*

6. MLD: median lethal dose (LD$_{50}$)

7. DPT (DTap or Tdap): a triple antigen with diphtheria toxoid, tetanus toxoid and pertussis vaccine

8. DTap: for children

9. Tdap: for adolescents and adults

SCAN ME

Check Your Answers

Review test

I. Multiple-choice questions (four selected one):

1. (   ) Which of the following diseases is characterized by a sore throat, low fever, and an adherent pseudomembrane on the tonsils, pharynx, and/or nasal cavity? (A) Diphtheria, (B) Pertussis, C, Mumps, (D) Rubella

2. (   ) In Taiwan, during which season is the endemic season of diphtheria? (A) spring, (B) summer, (C) fall, (D) winter

3. (   ) When do the late effects of diphtheria toxin adsorption appear after onset? (A) 1-2 wks, (B) 2-6 wks, (C) 8 wks, (D) 10-12 wks

4. (   ) How long is the incubation period of diphtheria usually? (A) within 24 hours, (B) 2-5 days, (C) 1 week, (D) it's variable

5. (   ) For the Schick test for diphtheria, what is the dose for the subcutaneous injection? (A) 1/5 MLD, (B) 1/10 MLD, (C) 1/50 MLD, (D) 1/250 MLD.

6. (   ) A 'Negative' result on the Schick test indicates what about the person? (A) lacks antibodies against diphtheria toxin, (B) hypersensitive to diphtheria toxin, (C) the person is immune, (D) susceptible and hypersensitive to diphtheria toxin

7. (   ) A 'Positive' result on the Schick test indicates what about the person? (A) lacks antibodies against diphtheria toxin, (B) hypersensitive to diphtheria toxin, (C) the person is immune, (D) susceptible and hypersensitive to diphtheria toxin

8. (   ) In what year did Taiwan no longer have confirmed cases of diphtheria? (A) 1948, (B) 1955, (C) 1981, (D) 2011

II. Simple answer:

1. Could you please provide information about the occurrence of diphtheria in Taiwan?

2. Could you please provide information about the transmission mode of diphtheria?

3. Could you please provide information about what the DPT 3-in-1 vaccine contains?

5-2

Pertussis (ICD-9 033.0; ICD-10 A37.0)
Parapertussis (ICD-9 033.1; ICD-10 A37.1)

Highlight

1. Pertussis

2. Whooping cough

3. Catarrhal stage

4. Paroxysmal stage

5. Quick short coughs

6. Repeated violent coughs

7. Inspiratory whoop

8. Convalescent stage

9. *Bordetella pertussis*

10. Respiratory isolation

Pertussis has likely been present in human populations for centuries, but the earliest recorded descriptions of its symptoms date back to the 16th century. The term "pertussis" comes from the Latin word "pertussis," meaning "violent cough." In the 18th century, physicians began to recognize and describe the distinct coughing fits associated with the disease. Pertussis, also known as whooping cough, a highly contagious disease caused by the bacterium *Bordetella pertussis*; it derived its name from the characteristic severe hacking cough followed by intake of breath that sounds like "whoop"; a similar, milder disease is caused by *B. parapertussis*. Although many medical sources describe the whoop as "high-pitched," this is generally the case with infected babies and children only, not adults.

It is a worldwide infectious disease; there are 30-50 million pertussis cases and about 300,000 deaths per year. Despite generally high coverage with the DTP and DTaP vaccines, pertussis is one of the leading causes of vaccine-preventable deaths world-wide. Most deaths occur in young infants who are either unvaccinated or incompletely vaccinated; three doses of the vaccine are necessary for complete protection against pertussis. Ninety percent of all cases occur in the developing world. Children tend to catch it more than adults.

Although it is now rare, as immunization is widespread, large epidemics occurred in the 1980s after concerns about vaccine safety resulted in low rates of acceptance. Morbidity is high in infants and in older children with respiratory or cardiac disease. Pertussis remains a significant global health concern, especially for infants and pregnant women, as they are particularly vulnerable to severe complications. International organizations and governments continue to work on expanding vaccination programs to reach more people.

Identification to the Pertussis:

Pertussis is an acute bacterial disease involving the respiratory tract. Whooping cough can cause fever and quick short coughs due to spasms of the glottis as the air leaves the lungs. The onset duration contains 3 stages: Catarrhal stage, Paroxysmal stage and Convalescent stage.

1. The initial catarrhal stage has an insidious onset with an irritating cough.

2. The paroxysmal stage is usually within 1 to 2 weeks and lasts for 1 to 2 months. Paroxysms are characterized by repeated violent coughs. Each series of paroxysms has many coughs without intervening inhalation and may be followed by a characteristic crowing or high-pitched inspiratory whoop. Paroxysms frequently end with the expulsion of clear, tenacious mucus.

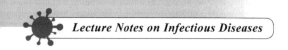

3. Convalescent stage: In the stage, the symptom and cough frequency are milder. Young infants and adults often do not have the typical whoop or cough paroxysm.

Pertussis can affect individuals of all ages, but its impact varies by age group. Infants, especially those too young to be fully vaccinated, are at the highest risk of severe complications and death. Adolescents and adults can also contract and transmit pertussis, although their symptoms may be milder. The fatality of pertussis in Taiwan is low; approximately 75% of deaths are among children under 1 year of age, most in those under 6 months. Morbidity and mortality are higher in females than males. In unimmunized populations, especially those with underlying malnutrition and multiple infections, pertussis is among the most lethal disease of infants and young children.

Parapertussis is a similar but usually milder disease clinically indistinguishable from pertussis. Parapertussis is usually seen in school-age children and occurs relatively infrequently.

🔹 Infectious agents:

Bordetella pertussis (the bacillus of pertussis stricto sensus), *Bordetella parapertussis* causes parapertussis.

B. pertussis was isolated in pure culture in 1906 by Jules Bordet and Octave Gengou, who also developed the first serology and vaccine. The complete *B. pertussis* genome of 4,086,186 base pairs was sequenced in 2002.

🔹 Occurrence:

Pertussis is endemic in virtually every part of the world, which often exhibits a seasonal pattern, with more cases reported during late summer and early fall. However, it can occur year-round. The disease is common to children everywhere, regardless of race, climate, or geographic location. There has been a marked decline in incidence and mortality rates during the past four decades, chiefly in communities fostering active immunization and where good nutrition and medical care are available.

Reservoir:

Men are believed to be the only host for pertussis. *Bordetella parapertussis* can also be isolated from sheep.

Mode of transmission:

Pertussis is highly contagious and spreads through respiratory droplets when an infected person coughs or sneezes. Close contact with an infected individual, especially within households, increases the risk of transmission. It is primary by direct contact with discharges from respiratory mucous membranes of infected persons by the airborne route, probably by droplets. The disease can also frequently bring home by an older sibling.

Incubation period:

Incubation period is commonly 7-14 days, almost uniformly within 10 days, and not exceeding 20 days.

Period of communicability:

It is highly communicable in the early catarrhal stage before paroxysmal cough stage. Thereafter, communicability gradually decreases and becomes negligible for ordinary non-familial contacts in about 3 weeks, despite persisting spasmodic cough with whoop.

▶ Susceptibility and resistance:

Susceptibility to pertussis is general, with no definitive evidence of effective transplacental immunity in infants. In particular, newborns, especially those who have not yet completed the full series of pertussis vaccinations (DTaP or Tdap), are notably vulnerable to pertussis due to their lack of sufficient immunity against the disease. Consequently, infants are highly susceptible to pertussis. Therefore, incidence rates are highest under 5 years of age.

Infants born to mothers who have received the Tdap vaccine during pregnancy receive passive immunity from maternal antibodies, providing some protection against pertussis in the early months of life. One attack confers definite and prolonged immunity, although second attacks can occasionally occur.

▶ Methods of control:

Vaccination is the primary means of developing resistance to pertussis. The DTaP (for children) and Tdap (for adolescents and adults) vaccines stimulate the immune system to produce antibodies against the pertussis bacterium, providing protection. In the 1990s, acellular pertussis vaccines (aP vaccines) were developed as an alternative to whole-cell vaccines. These vaccines contain purified components of the pertussis bacterium, reducing the risk of side effects associated with whole-cell vaccines. Pertussis vaccines are highly effective, strongly recommended, and save many infants lives every year. Though the protection they offer lasts only a few years, they are given so that immunity lasts through childhood, the time of greatest exposure and greatest risk. The immunizations are given in combination with tetanus and diphtheria immunizations, at ages 2, 4, and 6 months, and later at 15-18 months and 4-6 years and 11-year-old children. In recent years, the annual number of confirmed Pertussis cases is about 2 to 78 in

Taiwan (Fig. 5-3). According to the analysis of data from the notifiable infectious disease reporting system, the age distribution of confirmed cases indicated that most of the cases occurred in infants and adolescents. The Taiwan government provides free immunizations to children including 5-in-1 (diphtheria and tetanus toxoid with acellular pertussis, *Haemophilus influenzae* type b, and inactivated polio, **DTaP-Hib-IPV**), diphtheria and tetanus toxoids with acellular pertussis and inactivated polio vaccine (**DTaP-IPV**) (CDC, Taiwan, 2023).

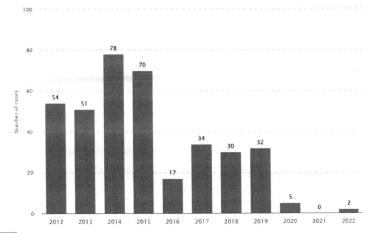

Figure 5-3   Number of confirmed cases of pertussis in Taiwan from 2012 to 2022
(https://www.statista.com/statistics/1079821/taiwan-pertussis-cases/)

When there is an outbreak, protection of health workers at high risk of exposure by the administration of a booster dose of 0.25 ml pertussis vaccine or a 14-day course of erythromycin may be considered. Respiratory isolation for known cases is necessary. Concurrent disinfection: discharges from nose and throat and articles soiled therewith terminal cleaning. Specific treatment: Antibiotics (e.g., erythromycin or TMP-SMX) may shorten the period of communicability.

General review

1. Pertussis, repeated violent coughs (whooping cough) is a worldwide infectious disease

2. An acute bacterial disease

3. The onset duration contains 3 stages: Catarrhal stage, Paroxysmal stage, Convalescent stage

4. Parapertussis is usually seen in school-age children

5. Infectious agent: *Bordetella pertussis*

6. Highly communicable in the early catarrhal stage before paroxysmal cough stage

7. DPT vaccine

SCAN ME

Check Your Answers

Review test

I.   Multiple-choice questions (four selected one):

1. (   ) The initial catarrhal stage of pertussis has an insidious onset, characterized by what symptoms? (A) irritating cough, (B) repeated violent coughs, (C) mild cough, (D) typical whoop

2. (   ) Which of the following methods are effective for controlling pertussis? (A) pertussis vaccine, (B) DPT vaccine, (C) A 14-day course of erythromycin, (D) all of the above

3. (   ) Which stage of pertussis infection is highly contagious? (A) early catarrhal stage, (B) before paroxysmal stage, (C) convalescent stage, (D) A and B

4. (   ) In clinical settings, which of the following vaccines is intended for children as part of pertussis control? (A) Tdap, (B) DTap, (C) DPT, (D) all of the above

5. (   ) Which stage of pertussis infection is characterized by repeated violent coughing fits? (A) Catarrhal stage, (B) Paroxysmal stage, (C) Convalescent stage, (D) Initial stage

6. (   ) Regarding the period of communicability of pertussis, how long does it take for the infection to transition from being highly infectious to becoming less contagious? (A) 5 to 7 days, (B) 2 weeks, (C) 3 weeks, (D) 3 months

7. (   ) Parapertussis infection is usually observed in which individuals? (A) infants, (B) school-age children, (C) pregnant women, (D) adolescents and adults

8. (   ) In what year did acellular pertussis vaccines (aP vaccines) were developed as an alternative to whole-cell vaccines? (A) 1970s, B, 1980s, (C) 1990s, (D) 2000s

II. Simple answer:

1. Could you please provide information about which stage of pertussis is the most contagious?

2. Could you please provide information about the characteristics and symptoms of pertussis infection?

3. Could you please provide information about the DPT immunization schedule for children?

5-3   Measles (ICD-9 055; ICD-10 B05)

😐 Highlight

1. Measles
2. Rubeola
3. Hard measles
4. Morbilli
5. Koplik spots
6. Malnourished children
7. *Morbillivirus* (Paramyxoviridae)
8. Respiratory isolation

Measles, also known as rubeola, hard measles, or morbilli which is a disease caused by a virus, specifically a paramyxovirus of the genus *Morbillivirus*. Measles is a highly contagious viral infection caused by the measles virus (MeV), which is spread through respiration (contact with fluids from an infected person's nose and mouth, either directly or through aerosol transmission), and is highly contagious—90% of people without immunity sharing a house with an infected person will catch it. Airborne precautions should be taken for all suspected cases of measles. It is a significant public health concern and has been the cause of numerous outbreaks throughout history.

Measles is a systemic viral infection whose main features are respiratory disease and rash. It is highly infectious among susceptible individuals and almost always produces clinical disease in those infected. In unprotected populations it tends to occur in large epidemics mainly affecting children, but the widespread use of effective immunization programmes has made it uncommon in many parts of the world. The important impact of measles contains: 1) It can be a severe and debilitating illness; 2) Secondary bacterial respiratory disease is common and may be severe; 3) Post-measles encephalitis is life-threatening and can leaves severe sequelae.

⏹ Identification to the Measles:

It is an acute, highly communicable viral disease. prodromal syndromes are fever, conjunctivitis, coryza, cough and Koplik spots on the buccal mucosa. Measles causes a red, blotchy rash that usually appears first on the face and behind the ears, then spreads downward to the chest and back and finally to the feet. A characteristic red blotchy rash appears on the 3rd to 4th days, beginning on the face, becoming generalized, lasting 4 to 7 days and sometimes ending in branny desquamation (Fig. 5-4). Measles is a more severe disease among the very young and in malnourished children, associated with hemorrhagic measles, protein-losing enteropathy, mouth sore, dehydration and severe skin infections, with a case fatality rate of 5-10% or more.

The symptoms of measles typically appear about 10-12 days after exposure and include:

1. High fever (104°F or 40°C)

2. Cough

3. Runny nose

4. Red, watery eyes (conjunctivitis)

5. A characteristic red rash that starts on the face and spreads to the rest of the body

Measles can lead to severe complications, especially in young children and immunocompromised individuals. These complications may include pneumonia, encephalitis, and in severe cases, it can be fatal.

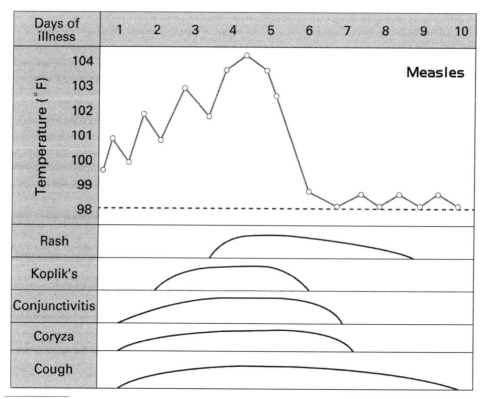

Figure 5-4   The characteristics and publications of Measles.
[Centigrade (°C) = (Fahrenheit (°F) − 32) × 5/9]
(www.life in the fastlane.com)

🔹 Infectious agent:

Measles virus. It is a member of the genus *Morbillivirus* of family Paramyxoviridae. It is a single-stranded RNA virus.

Occurrence:

Prior to widespread immunization, measles was common in childhood; so that over 90% of people had been infected by age 20; few persons went through life without an attack. Measles was endemic in large metropolitan communities, attaining epidemic proportions about every other year. In Taiwan, the endemics season are often during the winter months.

Reservoir:

Man.

Mode of transmission:

By droplet spread or direct contact with nasal or throat secretions of infected persons. Less commonly by airborne spread or by articles freshly soiled with secretions of nose and throat.

Incubation period:

About 10 days, varying from 8–13 days from exposure to onset of fever; about 14 days until rash appears.

Period of communicability:

It is from slightly before the beginning of the prodromal period to 4 days after appearance of the rash.

The period of communicability for measles can be divided into several phases:

1. **Prodromal phase**: This is the initial phase of illness, characterized by symptoms such as high fever, cough, runny nose, and red, watery eyes (conjunctivitis). During this phase, which typically lasts for about 2-4

days, the infected person is usually not yet aware that they have measles. However, they can already be contagious and capable of spreading the virus to others through respiratory droplets when coughing or sneezing.

2. **Early Rash phase**: After the prodromal phase, a characteristic red rash begins to appear on the face and spreads to the rest of the body over a period of a few days. During this phase, which can last for about 3-5 days, the individual remains highly contagious.

3. **Late Rash phase**: Even after the rash has fully developed, the individual can still be contagious for a few more days. This late rash phase can last for about 2-4 days. It's important to note that the person is considered contagious until all rash lesions have crusted over.

Susceptibility and resistance:

Practically all persons who have not had the disease or been immunized are susceptible. Acquired immunity after disease is usually permanent. Infants born of mothers who have had the disease are ordinarily immune for approximately the first 6-9 months or more depending on the amount of residual maternal antibody at the time of pregnancy.

Methods of control:

Vaccination: very high vaccination rate are required to prevent the spread of measles. Respiratory isolation: children with measles should be kept out of school until they are no longer infectious (5 days after the appearance of the rash). Unvaccinated children who have been in contact with a case of measles may be protected by vaccination, provided that it is given within 72 hrs of exposure.

In developed countries, most children are immunized against measles by the age of 18 months, generally as part of a three-part MMR vaccine (measles, mumps, and rubella). The vaccination is generally not given earlier than this because children younger than 18 months usually retain anti-measles immunoglobulins (antibodies) transmitted from the mother during pregnancy.

The MMR (Measles, Mumps, and Rubella) vaccine is an essential immunization for children to protect them against these three viral diseases. Below is the typical immunization schedule for MMR vaccination in children (CDC, Taiwan, 2023) (https://www.cdc.gov.tw/Category/List/_MJYeQXoPjzYik1sYwTj6Q) :

1. **First Dose**: The first dose of the MMR vaccine is typically administered when a child is around 12 to 15 months of age. This first dose provides primary protection against measles, mumps, and rubella.

2. **Second Dose**: A booster dose of the MMR vaccine is recommended for children to enhance and prolong immunity. The second dose is typically given at 5 to 6 years of age, often before a child enters kindergarten or elementary school. This second dose helps ensure long-lasting protection.

In Taiwan, measles had been listed as a reportable disease since 1985. A program to eradicate poliomyelitis, measles, rubella, congenital rubella syndrome (CRS), and neonatal tetanus (See Appendix: Introduction to Tetanus) was initiated in 1991. Through the implementation of the eradication program, the quality of the surveillance system was significantly strengthened and the vaccination coverage of measles containing vaccine was notably improved. Beginning 1993, measles has been brought under effective control in Taiwan. After the eradication program for poliomyelitis, neonatal tetanus, congenital rubella syndrome and measles was implemented in 1991 and two rounds of catch-up campaigns (1992-1994 and 2001-2004) were enforced of to intensify the surveillance system and to improve the vaccination coverage rate. Since 1993, only few confirmed measles cases were reported annually (Centers for Disease Control, R.O.C. Taiwan, 2018) (Fig. 5-5).

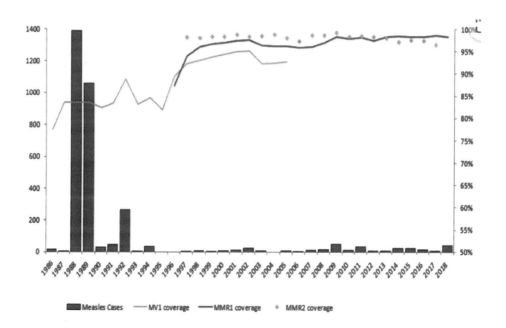

Figure 5-5   Measles cases and immunization coverage in Taiwan from
1986 to 2018 Measles Surveillance in Taiwan (Taiwan National
Infectious Disease Statistics System-Measles).
(https://www.cdc.gov.tw/En/Category/ListContent/bg0g_VU_Y
srgkes_KRUDgQ?uaid=GPRvsfwiREEPQXGGVv9tEA)

General review

1. Measles (rubeola, hard measles, or morbilli)

2. A paramyxovirus of the genus *Morbillivirus*

3. Acute, highly communicable viral disease

4. A severe and debilitating illness

5. Post-measles encephalitis

6. Koplik spots

7. Transmitted by droplet spread or direct contact

8. MMR vaccination

SCAN ME

Check Your Answers

Review test

I. Multiple-choice questions (four selected one):

1. ( ) Unvaccinated children who have been in contact with a case of measles may be protected by vaccination, provided that it is given within how long after exposure? (A) 12 hours, (B) 24 hours, (C) 48 hours, (D) 72 hours

2. ( ) How long should children with measles be kept out of school until they are no longer infectious? (A) 5 days, (B) 7 days, (C) 10 days, (D) 14 days

3. ( ) What is the fatality rate of untreated measles cases? (A) 1-3%, (B) 5-10%, (C) 30%, (D) exceeded 50%.

4. ( ) Which of the following represents the prodromal syndrome of measles? (A) fever, (B) Koplik spots on the buccal mucosa, (C) cough, (D) all of the above.

5. ( ) At what time does the red blotchy rash usually appear in a measles case? (A) first day, (B) second day, (C) 3rd-4th days, (D) 4th-7th days.

6. ( ) At what age is the first dose of the MMR vaccine typically administered to a child? (A) around 5 to 6 months of age, (B) around 12 to 15 months of age, (C) around 5 to 6 years of age, (D) around 12 to 15 years of age

7. ( ) At what age is the second dose of the MMR vaccine typically administered to a child? (A) around 5 to 6 months of age, (B) around 12 to 15 months of age, (C) around 5 to 6 years of age, (D) around 12 to 15 years of age

8. ( ) At what age is a booster dose of the MMR vaccine recommended for children to enhance and prolong immunity? (A) around 5 to 6 months of age, (B) around 12 to 15 months of age, (C) around 5 to 6 years of age, (D) around 12 to 15 years of age

II. Simple answer:

1. Could you please provide information on the occurrence of measles in Taiwan?

2. Could you please provide information on the important impacts of measles?

3. Could you please provide information on the prodromal symptoms of measles?

4. How long should children with measles be kept out of school until they are no longer infectious, and what is the name of this precaution?

5-4 Mumps (ICD-9 072; ICD-10 B26)

 Highlight

1. Infectious parotitis
2. Orchitis
3. Oophoritis
4. Mumps virus (genus *Paramyxovirus*)
5. MMR vaccine: a combination vaccine with mumps, measles and rubella live virus vaccine

Mumps is a viral infection caused by the mumps virus, which belongs to the Paramyxoviridae family. It primarily affects the salivary glands, leading to painful swelling of the cheeks and jaw, giving the infected person a characteristic "chipmunk" appearance. Mumps or epidemic parotitis is a viral disease of humans. The word "mumps" originally meant "to mumble" and came to be applied to the disease because of the side effects it causes. It was a common childhood disease worldwide and is still a significant threat to health in the third world. While symptoms are generally not severe in children, the symptoms in teenagers and adults can be more severe and complications such as infertility or subfertility are relatively common, although still rare in absolute terms. The disease is generally self-limited, running its course before waning, with no specific treatment apart from controlling the symptoms with painkillers.

Identification to the mumps:

The hallmark symptom of mumps is swollen salivary glands, which can be accompanied by other symptoms such as fever, headache, muscle aches, fatigue, and loss of appetite. The swelling typically occurs on one or both sides of the face and can be quite painful. The infection can lead to various complications in some cases, which include orchitis (inflammation of the testicles), oophoritis (inflammation of the ovaries), meningitis, encephalitis, and even hearing loss.

Orchitis, usually unilateral, occurs in 20-30% of males and oophoritis in about 5% of females past puberty. The CNS is frequently involved, either early or late in the disease, usually as an aseptic meningitis. Mumps infection during the 1st trimester of pregnancy may increase the rate of spontaneous abortions. There is no firm evidence that mumps during pregnancy causes congenital malformations.

Infectious agent:

Mumps virus, a member of the genus *Paramyxovirus*, antigenically related to the parainfluenza virus.

Occurrence:

About one-third of exposed susceptible persons have inapparent infections. Winter and spring are seasons of greatest prevalence. In Taiwan the decline has occurred in children 4-9 years old, but with effective pediatric and preschool immunization programs, the greatest risk of infection has shifted toward older children. Between 2012 and 2018, 5459 cases of mumps cases were reported to the Centers for Disease Control, Taiwan. The occurrence of mumps is influenced by seasonality (CDC, Taiwan, 2021) (Fig. 5-6).

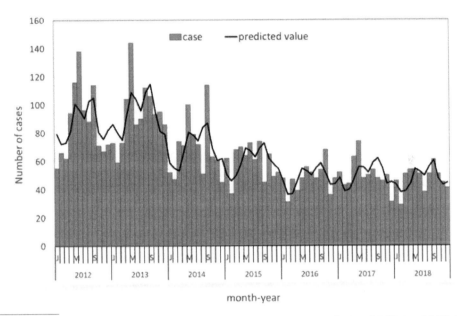

Figure 5-6 The actual and predicted mumps cases from 2012 to 2018 in Taiwan.
(https://www.ncbi.nlm.nih.gov/pmc/articles/PMC8447993/)

Reservoir:

Man (Infected person).

Mode of transmission:

It is by the way of airborne transmission or droplet spread, also direct contact with saliva of an infected person.

Incubation period:

Incubation period is about 16-18 days, range from 14 to 25 days.

Period of communicability:

The virus has been isolated from saliva from 6 days before overt parotitis up to 9 days after. The maximal infectiousness occurs about 48 hours before onset of illness. Urine may be positive for as long as 14 days after onset of illness. Inapparent infections can be communicable.

Susceptibility and resistance:

Susceptibility is general. Immunity is generally life-long and develops after inapparent as well as clinical attacks.

People who have not received the MMR (measles, mumps, and rubella) vaccine are highly susceptible to mumps infection. This includes infants and young children who have not yet been vaccinated. Those who have received only one dose of the MMR vaccine may still be susceptible to mumps, although the vaccine provides some level of protection. People with weakened immune systems, such as those with HIV/AIDS, certain cancers, or on immunosuppressive medications, may be more susceptible to mumps and its complications.

People who have previously had mumps develop natural immunity to the virus. Once a person has had mumps, they are usually immune to future mumps infections. High vaccination coverage within a population can lead to herd immunity, which indirectly protects unvaccinated or susceptible individuals. When a significant portion of the population is immune, the virus has fewer opportunities to spread, reducing the overall risk of mumps outbreaks.

Methods of control:

Public health efforts focus on achieving high vaccination rates to minimize the spread of mumps and prevent outbreaks. Maintaining up-to-date vaccination records and following recommended vaccination schedules are key strategies to protect individuals and communities from mumps and its complications. The most common preventative measure against mumps is immunization with a mumps vaccine (live attenuated vaccine). The vaccine may be given separately or as part of the MMR immunization vaccine which also protects against measles and rubella. The WHO recommends the use of mumps vaccines in all countries with well-functioning childhood vaccination programmes:

1. The first dose of the mumps-containing vaccine (MMR-1) should be administered at 12 to 15 months of age or later.

2. The second dose of the mumps vaccine (MMR-2) should be administered at either 5 years of age or upon entering the first grade of elementary school.

If persons or groups responsible for reporting found someone met mumps case definition or laboratory testing should notify local health department for one week. Current evidence suggests that patients diagnosed with mumps should be isolated for 9 days from the onset of symptoms. Susceptible people should avoid attending school (C.D.C., Taiwan, 2014).

General review

1. Mumps (epidemic parotitis)

2. An acute viral disease

3. Complications: ♂Orchitis; ♀ oophoritis; aseptic meningitis

4. High risk during pregnancy; spontaneous abortions

5. Mumps virus (*Paramyxovirus*; parainfluenza virus)

6. Occurrence in Taiwan during winter and spring

7. MMR live attenuated vaccine

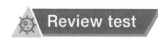

Review test

I. Multiple-choice questions (four selected one):

1. (   ) In the case of infectious parotitis, how long before the onset of illness does maximal infectiousness occur? (A) 12 hours, (B) 24 hours, (C) 48 hours, (D) 72 hours

2. (   ) In the case of mumps, how many days after the onset of illness can a patient's urine test still be positive? (A) 7 days, (B) 14 days, (C) 21 days, (D) it's variable and dependent on the patient

3. (   ) What is the likelihood of males developing unilateral orchitis as a complication of mumps? (A) 5%, (B) 10%, (C) 12-15%, (D) 20-30%

4. (   ) What is the likelihood of females developing oophoritis as a complication of mumps? (A) 5%, (B) 10%, (C) 12-15%, (D) 20-30%

5. (   ) Among the following options, who are highly susceptible to mumps infection if they are unvaccinated? (A) infants, (B) young children, (C) AIDS patient, (D) all of the above

6. (   ) In Taiwan, to whom should the first dose of the mumps-containing vaccine (MMR-1) be administered? (A) 6 months after birth, (B) 12 to 15 months of age, (C) 5 years of age, (D) all of the above

7. (   ) In Taiwan, to whom should the second dose of the mumps-containing vaccine (MMR-2) be administered? (A) 6 months after birth, (B) 12 to 15 months of age, (C) 5 years of age, (D) all of the above

8. ( ) How long should patients diagnosed with mumps be isolated from the onset of symptoms, according to current evidence? (A) 9 days, (B) 10 to 14 days, (C) 15 days, (D) 21 days

II. Simple answer:

1. Could you please provide information about the transmission of mumps?

2. Could you please provide information about the occurrence of mumps in Taiwan?

3. Could you please provide information about mumps infection complications?

5-5 Rubella (ICD-9 056; ICD-10 B06) Congenital Rubella Syndrome (ICD-9 771.0; ICD-10 P35.0)

 Highlight

1. German measles

2. CRS: congenital rubella syndrome

3. 1st trimester of pregnancy

4. Intrauterine death

5. Spontaneous abortion

6. Cataracts

7. Microphthalmia

8. Mental retardation

9. Rubella virus (family Togaviridae; genus *Rubivirus*)

10. Live attenuated rubella vaccine

Rubella, commonly known as German measles, is a disease caused by rubella virus. The name is derived from the Latin, meaning *little red*. Rubella is also known as German measles because the disease was first described by German physicians in the mid-eighteenth century. Friedrich Hoffmann made the first clinical description of rubella in 1740, which was confirmed by de Bergen in 1752 and Orlow in 1758. In 1969 a live attenuated virus vaccine was licensed. In the early 1970s, a triple vaccine containing attenuated measles, mumps and rubella (MMR) viruses was introduced.

This disease is often mild, and attacks often pass unnoticed. The disease can last one to five days. Children recover more quickly than adults. Infection of the mother by rubella virus during pregnancy can be serious; if the mother is infected within the first 20 weeks of pregnancy, the child may be born with congenital rubella syndrome (CRS), which entails a range of serious incurable illnesses. Spontaneous abortion occurs in up to 20% of cases. Rubella is a common childhood infection usually with minimal systemic upset although transient arthropathy may occur in adults. Serious complications are very rare. If it were not for the effects of transplacental infection on the developing fetus, rubella is a relatively trivial infection.

In most people the virus is rapidly eliminated however, it may persist for some months postpartum in infants surviving the CRS. These children were an important source of infection to other infants and, more importantly, pregnant female contacts.

◆ Identification to the rubella & congenital rubella syndrome:

Rubella is a mild febrile infectious disease with a diffuse punctate and macular rash sometimes resembling that of measles or scarlet fever.

Children may present few or no constitutional symptoms. Adults may experience a 1–5 day's prodrome of low-grade fever, headache, malaise, mild coryza, and conjunctivitis.

Rubella is important because of its ability to produce anomalies in the developing fetus. Congenital rubella syndrome occurs among 25% or more of infants born to women who acquired rubella during the 1st trimester of pregnancy; the risk of a single congenital defect falls to approximately 10% by the 16th week. Defects are rare when the maternal infection occurs after the 20th week of gestation. Fetuses infected early are at greatest risk of intrauterine death, spontaneous abortion and combinations of defects: deafness, cataracts, microphthalmia, microcephaly, mental retardation.

Infectious agent:

Rubella virus (family Togaviridae; genus *Rubivirus*).

Occurrence:

In the absence of generalized immunization rubella occurred worldwide at endemic levels with epidemic every 5–9 years. Large rubella epidemics resulted in very high levels of morbidity.

Universally endemic expect in remote and isolate communities, especially certain island groups which have epidemics every 10–15 years. The disease is prevalent in winter and spring. Taiwan has been epidemics in 1958–1959, 1968 and 1977.

Reservoir:

Man.

🔹 Mode of transmission:

Contact with nasopharyngeal secretions of infected persons. Infection is by droplet spread or direct contact with patients. Infants with congenital rubella may shed large quantities of virus in their pharyngeal secretions and urine, and severe as source of infection to their contacts.

🔹 Incubation period:

Incubation period is from16-18 days with a range of 14-23 days.

🔹 Period of communicability:

Period of communicability is for about 1 week before and at least 4 days after onset of rash. It is high communicable. Infant with congenital rubella may shed virus for months after birth.

🔹 Susceptibility and resistance:

Susceptibility is general after loss of transplacentally acquired maternal antibody. Individuals who have never been infected with the rubella virus and have not been vaccinated are susceptible to the disease. Rubella is more common in children and young adults who have not yet received the vaccine. They are often more susceptible to the virus. Pregnant women can become infected with rubella if they are not immune. Infection during pregnancy can lead to congenital rubella syndrome (CRS) in the unborn child.

Active immunity is acquired by natural infection or by vaccination and is usually permanent after natural infection and is expected to be long-term, probably lifelong, after vaccination.

Susceptibility and resistance to rubella are influenced by vaccination status, prior infection history, age, and individual health conditions. Vaccination is a highly effective way to develop immunity and prevent rubella, and it also plays a crucial role in reducing the overall prevalence of the disease in communities.

🔊 Methods of control:

Rubella control is needed primarily to prevent defects in the offspring of women who acquire the disease during pregnancy. A single dose of live attenuated rubella vaccine (Rubella Virus Vaccine, Live) elicits a significant antibody response in approximately 95% of susceptible. The vaccine in dried form and after reconstitution must be kept at 2-8°C or colder and protected from light to retain potency. Frozen vaccine must be kept at -10°C to -30°C to retain potency.

College and university students, healthcare personnel, non-pregnant women of childbearing age, childcare workers such as teachers and day care personnel, and international travelers are at increased risk for German measles, and these persons should receive two doses of MMR vaccine to ensure adequate protection (WHO, 2004). The rubella vaccine was introduced to Taiwan in 1986 for the third grader of junior high schoolgirls. In 1992, Taiwan CDC implemented universal vaccination of MMR vaccine to 12-month-old children. From 2001, Taiwan CDC began to provide the second dose of MMR regularly for 5-year-old children when they enter elementary school, the vaccination programme are according to the current immunization schedule in Taiwan (Tab. 5-1). The rubella cases reduced significantly. Since 1998, less than 60 confirmed rubella cases were reported annually (Fig. 5-7).

Table 5-1 Current Immunization Schedule in Taiwan (2019. 8 revised)

Age / Vaccine	< 24 hr after birth	1 month	2 months	4 months	5 months	6 months	12 months	15 months	18 months	21 months	27 months	5 years old	1st–6th grade Primary school students
Hepatitis B	HepB1	HepB2				HepB3							
DPT, Hib, Polio			DTaP-Hib-IPV1	DTaP-Hib-IPV2		DTaP-Hib-IPV 3			DTaP-Hib-IPV 4			DTaP-Hib-IPV 5	
Pneumococcal cognate vaccine			PCV13	PCV13			PCV13						
Varicella							Var						
MMR							MMR1					MMR2	
JEV								JEV1			JEV2		
Hepatitis A							HepA1		HepA2				
Influenza						Influenza (yearly)							

Note:

DTaP-Hib-IPV: Diphtheria, Tetanus, Pertussis, *Haemophilus influenzae* type b, Polio, 5 in 1 vaccine

PCV13: Pneumococcal 13-valent conjugate vaccine

MMR: Measles, Mumps, Rubella, 3 in 1 vaccine

JEV: Vero cell-derived Japanese encephalitis vaccine

In April 2019, hepatitis A vaccine program was expanded to children under 13 years of age from low-income and middle-to-low-income households. (https://www.cdc.gov.tw/Uploads/archives/3604cd18-8c64-4a49-a7c5-1b43df2f3f5b.pdf)

(CDC, Taiwan, 2023)

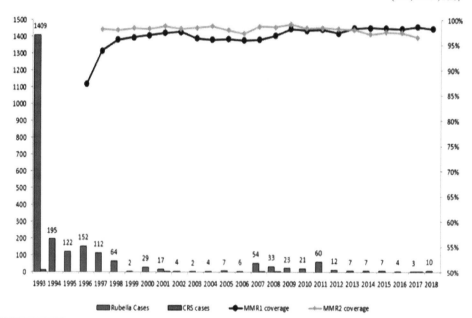

Figure 5-7 Rubella cases and immunization coverage in Taiwan from 1993 to 2018 Rubella (CRS) Surveillance in Taiwan. (http://www.cdc.gov.tw/english/info.aspx?treeid=E79C7A9E1 E9B1CDF&nowtreeid=E02C24F0DACDD729&tid=C07C33CE1 061D072)

General review

1. Rubella (German measles)

2. CRS: congenital rubella syndrome

3. Mild febrile infectious disease

4. High communicable

5. CRS: intrauterine death, spontaneous abortion

6. Combinations of defects: deafness, cataracts, microphthalmia, microcephaly, mental retardation

7. Rubella virus (family Togaviridae; genus *Rubivirus*)

8. Occurrence in Taiwan during winter and spring

SCAN ME

Check Your Answers

Review test

I. Multiple-choice questions (four selected one):

1. ( ) Congenital rubella syndrome occurs in 25% or more of infants born to women who contract rubella during which stage of pregnancy? (A) 1st trimester, (B) 2nd trimester, (C) 3rd trimester, (D) last trimester

2. ( ) Who should get the MMR vaccine among the following? (A) college and university students, (B) healthcare personnel, (C) non-pregnant women of childbearing age, (D) all of the above

3. ( ) At how many weeks of pregnancy is it rare for infants born to women who acquired rubella to have CRS defects? (A) 10th week, (B) 12th week, (C) 16th week, (D) 20th week

4. (   ) What is the proportion of infants born with CRS when women acquire rubella during the 1st trimester of pregnancy? (A) 5%, (B) 10%, (C) 20%, (D) 25%

5. (   ) What is the approximate reduction in the risk of a single congenital defect for women who acquired rubella during the 16th week of pregnancy? (A) 5%, (B) 10%, (C) 20%, (D) 25%

6. (   ) When was the triple vaccine containing attenuated measles, mumps, and rubella (MMR) viruses introduced for vaccination? (A) year of 1758, (B) year of 1969, (C) year of 1970s, (D) year of 1990s

7. (   ) In Taiwan, during which season is rubella highly prevalent? (A) winter, (B) spring, (C) autumn, (D) winter and spring

8. (   ) What is a potential serious consequence of a mother being infected with rubella during pregnancy? (A) Transient arthropathy in adults, (B) Spontaneous abortion in up to 20% of cases, (C) Rapid elimination of the virus, (D) Common childhood infection with minimal systemic upset

9. (   ) What is congenital rubella syndrome (CRS) associated with? (A) Rapid recovery in children, (B) Transient arthropathy in adults, (C) Serious, incurable illnesses in the child, (D) Minimal systemic upset in pregnant women

10. (   ) When is the risk of congenital rubella syndrome (CRS) highest if the mother is infected? (A) Within the first 20 weeks of pregnancy, (B) In the third trimester of pregnancy, (C) Postpartum period, (D) After the child turns one year old

11. (   ) What is mentioned as a common characteristic of rubella in most people? (A) Persistent infection in infants surviving CRS,

(B) Serious complications in the majority of cases, (C) Rapid elimination of the virus, (D) Trivial infection with minimal systemic upset

12. ( ) In what population are infants surviving congenital rubella syndrome (CRS) considered an important source of infection? (A) Elderly individuals, (B) Adolescents, (C) Other infants, (D) Young adults

13. ( ) When is the period of communicability for rubella, making it highly contagious? (A) 2 weeks after the onset of rash, (B) 1 week before and at least 4 days after onset of rash, (C) Only during the onset of rash, (D) 5 days after the onset of rash

14. ( ) For how long may infants with congenital rubella shed the virus after birth? (A) A few days, (B) Up to 2 weeks, (C) Several months, (D) Lifelong

15. ( ) When does susceptibility to rubella occur in individuals after the loss of transplacentally acquired maternal antibody? (A) Immediately after birth, (B) During the first year of life, (C) Before loss of maternal antibodies, (D) General after loss of maternal antibodies

16. ( ) Who is more susceptible to rubella, particularly if they have not received the vaccine? (A) Elderly individuals, (B) Children and young adults, (C) Middle-aged adults, (D) Adolescents

17. ( ) What risk does rubella infection pose for pregnant women? (A) Increased immunity, (B) No risk during pregnancy, (C) Development of lifelong immunity in the unborn child, (D) Congenital rubella syndrome (CRS) in the unborn child

18.( ) What is the primary goal of rubella control efforts? (A) Prevention of general rubella infections, (B) Reduction of transmission in the community, (C) Prevention of defects in the offspring of pregnant women with rubella, (D) Elimination of rubella in specific age groups

19.( ) What percentage of susceptible individuals does a single dose of live attenuated rubella vaccine elicit a significant antibody response in? (A) 75%, (B) 85%, (C) 95%, (D) 100%

20.( ) Who is considered at increased risk for German measles (rubella) and should receive two doses of MMR vaccine for adequate protection? (A) Elderly individuals, (B) Pregnant women, (C) College students and healthcare personnel, (D) Toddlers below 2 years old

21.( ) When was the rubella vaccine introduced to Taiwan for the third grader of junior high schoolgirls? (A) 1982, (B) 1986, (C) 1992, (D) 2001

II. Simple answer:

1. According to the WHO's recommendation in 2004, who should receive the MMR vaccine?

5-6 Meningococcal Meningitis
(ICD-9 036.0; ICD-10 A39.0)

 Highlight

1. Meningococcal meningitis
2. Cerebrospinal fever
3. Meningococcemia
4. Fulminating meningococcemia
5. *Neisseria meningitidis*
6. Benzylpenicillin
7. Meningococcal vaccines

Meningococcal septicemia, like many gram-negative blood infections, can cause disseminated intravascular coagulation (DIC), a condition where blood starts to clot throughout the body, sometimes causing ischemic tissue damage. DIC also causes bleeding, when the clotting factors are used up, causing the characteristic purpuric rash.

Meningococcal meningitis is a consequence of bacteria entering the cerebrospinal fluid (CSF) and irritating the meninges - the membranes that line the brain and spinal cord. Meningococcal infection is also known as cerebrospinal fever or meningococcemia. It is an important disease to cause of morbidity and mortality in children and young adults. The signs of meningitis of infants are fever, vomiting, cry or whimpering, fretful, neck retraction with arching of back, blank and staring expression, difficult to wake, pale, blotchy complexion (Fig. 5-8). The signs of meningitis of children or adults are stiff neck, headache, fever, vomiting, light sensitivity, drowsiness, joint pain, and fitting (Fig. 5-9). About 80% of cases have signs of meningitis, which often leads to a prompt diagnosis.

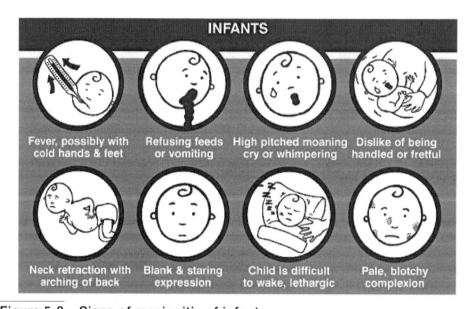

Figure 5-8   Signs of meningitis of infants.

(www.som.flinders.edu.au/Fuswikis/dsrswikiol/doku.php?id)

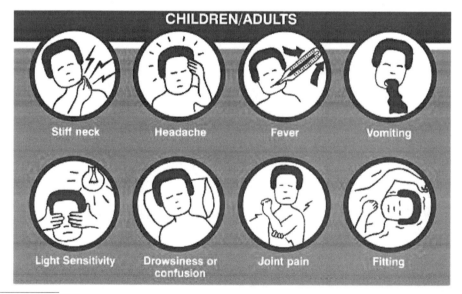

Figure 5-9   Signs of meningitis of children or adults.

(www.eastmed.co.nz/meningitis-children-adults-symptoms-
signs-vaccination-vaccine.php)

🔹 Identification to the Meningococcal meningitis:

It is an acute bacterial disease characterized by sudden onset with fever, intense headache, nausea and often vomiting, stiff neck, and frequently a petechial rash with pink macules or, very rarely, vesicles. Formerly case fatality rates exceeded 50% but with early diagnosis, modern therapy and supportive measures, the case fatality rate should be less than 10%. It is caused by the bacterium *Neisseria meningitidis*, also known as meningococcus. This bacterium can lead to two main types of infections:

1. **Meningitis**: This is the most common manifestation of the disease. Meningitis is an inflammation of the meninges, causing symptoms such as severe headache, fever, stiff neck, and sensitivity to light. If not promptly treated, it can progress rapidly and lead to seizures, coma, and death.

2. **Septicemia (Blood Infection)**: Meningococcal bacteria can also cause septicemia, which is a severe bloodstream infection. Symptoms of septicemia include fever, rash, rapid breathing, and cold extremities. This form of the disease can be extremely dangerous and may result in organ failure and death if not treated promptly.

Meningococcal infection may be restricted to the nasopharynx, asymptomatic or with only local symptoms. In fulminating meningococcemia the death rate remains high despite even prompt antibacterial treatment.

🔹 Infectious agent:

Neisseria meningitidis, the meningococcus. 50% of cases were caused with group B, 20% were caused with group C. Group A organisms have caused the major epidemics of the world (Epidemics currents about 8–12 years). Serogroups have been recognized as pathogens in recent years, e.g., groups W-135, X, Y and Z. (May be less virulent, but fatal infections and 2nd cases have occurred with all). As for 2017, the predominant serogroups causing infection in Taiwan are serogroups B, C, and Y. The first one is serogroup B, accounting for 67% of ratio. And then, the second is serogroup C (11%), following by serogroup Y (3%) (Fig. 5-10).

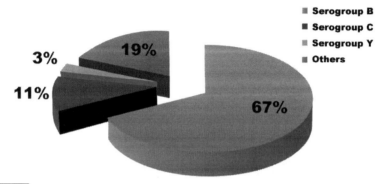

Figure 5-10 Serogroup distribution of Meningococcal Meningitis in Taiwan, 2011-2017.
(http://www.cdc.gov.tw/english/info.aspx?treeid=E79C7A9E1 E9B1CDF&nowtreeid=E02C24F0DACDD729&tid=E3F090F82D B3B457)

Occurrence:

Meningococcal infections are common in both temperate and tropical climates, with sporadic cases throughout the year in both urban and rural areas. Greatest incidence occurs during winter and spring. Epidemic meningococcal diseases in Taiwan were from 1919 and 1933–1946. Since 2011, approximately 3-8 people contract meningococcal meningitis each year in Taiwan. Most of all are sporadic cases. The annual incidence of meningococcal meningitis per 100,000 population in Taiwan has varied between 0.009 to 0.204. The case fatality rate (CFR) declined from 18.1% for patients in 1993 to 2002 to 9.8% in 2003 to 2020 (Fig. 5-11). And that is most common in the younger under age 1 and the elder over age 75. The number of cases peaks in December and January.

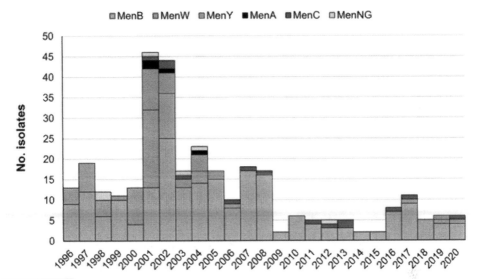

Figure 5-11 Distribution of serogroups for *N. meningitidis* isolates in Taiwan, 1996 to 2020 (n = 323).

(https://pubmed.ncbi.nlm.nih.gov/35862973/)

Reservoir:

Man.

Mode of transmission:

By direct contact, including droplets and discharges from nose and throat of infected persons. During epidemics, over half the men in a military unit may be healthy carriers of pathogenic meningococci. Up to 5-10% of people may be asymptomatic carriers with nasopharyngeal colonization by *N. meningitides*. Less than 1% of those colonized will progress to invasive disease. Carrier rate of 25% have been documented in some populations in the absence of any cases of meningococcal diseases.

🔋 Incubation period:

Varies from 2-10 days, commonly 3-4 days.

🔋 Period of communicability:

Meningococcal meningitis is highly contagious and can spread through respiratory droplets when an infected person coughs, sneezes, or comes into close contact with others. Crowded living conditions, such as college dormitories or military barracks, can increase the risk of outbreaks. In particular, the risk of infection and disease among close contacts is relatively high, with the disease attack rate among household contacts being 500 to 800 times that of the general population. Contacts are at the highest risk within 10 days of exposure to the patient's oral and nasal secretions. It started 10 days before the onset of the case and continued until 24 hours after the initiation of appropriate antibiotic treatment, at which point the mouth and nose were no longer contaminated with meningococci.

🔋 Susceptibility and resistance:

Susceptibility to the clinical disease is low and decreases with age. The chronic and temporary carriers may induce specific immunity.

Infants and young children, as well as teenagers and young adults, are more susceptible to meningococcal infections. College students living in dormitories are at a higher risk due to close living conditions. People with weakened immune systems, such as those with certain medical conditions or on immunosuppressive medications, are more susceptible. Being in close contact with someone who has a meningococcal infection, such as living in the same household or kissing an infected person, can increase the risk of transmission. Traveling to regions with higher rates of meningococcal disease can increase susceptibility. Some countries have higher rates of the disease, particularly during certain seasons.

🔋 Methods of control:

Five serogroups, A, B, C, Y and W135 are responsible for virtually all cases of the disease in humans. Almost all meningococci are extremely sensitive to benzylpenicillin. This policy saves lives, as the disease can progress alarmingly in the time it takes to reach hospital. The most important form of prevention is a vaccine against *Neisseria meningitidis*. Different countries have different strains of the bacteria and therefore use different vaccines. There are 3 types of meningococcal vaccines available in the United States:

1. Meningococcal conjugate or MenACWY vaccines (Menveo® and MenQuadfi®)

2. Serogroup B meningococcal or MenB vaccines (Bexsero® and Trumenba®)

3. Pentavalent meningococcal or MenABCWY vaccine (Penbraya™)

All 11- to 12-year-olds should get a MenACWY vaccine, with a booster dose at 16 years old. Teens and young adults (16 to 23 years old) also may get a MenB vaccine. Those who are getting MenACWY and MenB vaccines at the same visit may instead get a MenABCWY vaccine. CDC also recommends meningococcal vaccination for other children and adults who are at increased risk for meningococcal disease (CDC, U.S., 2023).

Additionally, basic hygiene measures, such as handwashing and not sharing drinking cups, can reduce the incidence of infection by limiting exposure.

When a case is confirmed, all close contacts with the infected person can be offered antibiotics to reduce the likelihood of the infection spreading to other people.

🔬 General review

1. Meningococcal infection (cerebrospinal fever or meningococcemia)

2. An acute bacterial disease (sudden onset, case fatality rates exceeded 50%)

3. Fulminating meningococcemia

4. *Neisseria meningitidis*

5. Serogroup A organisms are the major epidemics of the world

6. 50% of cases were caused with serogroup B

7. Vaccines are available against groups A, B, C, Y and W135 strains

8. Meningococci are extremely sensitive to benzylpenicillin

SCAN ME

Check Your Answers

🦠 Review test

I. Multiple-choice questions (four selected one):

1. ( ) What was the former case fatality rate of meningitis? (A) 10%, (B) 25%, (C) 35%, (D) exceeded 50%.

2. ( ) Among the cases of meningitis, 50% of the patients were caused by which serogroup of *Neisseria meningitidis*? (A) group A, (B) group B, (C) group C, (D) group W-135

3. ( ) How long does it typically take for meningococci to disappear from the nasopharynx after the initiation of treatment? (A) 24 hrs, (B) 36 hrs, (C) 48 hrs, (D) 72 hrs

4. ( ) Which of the following drugs are almost all meningococci extremely sensitive to? (A) penicillin, (B) amoxicillin, (C) benzylpenicillin, (D) all of the above.

5. (　) What proportion of people may be asymptomatic carriers with nasopharyngeal colonization by *N. meningitidis*? (A) 5-10%, (B) 15%, (C) 20%, (D) 25%

6. (　) What proportion of carriers have been documented in some populations in the absence of any cases of meningococcal disease? (A) 5-10%, (B) 15%, (C) 20%, (D) 25%

7. (　) What is the primary mode of transmission for meningococcal meningitis? (A) Foodborne, (B) Vector-borne, (C) Respiratory droplets, (D) Blood transfusion

8. (　) During what timeframe are contacts at the highest risk of meningococcal meningitis after exposure to an infected person's oral and nasal secretions? (A) 24 hours, (B) 5 days, (C) 10 days, (D) 14 days

9. (　) Who is more susceptible to meningococcal infections? (A) Elderly individuals, (B) Adolescents and young adults, (C) Middle-aged individuals, (D) All age groups equally

10. (　) What factor increases the risk of meningococcal infection in college students? (A) Distance from campus, (B) On-campus dining, (C) Close living conditions in dormitories, (D) Participation in sports clubs

II. Simple answer:

1. Could you please provide me with information about the high-incidence season of cerebrospinal fever in Taiwan?

2. What are the three types of meningococcal vaccines available in the United States, and which age group is recommended to receive a MenB vaccine?

3. Could you please provide information about the five major signs of meningitis in infants?

4. Could you please provide information about the five major signs of meningitis in children or adult?

5-7 Scarlet Fever (ICD-9 034.1; ICD-10 A38)

 Highlight

1. Scarlet fever
3. Streptococcal sore throat
3. Impetigo
4. Erysipelas
5. Puerperal fever
6. Strawberry tongue
7. Otitis media
8. Peritonsillar abscess
9. Acute rheumatic fever
10. Acute glomerulonephritis
11. Sydenham's chorea
12. *Streptococcus pyogenes*, group A streptococci

Scarlet fever is a bacterial infection that primarily affects children and, less commonly, adults. It is caused by the bacterium *Streptococcus pyogenes*, which is the same bacterium responsible for strep throat. Scarlet fever gets its name from the characteristic red rash that often accompanies it. The alternative names of Scarlet fever are Streptococcal sore throat, Impetigo, Erysipelas or Puerperal fever.

Scarlet fever is a disease caused by an exotoxin released by *Streptococcus pyogenes* Group A occurs rarely with impetigo or other streptococcal infections. It is characterized by sore throat, fever, a "strawberry tongue", and a fine sandpaper rash over the upper body that may spread to cover almost the entire body. Scarlet fever is not rheumatic fever, but may progress into that condition. The rate of development of rheumatic fever in individuals with untreated streptococcal infection is estimated to be 3%. The rate of development is far lower in individuals who have received antibiotic treatment.

Identification to the scarlet fever:

Scarlet fever is a form of streptococcal disease characterized by a skin rash; it occurs when the infecting strain of streptococcus is a toxin-producer, and the patient is sensitized but not immune to the toxin.

The symptoms of scarlet fever typically start with signs that are similar to those of strep throat, including a sore throat, fever, and swollen tonsils. One of the distinguishing features is a red rash that usually appears a day or two after the sore throat. This rash feels rough to the touch and resembles a sunburn, giving the skin a reddish appearance. It often starts on the chest and spreads to other parts of the body. The rash is usually a fine erythema, commonly punctate, blanching on pressure, often felt (like sandpaper) better than seen and appearing most often on the neck, chest, in folds of the axilla, elbow and groin, and on inner surfaces of the thighs. Typically, the rash does not involve the face, but there is flushing of the checks and circumoral pallor.

It can also cause simple angina, erysipelas, and serious toxin-mediated syndromes like necrotizing fasciitis and the so-called streptococcal toxic shock-like syndrome. The virulence of group A streptococcus seems to be increasing lately. The exanthem, or widespread rash, of scarlet fever is thought to be due to erythrogenic toxin production by specific streptococcal strains in a nonimmune patient. Besides erythrogenic toxins, the Group A streptococcus produces several other toxins and enzymes. Two of the most important are the streptolysins O and S. Streptolysin O, a hemolytic, thermolabile and immunogenic toxin, is the base of the anti-streptolysin O titer, an assay for scarlet fever and erysipelas.

The complications of scarlet fever may be a minimum of symptoms. Coincident or subsequent otitis media or peritonsillar abscess may occur. Acute rheumatic fever or acute glomerulonephritis or chorea may appear in 1-5 weeks; rheumatic heart disease is a later complication. Clinical characteristics may include all those symptoms occurring with a streptococcal sore throat (or it may be associated with a wound, skin or puerperal infection) as well as enanthem, strawberry tongue, and exanthem (Fig. 5-12).

Infectious agent:

Streptococcus pyogenes, group A streptococci of approximately seventy-five serologically distinct types which may greatly in geographic and time distributions. While β-hemolysis is characteristic of group A streptococci.

Occurrence:

Streptococcal sore throat and scarlet fever are common in temperate zones, well recognized in semitropical areas and less frequently recognized in tropical climates. The highest incidence of scarlet fever occurs in young children in late summer, fall and winter in Taiwan. Occurrence is sporadic in northern Taiwan, even during epidemics of streptococcal infection.

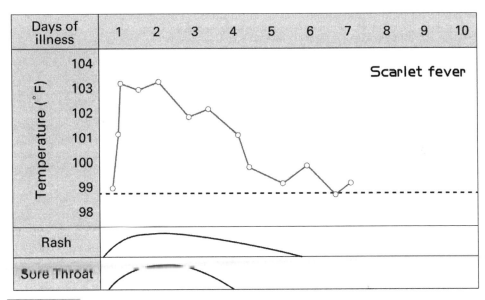

Figure 5-12 Clinical characteristics and symptoms of Scarlet fever: Skin
rush and streptococcal sore throat as well as enanthem,
strawberry tongue, and exanthem. [Centigrade (°C) =
(Fahrenheit (°F) − 32) x 5/9]
(nu107018 www.fotosearch.com)

Reservoir:

Man.

Mode of transmission:

Scarlet fever is primarily transmitted through direct or close contact with
an infected patient or carrier, either via respiratory droplets released when
an infected person coughs or sneezes or by coming into contact with
contaminated objects or surfaces. Close contact with an infected person
increases the risk of contracting scarlet fever. Household members,
schoolmates, and others who spend time in close proximity to an infected

individual are at a higher risk of exposure. It is rarely by indirect contact through objects or hands. Nasal carriers are particularly likely to transmit disease.

Incubation period:

Incubation period is short, usually 1-3 days, rarely longer.

Period of communicability:

In untreated uncomplicated cases are 10-21 days; in untreated conditions with purulent discharges, weeks or months. With adequate penicillin therapy, transmissibility generally is terminated within 24-48 hours.

Susceptibility and resistance:

Susceptibility to scarlet fever is general, scarlet fever is most seen in children between the ages of 5 and 15. Children in this age range are often more susceptible to the infection, but it can occur in individuals of any age. Although many persons develop either antitoxic or type-specific antibacterial immunity, or both, through inapparent infection. Antibacterial immunity develops only against the specific M-type of group A streptococcus that induced infection and may lost for years. One attack of erysipelas appears to predispose individuals to subsequent attacks.

Methods of control:

Infected individuals, especially children, should be kept home from school or daycare until they have received antibiotic treatment for at least 24 hours and are no longer contagious.

1. Educate the public in mode of transmission, in the relationship of streptococcal infection to acute rheumatic fever, Sydenham's chorea,

rheumatic heart disease and glomerulonephritis, and the necessity for completing the full course of antibiotics therapy prescribed for streptococcal infection.

2. Long-term antimicrobial prophylaxis: monthly injections of long-acting benzathine penicillin G or daily penicillin or sulfadiazine orally for persons to whom recurrent streptococcal infections.

3. Boil or pasteurized milk and exclude infected persons from handling milk likely to become contaminated. Other foods such as deviled eggs should be prepared just prior to serving or be adequately refrigerated in small quantities at lower than 5°C.

4. Encourage regular handwashing with soap and water for at least 20 seconds, especially before eating, after using the bathroom, and after coughing or sneezing. Hand sanitizers with 70% alcohol can also be used when soap and water are not available.

General review

1. Scarlet fever alternative names are Streptococcal sore throat, Impetigo, Erysipelas, and Puerperal fever)

2. Streptococcal disease characterized by a sensitized skin rash

3. Publications as enanthem, strawberry tongue, and exanthem

4. Typically, the rash is flushing of the checks and circumoral pallor

5. Complications: otitis media, peritonsillar abscess, acute rheumatic fever, acute glomerulonephritis, chorea

6. The highest incidence of scarlet fever occurs in young children in late summer, fall and winter in northern Taiwan

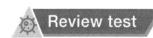

Review test

I. Multiple-choice questions (four selected one):

1. (　) Which of the following complications does not include scarlet fever? (A) otitis media, (B) peritonsillar abscess, (C) acute rheumatic fever, (D) enanthem and exanthem

2. (　) In which season was the highest incidence of erysipelas found in Taiwan? (A) late summer, (B) autumn, (C) winter, (D) all of the above

3. (　) One of the complications of scarlet fever is acute glomerulonephritis. How long may it appear after the onset? (A) 2 weeks, (B) 4 weeks, (C) 2 months, (D) 1-5 weeks.

4. (　) Which of the following is a later complication of scarlet fever? (A) rheumatic heart disease, (B) peritonsillar abscess, (C) chorea, (D) acute glomerulonephritis

5. (　) What is the typical incubation period of scarlet fever? (A) 1-3 days, (B) 5-7 days, (C) 10-12 days, (D) variable

6. (　) What are the characteristic of Group A streptococci? (A) pyogenesis, (B) strawberry tongue, (C) β-hemolysis, (D) all of the above

II. Simple answer:

1. In Taiwan, during which season is the incidence of scarlet fever the highest?

2. Could you please provide information about the transmission of scarlet fever?

5-8 Chickenpox / Herpes Zoster

(ICD-9 052-053; ICD-10 B01-B02)

 Highlight

1. Varicella

2. Herpes zoster

3. Shingles

4. Skin eruption (maculopapular)

5. Erythematous

6. VZV: Varicella-Zoster virus

7. Vesiculopustular

8. Immunosuppressants

9. VZIG: Varicella-Zoster Immune Globulin

Chickenpox is a highly contagious illness caused by primary infection with varicella zoster virus (VZV), which belongs to the herpesvirus family. It generally begins with conjunctival and catarrhal symptoms and then characteristic spots appearing in two or three waves, mainly on the body and head rather than the hands and becoming itchy raw pockmarks, small open sores which heal mostly without scarring. Chickenpox is an acute generalized viral disease with sudden onset of slight fever (37.5-39°C), mild constitutional symptoms and a skin eruption which is maculopapular for a few hours, vesicular for 3-4 days, and leaves a granular scab. The disease is rarely fatal; the most common cause of death in adults is primary viral pneumonia; among children, it is septic complications and encephalitis. Pregnant women and those with a suppressed immune system are at highest risk of serious complications. The most common late complication of chicken pox is shingles, caused by reactivation of the varicella zoster virus decades after the initial episode of chickenpox.

Herpes zoster (or simply zoster), commonly known as shingles, is a viral disease characterized by a painful skin rash with blisters in a limited area on one side of the body. The initial infection with VZV causes the acute (short-lived) illness chickenpox, and generally occurs in children and young people. Once an episode of chickenpox has resolved, the virus is not eliminated from the body but can go on to cause shingles—an illness with very different symptoms—often many years after the initial infection.

Varicella zoster virus can become latent in the nerve cell bodies and less frequently in non-neuronal satellite cells of dorsal root, cranial nerve or autonomic ganglion, without causing any symptoms. In an immunocompromised individual, perhaps years or decades after a chickenpox infection, the virus may break out of nerve cell bodies and travel down nerve axons to cause viral infection of the skin in the region of the nerve. The virus may spread from one or more ganglia along nerves of an affected segment and infect the corresponding dermatome causing a painful rash. Although the rash usually heals within two to four weeks, some sufferers experience residual nerve pain for months or years, a condition called postherpetic neuralgia. Exactly how the virus remains latent in the body, and subsequently re-activates is not understood.

Identification to the chickenpox:

Vesicles with an erythematous base are restricted to skin areas supplied by sensory nerves of a single or associated group of dorsal root ganglia. In the immunosuppressed, extensive skin lesions may appear outside the dermatome (shingles). Clinical chickenpox has been a frequent antecedent of Reye syndrome. Zoster occurs mainly in older adults although there is some evidence that almost 10% of children being treated for a malignant neoplasm are prone to develop herpes zoster. Common symptoms of chickenpox include:

1. **Itchy rash**: The hallmark of chickenpox is a red, itchy rash that typically starts on the face, chest, and back and then spreads to other parts of the body.

2. **Fever**: Many individuals with chickenpox develop a mild to moderate fever (37.5-39℃).

3. **Fatigue and general discomfort**: It is common to feel tired and unwell during the illness.

Complicated Varicella: Complications from varicella can occur, but they are not common in healthy people who get the disease. People who may get a serious case of varicella and may be at high risk for complications include infants, adults, pregnant women, people with weakened immune systems because of illness or medications. Serious complications from varicella include bacterial infections of the skin and soft tissues, pneumonia, infection or inflammation of the brain (encephalitis, cerebellar ataxia), blood stream infections (sepsis), dehydration. Some people with serious complications from varicella can become so sick that they need to be hospitalized. Varicella can also cause death. Complicated varicella surveillance in Taiwan is rare (Fig. 5-13).

🔹 Infectious agent:

Human α herpesvirus 3 (varicella-zoster virus, VZV), which is a member of the *Herpesvirus* group.

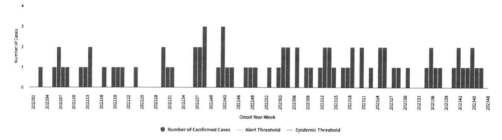

Figure 5-13 The complicated varicella surveillance in Taiwan (CDC, Taiwan, 2023)

Occurrence:

Worldwide, infection with human α herpesvirus 3 is nearly universal. In metropolitan communities, about 75% of the population has had chickenpox by age 15 and at least 90% by young adulthood. The infection rate in a family is more than 85%. In temperate zones chickenpox occurs most frequently in winter and early spring.

Reservoir:

Man.

Mode of transmission:

It is from person to person by direct contact, droplet, or airborne spread of secretions of respiratory tract of chickenpox cases or of the vesicle fluid of patients with herpes zoster. Chickenpox is one of the most readily communicable of disease, especially in the early stages of the eruption. Scabs from varicella lesions are not infective.

Incubation period:

After exposure to the virus, it can take 2 to 3 weeks for symptoms to appear. Incubation period is commonly 13-17 days.

🔹 Period of communicability:

1. **Prodromal phase**: Chickenpox is contagious even before the rash appears. The virus can be transmitted during the prodromal phase, which is as long as 5 but usually 1–2 days before onset of rash. This phase may include symptoms such as fever, fatigue, and malaise. It's during this time that the infected person can unknowingly spread the virus to others.

2. **Rash development**: Once the characteristic chickenpox rash begins to appear, the person remains contagious. The fluid-filled blisters in the rash contain the varicella-zoster virus, and if these blisters rupture, the virus can be released into the environment.

3. **Until all lesions crust over**: The period of communicability continues until all the chickenpox lesions (blisters) have crusted over. This means that once the blisters have dried up and formed scabs, the person is no longer considered contagious.

🔹 Susceptibility and resistance:

Susceptibility to chickenpox is universal among those not previously infected, ordinarily a more severe disease of adults than of children. One infection confers long immunity. Infection apparently remains latent and may recur years later as herpes zoster in a proportion of older adults, sometimes in children.

People who is most likely to get shingles. The follows are at high risk:

1. Conditions that affect the immune system, including HIV infection.

2. Periods of increased stress.

3. Excess alcohol intake.

4. Long term courses of steroids.

5. Chemotherapy or radiotherapy - cancer treatments.

6. Medicines used after organ transplants (immunosuppressants).

Methods of control:

A varicella vaccine has been available since 1995 to inoculate against the disease. Some countries require the varicella vaccination or an exemption before entering elementary school. In Taiwan, the chickenpox vaccination (VZIG) schedule is as follows: Children aged 12 months or older are eligible for the first dose of the publicly funded vaccine. Children between the ages of 4 and 6 have the option to receive the second dose at their own expense. For individuals aged 13 and above, who have neither been vaccinated nor had chickenpox, a two-dose regimen is recommended. These two doses should be administered four to eight weeks apart, and the cost of vaccination is borne by the individual. This vaccination strategy aims to provide protection against chickenpox for people of different. Protection is not lifelong and further vaccination is necessary five years after the initial immunization (CDC, Taiwan, 2019).

Varicella-zoster immune globulin (VZIG) does not provide long-term immunity but offers short-term protection. Its effectiveness is highest when administered shortly after exposure, ideally within 96 hours but may still be beneficial if given within 10 days of exposure. VZIG is a live attenuated varicella virus vaccine among normal children has shown a very high level of protection. While VZIG is primarily associated with chickenpox, it can also be used in some cases to manage shingles in individuals at high risk of complications, such as those with weakened immune systems.

General review

1. Chickenpox, Varicella, Herpes zoster, Shingles

2. Varicella zoster virus (VZV), highly contagious

3. The early stages of the eruption

4. Occurrence in winter and early spring / Taiwan

5. Transmitted by direct contact, droplet

6. Scabs from varicella lesions are not infective

7. Varicella-Zoster Immune Globulin (VZIG)

8. Live attenuated varicella virus vaccine

SCAN ME

Check Your Answers

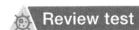 Review test

I. Multiple-choice questions (four selected one):

1. (   ) In Taiwan, in which age group of people does varicella mainly occur? (A) children and young people, (B) adults, (C) old people, (D) all of the above

2. (   ) The following who is most likely to get shingles? (A) HIV infected person, (B) immunosuppressants person, (C) long term courses of steroids, (D) all of the above

3. (   ) In metropolitan communities, what percentage of the population has had chickenpox by age 15? (A) 25%, (B) 75%, (C) 85%, (D) 90%

4. (   ) In metropolitan communities, what percentage of the population has had chickenpox by young adulthood? (A) 25%, (B) 75%, (C) 85%, (D) 90%

5. (   ) What percentage is the infection rate of chickenpox in a family? (A) 25%, (B) 75%, (C) 85%, (D) 90%.

6. (   ) Which of the following varicella lesions are not infectious? (A) scabs, (B) cluster of small bumps, (C) break open crust, (D) blisters

7. (   ) The effectiveness of VZIG is highest when administered shortly after exposure to chickenpox. How long after exposure should it be administered? (A) 24 hours, (B) 48 hours, (C) 96 hours, (D) 10 days.

8. (   ) What is the most common late complication of chickenpox? (A) Septic complications, (B) Encephalitis, (C) Shingles, (D) Primary viral pneumonia

9. (   ) What is the initial infection caused by the varicella-zoster virus in children and young people? (A) Encephalitis, (B) Shingles, (C) Chickenpox, (D) Septic complications

10. (   ) What is the typical duration of the vesicular stage in the skin eruption of chickenpox? (A) A few hours, (B) 3-4 days, (C) Several weeks, (D) Months

11. (   ) Which viral disease is characterized by a painful skin rash with blisters in a limited area on one side of the body? (A) Chickenpox, (B) Encephalitis, (C) Primary viral pneumonia, (D) Shingles

12 (   ) What is the hallmark of chickenpox? (A) High fever, (B) Itchy rash, (C) Fatigue, (D) General discomfort

13. (   ) In which order does the chickenpox rash typically spread? (A) Chest, face, and back, (B) Face, chest, and back, (C) Back, chest, and face, (D) Back, face, and chest

14. ( ) What is a common symptom of chickenpox besides the itchy rash? (A) High fever, (B) Fatigue, (C) General discomfort, (D) All of the above

15. ( ) Who is at high risk for serious complications from varicella? (A) Healthy adults, (B) Infants, (C) Teenagers, (D) Individuals with mild symptoms

16. ( ) During which phase of chickenpox is the infected person most likely to spread the virus to others? (A) Rash development, (B) Prodromal phase, (C) Until all lesions crust over, (D) After receiving the vaccination

17. ( ) When does the period of communicability for chickenpox end? (A) Once the rash appears, (B) During the prodromal phase, (C) Until all lesions crust over, (D) After receiving the second dose of the vaccine

18. ( ) In Taiwan, when are children between the ages of 4 and 6 eligible for the second dose of the chickenpox vaccine? (A) After the first dose, (B) At their own expense, (C) At age 6, (D) Between 13 and above

19. ( ) For individuals aged 13 and above who have neither been vaccinated nor had chickenpox, how many doses of the chickenpox vaccine are recommended in Taiwan? (A) One dose, (B) Two doses, (C) Three doses, (D) Four doses

20. ( ) What is the primary purpose of Varicella-zoster immune globulin (VZIG)? (A) Long-term immunity, (B) Short-term protection, (C) Treatment of shingles, (D) Booster for the chickenpox vaccine

II. Simple answer:

1. Could you please provide information about the individuals who are most likely to develop shingles?

2. Please provide information on effective methods for controlling chickenpox.

3. Could you please provide information about the current varicella vaccine schedule for children in our country, including the first and second doses?

4. In temperate zones, during which season does chickenpox occurs most frequently?

5-9 Tuberculosis (ICD-9 010-018; ICD-10 A15-A19)

 Highlight

1. Tuberculosis
2. Mycobacterial disease
3. Pulmonary or tracheobronchial lymph node calcifications
4. Hemoptysis
5. PPD: Purified Protein Derivative-Standard
6. *Mycobacterium tuberculosis* (humans)
7. *M. africanum* (humans)
8. *M. bovis* (cattle)
9. DOTS: direct observation of treatment for short course (3-6 months).
10. BCG vaccination

Tuberculosis (abbreviated as TB for *tubercle bacillus* or tuberculosis) is a common and deadly infectious disease caused by mycobacteria, mainly *Mycobacterium tuberculosis*. Tuberculosis most commonly attacks the lungs (as pulmonary TB) but can also affect the central nervous system, the lymphatic system, the circulatory system, the genitourinary system, bones, joints and even the skin.

Over one-third of the world's population has been exposed to the TB bacterium, and new infections occur at a rate of one per second. Not everyone infected develops the full-blown disease; asymptomatic, latent TB infection is most common. However, one in ten latent infections will progress to active TB disease, which, if left untreated, kills more than half of its victims. In some cases, TB bacteria can become resistant to the standard antibiotics. This is called drug-resistant TB, and it requires more complex and prolonged treatment.

Tuberculosis has significant mortality and morbidity statistics globally. Here are some key statistics updates (WHO, 2021):

1. **Mortality**
   - Global TB Deaths: In 2020, approximately 1.5 million people died from TB worldwide. This figure had been slowly declining over the years, but the COVID-19 pandemic in 2020 may have disrupted TB services and led to an increase in TB-related deaths in some regions.
   - TB Mortality by Region: TB mortality is not evenly distributed globally. The majority of TB deaths occur in low- and middle-income countries, particularly in regions such as sub-Saharan Africa and Southeast Asia.
   - TB and HIV Co-Infection: TB is a leading cause of death among people living with HIV (PLHIV). In 2020, an estimated 685,000 TB deaths occurred among PLHIV.

2. Morbidity

- Global TB Incidence: In 2020, there were an estimated 9.9 million new TB cases globally. This includes both drug-sensitive and drug-resistant TB cases.

- TB Incidence by Region: The burden of TB varies by region. High-incidence regions include parts of sub-Saharan Africa, Southeast Asia, and the Western Pacific.

- Drug-Resistant TB: There were an estimated 465,000 new cases of rifampicin-resistant TB (a marker for multidrug-resistant TB or MDR-TB) in 2020. Out of these, around 78% had MDR-TB.

- TB in Children: TB in children is a significant concern, and in 2020, there were an estimated 1.15 million new TB cases among children under 15 years old.

The emergence of drug-resistant strains of TB is a concerning public health issue. Drug-resistant TB occurs when the bacteria responsible for TB become resistant to the drugs that are typically used to treat the infection. There are several levels of drug resistance in TB, including:

1. **Multidrug-Resistant TB (MDR-TB)**: This form of TB is resistant to at least two of the most potent first-line drugs, isoniazid and rifampicin. MDR-TB requires more complex and lengthy treatment regimens with second-line drugs, which are often less effective, more toxic, and more expensive.

2. **Extensively Drug-Resistant TB (XDR-TB)**: XDR-TB is a severe form of drug-resistant TB that is resistant to not only isoniazid and rifampicin but also to at least one of the second-line injectable drugs (e.g., amikacin, kanamycin, or capreomycin) and to any fluoroquinolone (e.g., ciprofloxacin or levofloxacin). Treatment of XDR-TB is even more challenging and may require novel drugs.

Identification to the tuberculosis:

Tuberculosis is a mycobacterial disease important as a cause of disability and death in many parts of the world. The initial infection usually goes unnoticed; tuberculin sensitivity appears within a few weeks; lesions commonly heal, leaving no residual changes except pulmonary or tracheobronchial lymph node calcifications. Mycobacteria may progress directly to pulmonary tuberculosis or, by lymphohematogenous dissemination of bacilli, to produce pulmonary, miliary, meningeal or other extrapulmonary involvement. Serious outcome of the initial infection is more frequent in infants, adolescents and young adults. There are two main forms of TB: latent TB infection (LTBI) and active TB disease:

1. **Latent TB Infection (LTBI)**: In this form, the bacteria are present in the body but are not causing symptoms. People with LTBI are not contagious, but they are at risk of developing active TB in the future.

2. **Active TB Disease**: This is when the bacteria become active and cause symptoms. Active TB is contagious and can spread to others.

When the disease becomes active, 75% of the cases are pulmonary TB. Symptoms include chest pain, coughing up blood, and a productive, prolonged cough for more than three weeks. Systemic symptoms include fever, chills, night sweats, appetite loss, weight loss, pallor, and often a tendency to fatigue very easily. In the other 25% of active cases, the infection moves from the lungs, causing other kinds of TB more common in immunosuppressed persons and young children. Extrapulmonary infection sites include the pleura, the central nervous system in meningitis, the lymphatic system in scrofula of the neck, the genitourinary system in urogenital tuberculosis, and bones and joints in Pott's disease of the spine. An especially serious form is disseminated TB, more commonly known as miliary tuberculosis (Fig. 5-14). Although extrapulmonary TB is not contagious, it may co-exist with pulmonary TB, which is contagious.

Tuberculin skin test

For without BCG vaccinated scarred person. People who are or have been infected with *Mycobacterium tuberculosis* and *M. bovis* will almost always react to a low dose tuberculin skin test, i.e., bio-equivalent to 5 International Unit (IU) (or 5 Tuberculin Units-5TU) of the International Standard of Purified Protein Derivative-Standard (PPD).

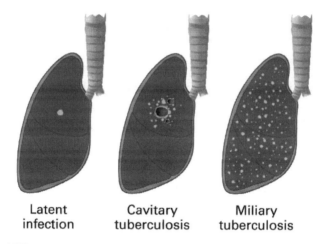

| Latent | Cavitary | Miliary |
| infection | tuberculosis | tuberculosis |

Figure 5-14 Miliary tuberculosis is characterized by a chronic, contagious bacterial infection caused by *Mycobacterium tuberculosis* that has spread to other organs of the body by the blood or lymph system.
(The figure has been made in authorized to use the Image DJ Corporation. Copyright: Alila Medical Media.)

Classifying the tuberculin test

Read reaction 48-72 hours after injection; if indurations <10 mm: Negative, should vaccinated BCG, if indurations ≥ 10 mm: Positive, means persons with clinical conditions that place them at high risk.

Infectious agent:

Mycobacterium tuberculosis and *M. africanum* are primarily from humans. *M. bovis* is primarily from cattle. *Mycobacterium tuberculosis* is a slow-growing bacterium with a thick, waxy cell wall that makes it resistant to many antibiotics and the body's immune response.

Occurrence:

Worldwide, numerous countries have shown downward trends of mortality and morbidity for many years. In low incidence area, most tuberculosis is endogenous, i.e., it is a reactivation from latent foci remaining from the initial infection, notably household associates, may lead to a 30% risk of becoming infected, and 1–5% chance of the infection progressing to diseases within a year. In 2020, the World Health Organization (WHO) estimated that there were 100,000 cases of tuberculosis, with 10,000 people dying from tuberculosis, making it the second-largest infectious disease killer, second only to COVID-19. As for Taiwan, in 2019, there were 7,062 cases of tuberculosis (100 cases per 300,000 people) and 10 deaths related to tuberculosis (1.9 cases per 4.46 million people). Compared to 2011, the incidence rate decreased by 28.8%. Clearly, the incidence rate has been consistently declining (CDC, Taiwan, 2022) (Fig. 5-15).

Reservoir:

Primarily man; in some areas are also diseased cattle.

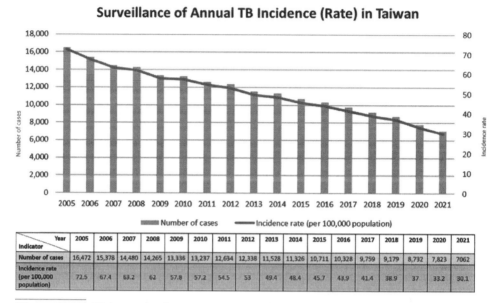

Surveillance of Annual TB Incidence (Rate) in Taiwan

Legend: Number of cases   Incidence rate (per 100,000 population)

Year / Indicator	2005	2006	2007	2008	2009	2010	2011	2012	2013	2014	2015	2016	2017	2018	2019	2020	2021
Number of cases	16,472	15,378	14,480	14,265	13,336	13,237	12,634	12,338	11,528	11,326	10,711	10,328	9,759	9,179	8,732	7,823	7062
Incidence rate (per 100,000 population)	72.5	67.4	63.2	62	57.8	57.2	54.5	53	49.4	48.4	45.7	43.9	41.4	38.9	37	33.2	30.1

Figure 5-15 Tuberculosis case number and incidence, 2005-2021 Taiwan. (https://www.cdc.gov.tw/En/Category/ListContent/bg0g_VU_Ysrgkes_KRUDgQ?uaid=0WialNbsh7SEGERJLa29FA)

▶ Mode of transmission:

When people suffering from active pulmonary TB cough, sneeze, speak, kiss, or spit, they expel infectious aerosol droplets 0.5 to 5 μm in diameter. A single sneeze, for instance, can release up to 40,000 droplets. Each one of these droplets may transmit the disease since the infectious dose of tuberculosis is very low and the inhalation of just a single bacterium can cause a new infection.

Prolonged close exposure to an infectious case may lead to infection of contacts. Direct invasion through mucous membranes or breaks in the skin may occur but is extremely rare.

🔹 Incubation period:

Incubation period is from infection to demonstrable primary lesion or significant tuberculin reaction, about 4–12 weeks. While the subsequent risk of progressive pulmonary or extrapulmonary tuberculosis, which is greatest within 6–12 months after infection. It may persist for a lifetime as a latent infection.

🔹 Period of communicability:

Theoretically, the communicability is as long as infectious tubercle bacilli are being discharged in the sputum. The degree of communicability depends on the number of bacilli discharged, the virulence of the bacilli and opportunities for their aerosolization by coughing, sneezing, talking or singing. Extrapulmonary tuberculosis is generally not communicable.

🔹 Susceptibility and resistance:

Susceptibility is general; the most hazardous period for development of clinical disease is the first 6-12 months after infection. The risk of developing disease is highest in children under 3 years old, and high again in 60-year-old man. Susceptibility to disease is increased among underweight or undernourished persons; among persons with diabetes, or gastrectomies; and among alcoholics and the immunosuppressed.

🔹 Methods of control:

TB prevention and control takes two parallel approaches. In the first, people with TB and their contacts are identified and then treated. Identification of infections often involves testing high-risk groups for TB. In the second approach, children are vaccinated to protect them from TB. Unfortunately, no vaccine is available that provides reliable protection for adults. However, in tropical areas where the incidence of atypical mycobacteria is high, exposure to nontuberculous mycobacteria gives some protection against TB.

The effective control methods are as follows:

1. Report to local health authority.

2. Isolation: control of infectivity is best achieved by prompt specific drug therapy.

3. DOTS: direct observation of treatment for short course (3–6 months).

4. BCG (Bacillus Calmette-Guérin) vaccination of uninfected (tuberculin-negative) persons can induce tuberculin sensitivity in > 90% of vaccines, that protection may persist for as long as 20 years, especially in children.

5. Concurrent disinfection: microbial decontamination of air by ventilation; this may be supplemented by UV light.

General review

1. Tuberculosis (deadly infectious disease) caused by mycobacteria (*Mycobacterium tuberculosis*)

2. Drug-resistant TB (XDR-TB)

3. Cause of disability and death

4. Symptoms: fatigue, fever, weight loss, cough, chest pain, hemoptysis and hoarseness

5. Extrapulmonary TB includes TB meningitis, acute hematogenous (miliary) TB

6. *M. bovis* will almost always react to a low dose tuberculin skin test

7. Classifying the tuberculin test

8. *Infective agents:* M. tuberculosis and *M. africanum*

9. Communicability: aerosolization by coughing, sneezing, talking or singing

10. DOTS: direct observation of treatment for short course (3-6 months)

11. BCG vaccination

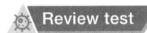 **Review test**

SCAN ME

Check Your Answers

I. Multiple-choice questions (four selected one):

1. ( ) DOTS is one of the effective control methods for tuberculosis. What does 'short course' mean? (A) 3 weeks, (B) 6 weeks, (C) 3 months, (D) 3-6 months

2. ( ) Among the following options, which one is susceptible to tuberculosis infection? (A) undernourished persons, (B) diabetes, (C) gastrectomies, (D) all of the above

3. ( ) How much dose of the tuberculin skin test will people who are or have been infected with M. tuberculosis and M. bovis almost always react to? (A) 5 IU, (B) 10 TU, (C) 15 IU, (D) 15 TU

4. ( ) What does it mean when the injection site for the tuberculin skin test (PPD) shows redness and swelling of less than 10 mm for classification? (A) negative, B false negative, (C) positive, (D) false positive

5. ( ) What does it mean when the injection site for the tuberculin skin test (PPD) shows redness and swelling of more than 10 mm for classification? (A) negative, B should vaccinate BCG, (C) positive, (D) false positive

6. ( ) What percentage of risk does having household associates with T.B. lead to for becoming infected? (A) 1-5%, (B) 10%, (C) 30%, (D) exceeded 50%

7. ( ) Having household associates may lead to a high risk of becoming infected. What percentage of that risk progresses to disease within a year? (A) 1-5%, (B) 10%, (C) 30%, (D) exceeded 50%

8. ( ) What is the main characteristic of Latent TB Infection (LTBI)? (A) Contagious with symptoms, (B) Bacteria causing symptoms, (C) Contagious without symptoms, (D) Risk of developing active TB is minimal

9. ( ) When the bacteria causing TB to become active and contagious, what is this form called? (A) Latent TB Infection (LTBI), (B) Non-contagious TB, (C) Pre-active TB, (D) Active TB Disease

10.( ) What percentage of active TB cases are classified as pulmonary TB? (A) 25%, (B) 50%, (C) 75%, (D) 100%

11.( ) In the 25% of active TB cases where the infection moves from the lungs, which system or organ is commonly affected in urogenital tuberculosis? (A) Pleura, (B) Central nervous system, (C) Genitourinary system, (D) Bones and joints

12.( ) What does an induration size of less than 10 mm indicate in the tuberculin test? (A) Positive result, (B) Negative result, (C) Vaccinated with BCG, (D) High risk of clinical conditions

13.( ) If an individual has an induration size of 10 mm or more in the tuberculin test, what does it typically suggest? (A) Negative result, (B) Positive result, (C) Vaccinated with BCG, (D) Low risk of clinical conditions

14. (　) Which of the following is a key component of the second approach to TB prevention and control? (A) Prompt drug therapy for infected individuals, (B) Vaccination of children, (C) Direct observation of treatment for short course (DOTS), (D) Isolation of TB patients

15. (　) What does BCG vaccination induce in uninfected (tuberculin-negative) persons? (A) Tuberculin insensitivity, (B) Microbial decontamination, (C) Tuberculin sensitivity, (D) Atypical mycobacteria exposure

16. (　) How long may protection persist in individuals who receive BCG vaccination, especially in children? (A) 1 year, (B) 5 years, (C) 10 years, (D) 20 years

17. (　) What is the primary method for controlling infectivity in TB patients? (A) Concurrent disinfection, (B) Isolation, (C) Direct observation of treatment, (D) BCG vaccination

II. Simple answer:

1. What does DOTS mean, and for what type of disease treatment is it used?

2. Could you please provide information about the methods for controlling tuberculosis?

3. Could you please provide information about screening methods for tuberculosis?

5-10   Legionellosis (ICD-9 482.8; ICD-10 A48.1)

Highlight

1. Legionnaires' disease
2. Pontiac fever
3. Community-acquired pneumonia
4. *Legionella pneumophila*
5. Air conditioning system
6. Respiratory failure

The first recognized outbreak occurred on July 27, 1976, at the Bellevue Stratford Hotel in Philadelphia, Pennsylvania, where members of the American Legion, a United States military veterans association, had gathered for the American Bicentennial. Within two days of the event's start, veterans began falling ill with a then-unidentified pneumonia. They had high breathing rates and chest pains. Numbers differ, but perhaps as many as 221 people were given medical treatment and 34 deaths occurred.

Legionellosis is an infectious disease caused by bacteria belonging to the genus *Legionella*. Over 90% of legionellosis cases are caused by *Legionella pneumophila*, a ubiquitous aquatic organism that thrives in warm environments (25 to 45°C with an optimum around 35°C). Legionellosis takes two distinct forms:

1. Legionnaires' disease is the more severe form of the infection and produces pneumonia. Legionnaires' disease is important in metropolitans because it is often unrecognized until a late stage, it does not respond well to conventional treatment for community-acquired pneumonia, and it can be life-threatening. It commonly occurs in clusters or outbreaks of cases.

2. Pontiac fever is a relatively mild and self-limiting illness caused by the same bacteria responsible for Legionnaires' disease—Legionella species, primarily *Legionella pneumophila*. However, unlike Legionnaires' disease, Pontiac fever does not lead to pneumonia and is characterized by flu-like symptoms.

Identification to the legionellosis:

Legionellosis is an acute bacterial disease with currently recognized distinct clinical epidemiologic manifestations: Legionnaires' disease (ICD-10 A48.1) and Pontiac fever (ICD-10 A48.2). Both are characterized initially by anorexia, malaise, myalgia, and headache. Within a day, there is usually a rapidly rising fever associated with chills.

Legionnaires' disease is a nonproductive cough is common; abdominal pain and diarrhea occur in many patients. Body temperatures commonly reach 39–40.5°C. Chest x-ray may show patchy areas of consolidation which may progress to bilateral involvement and ultimately to respiratory failure. The overall case fatality rate has been as 15% in hospitalized cases of Legionnaires' disease (Fig. 5-16).

Pontiac fever is an acute febrile illness that resembles a flu-like syndrome. It is generally characterized by sudden onset of symptoms that can include fever, chills, headache, muscle aches, and general malaise. Unlike Legionnaires' disease, it does not cause pneumonia or severe respiratory symptoms; patients recover spontaneously in 1 week without treatment.

Infectious agent:

Legionella pneumophila, a poorly staining gram-negative rod that is difficult to grow *in vitro*. Serogroups 1-14 are currently recognized.

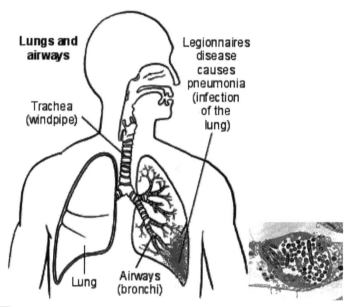

Lungs and airways

Legionnaires disease causes pneumonia (infection of the lung)

Trachea (windpipe)

Lung

Airways (bronchi)

Figure 5-16   Legionnaires' disease is a nonproductive cough, Chest x-ray may show patchy areas of consolidation. (www.patient.co.uk)

🔋 Occurrence:

Legionellosis is neither new nor localized. The earliest documented case occurred in 1947 and the earliest documented outbreak in 1957 in Minnesota, USA. Since then, the disease has been identified in most countries as well as in Australia, African countries, Canada, South America, European countries, and Taiwan. Sporadic cases and outbreaks are recognized more commonly in summer and autumn.

Outbreaks of legionellosis usually occur with low attack rates (0.1–5%) in the population at risk. Epidemic Pontiac fever has had a high attack rate (about 95%) in several outbreaks.

In recent years, the annual number of confirmed Legionnaires' disease cases is about 383 in Taiwan (Fig. 5-17). Legionnaires' disease epidemic also occurred in hospitals, resorts, hotels and gyms. The monthly distribution of Legionnaires' disease cases shows that the number of cases peaks in the summer. Regarding the age distribution of Legionnaires' disease cases, Taiwan has the same trend with other countries, with the incidence increasing with age. The elders are at a higher risk of Legionnaires' disease, and this will be a main target of disease prevention (C.D.C., Taiwan).

Reservoir:

Probably aqueous; soil has been suspected. Hot water systems and air-conditioning cooling towers or evaporative condensers have been implicated epidemiologically.

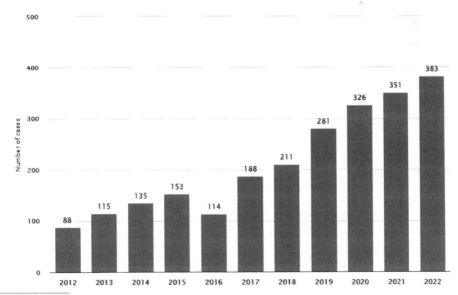

Figure 5-17 Number of confirmed cases of legionnaires' diseases in Taiwan from 2012 to 2022.
(https://www.statista.com/statistics/1079808/taiwan-legionnaires-disease-cases/)

Mode of transmission:

Epidemiological evidence supports air borne transmission; other modes are possible, including aspiration of water. Potential sources of such contaminated water include cooling towers used in industrial cooling water systems as well as in large central air conditioning systems, evaporative coolers, hot water systems, showers, whirlpool spas, architectural fountains, room-air humidifiers, ice making machines, misting equipment, and similar disseminators that draw upon a public water supply.

The disease may also be spread in a hot tub if the filtering system is defective. Freshwater ponds, creeks, and ornamental fountains are also potential sources of *Legionella*. Drinking water contaminated with Legionella is not a common source of infection, as the bacteria typically cause problems when they are inhaled into the lungs.

Incubation period:

The incubation period of Legionnaires' disease is probably 2–10 days, most often 5–6 days; Pontiac fever is probably 5–66 hours, most often 24–48 hours.

Period of communicability:

Person-to-person transmission has not been documented.

Susceptibility and resistance:

Susceptibility is general but the disease is rare in those under 20 years of age. Several outbreaks of Legionellosis have occurred among hospitalized patients. More serious illness tends to occur with increasing age, especially in smokers and the immunocompromised. The male/female ratio is about

2.5:1; and the average age of cases is in the 50 years old. There are no known specific risk factors that significantly increase susceptibility to Pontiac fever. In most cases, Pontiac fever does not lead to severe complications, and individuals typically recover within a few days to a week without specific medical intervention.

Methods of control:

It is necessary to disinfection of cooling tower waters and adequate treatment of water supplies. Here are key control methods to prevent Legionnaires' disease:

1. Cooling towers should be drained when not in use, and mechanically cleaned periodically to remove scale and sediment.

2. Appropriate biocides should be used to limit the growth of slime-forming organisms.

3. Tap water should not be used in respiratory therapy devices.

4. Maintaining hot water system temperature at 50 °C or higher may reduce the risk of transmission.

5. Use appropriate disinfection methods such as chlorine, chlorine dioxide, copper-silver ionization, or ultraviolet (UV) light to control Legionella in water systems.

These control methods are particularly important in high-risk settings such as hospitals, hotels, cooling towers, and large buildings.

General review

1. Legionellosis (Legionnaires' disease)

2. Community-acquired pneumonia

3. An acute bacterial disease

4. Legionnaires' disease (fatality rate 15%)

5. Pontiac fever (recover spontaneously)

6. *Legionella pneumophila*

7. Occurrence in summer and fall / Taiwan

8. Reservoir: air-conditioning cooling towers

9. Person-to-person transmission has not been documented

SCAN ME

Check Your Answers

Review test

I. Multiple-choice questions (four selected one):

1. ( ) What is the case fatality rate for hospitalized Legionnaires' disease cases? (A) 0.1-5%, (B) 10%, (C) 15%, (D) exceeded 90%.

2. ( ) Pontiac fever is not associated with pneumonia or death. How long does it take for patients to naturally recover without treatment? (A) 72 hours, (B) 1 week, (C) 2 weeks, (D) 4 weeks.

3. ( ) What is the typical incubation period for Legionnaires' disease? (A) 24-48 hours, (B) 72 hours, (C) 2-10 days, (D) 10-14 days

4. ( ) What is the typical incubation period for Pontiac fever? (A) 24-48 hours, (B) 72 hours, (C) 2-10 days, (D) 10-14 days

5. ( ) What is the attack rate in the population at risk during outbreaks of Legionellosis? (A) 0.1-5%, (B) 20-35%, (C) 50%, (D) 95%

6. ( ) What is the attack rate during several outbreaks of Epidemic Pontiac fever? (A) 0.1-5%, (B) 20-35%, (C) 50%, (D) 95%

7. (   ) Which form of legionellosis produces pneumonia and can be life-threatening? (A) Pontiac fever, (B) Severe Legionnaires' disease, (C) Legionella species, (D) Metropolitans fever

8. (   ) Why is Legionnaires' disease important in metropolitans? (A) It responds well to conventional treatment, (B) It commonly occurs as an isolated case, (C) It is often unrecognized until a late stage, (D) It does not lead to pneumonia

9. (   ) What distinguishes Pontiac fever from Legionnaires' disease? (A) Pontiac fever is life-threatening, (B) Pontiac fever does not lead to pneumonia, (C) Legionnaires' disease has flu-like symptoms, (D) Both are severe forms of the infection

10. (   ) In which type of setting does Legionnaires' disease commonly occur? (A) Isolated rural areas, (B) Clusters or outbreaks, (C) Suburban neighborhoods, (D) Tropical climates

11. (   ) Which of the following is a characteristic feature of Pontiac fever? (A) Pneumonia, (B) Sudden onset of symptoms, (C) Severe respiratory symptoms, (D) Requires treatment for recovery

12. (   ) How long does it typically take for patients with Pontiac fever to recover without treatment? (A) 24 hours, (B) 1 week, (C) 2 weeks, (D) 1 month

13. (   ) Unlike Legionnaires' disease, Pontiac fever does not cause: (A) Pneumonia, (B) Headache, (C) General malaise, (D) Chills

14. (   ) What type of transmission is supported by epidemiological evidence for Pontiac fever? (A) Waterborne transmission, (B) Vector-borne transmission, (C) Person-to-person transmission, (D) Airborne transmission

15. ( ) What is the purpose of using appropriate biocides in water systems? (A) Increase the growth of slime-forming organisms, (B) Enhance water system scale, (C) Limit the growth of slime-forming organisms, (D) Reduce the water temperature

16. ( ) What temperature range is recommended for maintaining hot water systems to reduce the risk of Legionella transmission? (A) Below 30°C, (B) Between 30°C and 40°C, (C) 50°C or higher, (D) Exactly 60°C

17. ( ) Which of the following is NOT mentioned as a disinfection method to control Legionella in water systems? (A) Chlorine, (B) Copper-silver ionization, (C) Tap water, (D) Ultraviolet (UV) light

II. Simple answer:

1. Could you please provide information about how Legionnaires' disease is transmitted?

2. Could you please provide information about controlling Legionnaires' disease?

3. Could you please provide information about the reservoir for Legionella pneumophila?

4. Could you please provide the probable reservoirs for Legionnaires' disease?

5-11 Influenza (ICD-9 487; ICD-10 J10, J11)

 Highlight

1. Influenza
2. Epidemics of influenza A (1-3 years)
3. Epidemics of influenza B (3-4 years)
4. Incidence of infection is often highest in school-age children
5. Control: Active immunization

The first convincing record of an influenza pandemic was of an outbreak in 1580, which began in Asia and spread to Europe via Africa. The most famous and lethal outbreak was the so-called Spanish flu pandemic (type A influenza, H1N1 subtype), which lasted from 1918 to 1919. Older estimates say it killed 40-50 million people, while current estimates say 50 million to 100 million people worldwide were killed.

Influenza, commonly known as flu, is an infectious disease of birds and mammals caused by RNA viruses of the family Orthomyxoviridae (the influenza viruses). The name *influenza* comes from the Italian: *influenza*, meaning "influence", (Latin: *influentia*). In humans, common symptoms of the disease are the chills, then fever, sore throat, muscle pains, severe headache, coughing, weakness and general discomfort. In more serious cases, influenza causes pneumonia, which can be fatal, particularly in young children and the elderly. Influenza can also lead to epidemics and pandemics. An epidemic is when there's a sudden increase in the number of cases in a specific region, while a pandemic is a global outbreak of a new strain of influenza virus that affects a large portion of the world's population.

Although it is sometimes confused with the common cold; colds usually have a gradual onset, which may start to feel mildly unwell, and symptoms develop slowly over a few days. Colds are usually milder and less likely to cause severe symptoms or complications. Influenza is a much more severe disease and is caused by a different type of virus. Influenza can produce nausea and vomiting, especially in children, but these symptoms are more characteristic of the unrelated gastroenteritis, which is sometimes called "stomach flu" or "24-hour flu".

❶ Identification to the Influenza:

Influenza is a moderate to severe illness most often caused by influenza A or B virus. It is highly infectious to susceptible, and with its short incubation period it can cause overwhelming epidemics. Influenza is an acute viral disease of respiratory tract characterized by fever, chillness, headache, myalgia, prostration (fatigue), coryza and mild sore throat. Cough is often severe and protracted. The disease is usually self-limited, with recovery in 2-7 days.

There are several subtypes of influenza A viruses, which are the most common cause of seasonal and pandemic flu. Influenza B viruses also exist and are responsible for seasonal flu but have a more limited range of subtypes.

1. Influenza A viruses are further categorized into subtypes based on their H and N proteins; "H" means haemagglutinin, "N" means Neuraminidase. Some common influenza A subtypes include:

   ❍ H1N1: This subtype caused the Spanish flu pandemic in 1918 and the 2009 H1N1 pandemic. It can lead to severe respiratory illness.

- H1N2: This subtype is less common in causing pandemics but can lead to seasonal flu outbreaks with symptoms similar to other influenza strains. It can lead to endemic in humans and pigs.

- H2N2: It caused a pandemic known as the "1957 influenza pandemic" or "Asian flu pandemic." This pandemic had a global impact, with outbreaks occurring in various parts of the world.

- H3N2: This subtype has been responsible for seasonal flu epidemics (Hong Kong Flu), and it can lead to more severe illness, particularly in older adults and young children.

- H5N1: Also known as avian influenza or bird flu, this subtype primarily infects birds but can occasionally infect humans. It has a high mortality rate in humans. It was a pandemic threat in the 2007-08 flu season.

- H7N9: Another avian influenza subtype, H7N9, has caused sporadic outbreaks in China. It can lead to severe respiratory illness in humans.

- H9N2: This subtype is primarily found in poultry and wild birds but has been known to infect humans. Human cases are usually mild.

2. Influenza B viruses are categorized into two lineages: Victoria and Yamagata. Influenza B can cause seasonal flu, but it typically leads to milder illness compared to some subtypes of influenza A. It's important to note that unlike influenza A viruses, influenza B viruses do not have subtypes based on H and N proteins.

🔟 Infectious agent:

The influenza virus is an RNA virus of the family Orthomyxoviridae, which comprises five genera: influenzavirus A, influenzavirus B, influenzavirus C, Isavirus, and Thogotovirus. There are three types of influenza virus: The influenza A and B viruses that routinely spread in people (human influenza viruses) are responsible for seasonal influenza epidemics each year. Type A influenza viruses are further classified into subtypes according to the combinations of various virus surface proteins. Among many subtypes of influenza A viruses, influenza A (H1N1) and A (H3N2) subtypes are currently circulating among humans. Currently circulating influenza B viruses belong to one of the two following lineages: B/Yamagata and B/Victoria. Type C influenza cases occur much less frequently than A and B (C.D.C., Taiwan).

Influenza viruses can change over time through a process called antigenic drift or antigenic shift. This is why the flu vaccine needs to be updated regularly to provide protection against the most prevalent strains.

🔟 Occurrence:

Influenza can also lead to epidemics and pandemics. An epidemic is when there's a sudden increase in the number of cases in a specific region, while a pandemic is a global outbreak of a new strain of influenza virus that affects a large portion of the world's population. Clinical attack rate epidemics range from 10-20% in the general community to more than 50% in closed populations (e.g., nursing home, schools). Epidemics of influenza A have appeared in Taiwan at intervals of roughly 1-3 years, influenza B usually every 3-4 years. Mixed epidemics also occur. In temperate zones, epidemics tend to occur in winter; in the tropics often occur in rainy seasons. Influenza occurs globally with an annual attack rate estimated at 5-10% in adults and 20-30% in children. In Taiwan, among outpatient cases of influenza, about 0.5% requires hospitalization, of which 7% of the patients with serious complications need intensive care, and of which the mortality rate is about 20% (Fig. 5-18).

Influenza viral infections also occur in swine, horse, and many domestic and wild avian species in many parts of the world (Fig. 5-19).

🄳 Reservoir:

Men are the primary reservoir for human infections; birds and mammalian reservoirs such as swine are likely sources of new human subtypes thought to emerge through genetic re-assortment.

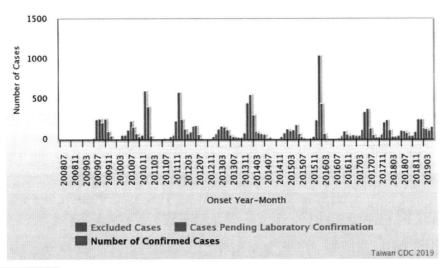

Severe Complicated Influenza , Nationwide, Indigenous and Imported , Month 07/2008 - Month 06/2019

Figure 5-18   Severe Complicated Influenza in Taiwan, 2008/7-2019/6
(CDC, Taiwan, 2020).
(https://www.cdc.gov.tw/En/Category/ListContent/bg0g_V
U_Ysrgkes_KRUDgQ?uaid=Zvnt3Ff941PorUmUD0-leA)

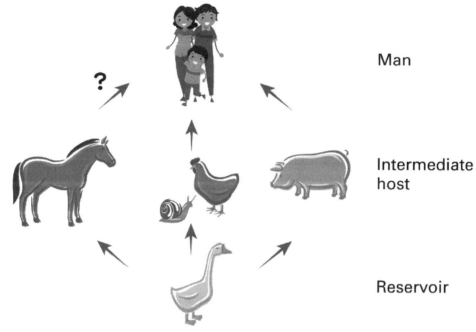

Man

Intermediate host

Reservoir

Figure 5-19   Influenza viral infections also occur in swine, horse, and many domestic and wild avian species in many parts of the world.

Mode of transmission:

It is by direct contact through droplet infection, airborne spread among crowded populations in enclosed spaces.

Typically, influenza is transmitted from infected mammals through the air by coughs or sneezes, creating aerosols containing the virus, and from infected birds through their droppings. Influenza can also be transmitted by saliva, nasal secretions, feces, and blood.

Incubation period:

Incubation period is short, usually 24-72 hours.

🔹 Period of communicability:

Probably limited to 3-5 days from clinical onset, child perhaps prolong to 7 days.

🔹 Susceptibility and resistance:

With a new subtype, susceptibility is universal. Incidence of infection is often highest in school-age children. Influenza is particularly dangerous for highly susceptible individuals, including:

1. **Elderly individuals**: They are at a higher risk of severe complications and hospitalization.

2. **Young children**: Especially those under 2 years old.

3. **Pregnant women**: They are more susceptible to severe illness.

4. **People with underlying health conditions**: Such as asthma, heart disease, diabetes, or compromised immune systems.

🔹 Methods of control:

Active immunization gives effective protection against infections, which protection rate are 70-80%.

Vaccinations against influenza are usually given to people in developed countries with a high risk of contracting the disease and to farmed poultry. The most common human vaccine is the trivalent influenza vaccine that contains purified and inactivated material from three viral strains. Typically, this vaccine includes material from two influenza A virus subtypes and one influenza B virus strain. A vaccine formulated for one year may be ineffective in the following year, since the influenza virus changes rapidly over time, and different strains become dominant. For trivalent vaccines for use in the 2023-2024 northern hemisphere influenza season, the WHO recommends the following:

1. **Egg-based vaccines (3 in 1)**

   an A/Victoria/4897/2022 (H1N1) pdm09-like virus;

   an A/Darwin/9/2021 (H3N2)-like virus; and

   a B/Austria/1359417/2021 (B/Victoria lineage)-like virus.

2. **Cell culture- or recombinant-based vaccines (3 in 1)**

   an A/Wisconsin/67/2022 (H1N1) pdm09-like virus;

   an A/Darwin/6/2021 (H3N2)-like virus; and

   a B/Austria/1359417/2021 (B/Victoria lineage)-like virus.

Antiviral drugs can be used to treat influenza, with neuraminidase inhibitors being particularly effective. Antiviral drugs such as oseltamivir (trade name Tamiflu) and zanamivir (trade name Relenza) are neuraminidase inhibitors that are designed to halt the spread of the virus in the body. These drugs are often effective against both influenza A and B. Amantadine hydrochloride or Rimantadine, 100 mg (b.i.d x III) is effective in the chemoprophylaxis of influenza A.

General review

1. Influenza

2. Flu

3. Influenza A viruses:

4. H1N1= Haemagglutinin type1, Neuraminidase type1

5. Influenza B viruses: Victoria and Yamagata

6. Epidemics of influenza A

7. Epidemics of influenza B

SCAN ME

Check Your Answers

Review test

I. Multiple-choice questions (four selected one):

1. (　) How many years, on average, do the epidemics of influenza A appear in Taiwan at intervals? (A) 1-3 years, (B) 3-4 years, (C) 3-5 years, (D) dependent on the weather.

2. (　) How many years, on average, do the epidemics of influenza B appear in Taiwan at intervals? (A) 1-3 years, (B) 3-4 years, (C) 3-5 years, (D) dependent on the weather.

3. (　) How long is the incubation period of epidemic influenza? (A) within 24 hours, (B) 24-48 hours, (C) 24-72 hours, (D) 5-8 days, (E) 2-10 days.

4. (　) How long is the communicable period of epidemic influenza? (A) 24-72 hours, (B) 3-5 days, (C) 5-8 days, (D) 1 week

5. (　) In which year was the first convincing record of an influenza pandemic outbreak made? (A) 1580, (B) 1680, (C) 1780, (D) 1880

6. (　) What is the main difference between an epidemic and a pandemic? (A) The severity of symptoms, (B) The region affected, (C) The type of virus, (D) The onset of symptoms

7. (　) How do colds differ from influenza? (A) Colds have a sudden onset of symptoms, (B) Influenza is caused by the same virus that causes colds, (C) Influenza symptoms develop slowly over a few days, (D) Colds are more severe and likely to cause complications

8. (　) What is a common misconception regarding influenza symptoms in children? (A) Influenza symptoms in children are

usually mild, (B) Nausea and vomiting are not associated with influenza in children, (C) Gastroenteritis is sometimes confused with influenza in children, (D) Influenza is often referred to as the "24-hour flu" in children

9. (   ) What do the letters "H" and "N" represent in the categorization of influenza A viruses? (A) High and Normal, (B) Haemagglutinin and Neuraminidase, (C) Host and Nucleus, (D) Hemoglobin and Nucleotide

10. (   ) Which influenza A subtype caused the Spanish flu pandemic in 1918 and the 2009 H1N1 pandemic? (A) H1N2, (B) H2N2, (C) H1N1, (D) H5N1

11. (   ) What is the significance of H5N1, also known as avian influenza or bird flu? (A) It primarily infects pigs, (B) It caused the 1957 influenza pandemic, (C) It has a high mortality rate in humans, (D) It is less common in causing pandemics

12. (   ) Influenza B viruses are categorized into which two lineages? (A) Alpha and Beta, (B) Victoria and Yamagata, (C) Gamma and Delta, (D) A and B

13. (   ) What is a characteristic difference between influenza A and influenza B viruses? (A) Influenza B viruses have higher mortality rates, (B) Influenza A viruses have subtypes based on H and N proteins, (C) Influenza B viruses caused the 2009 H1N1 pandemic, (D) Influenza A viruses do not have subtypes.

14. (   ) What is the process responsible for the change in influenza viruses over time? (A) Immunization, (B) Antigenic Drift, (C) Viral Drift, (D) Immune Response

15. (　) Why does the flu vaccine need to be updated regularly? (A) To boost immunity, (B) To prevent epidemics, (C) To address antigenic drift or shift, (D) To decrease clinical attack rates

16. (　) What characterizes an epidemic of influenza? (A) Global outbreak, (B) Sudden increase in cases in a specific region, (C) Long-term, gradual increase in cases, (D) Affecting a small, isolated population

17. (　) In closed populations such as nursing homes or schools, what range of clinical attack rate epidemics is mentioned? (A) 5-10%, (B) 20-30%, (C) 30-40%, (D) 50-60%

18. (　) Who is particularly at a higher risk of severe complications and hospitalization due to influenza? (A) Young adults, (B) Pregnant women, (C) Middle-aged individuals, (D) Teenagers

19. (　) Why are young children, especially those under 2 years old, considered highly susceptible to influenza? (A) They have stronger immune systems, (B) They are more likely to receive the flu vaccine, (C) Their immune systems are still developing, (D) They are less exposed to influenza viruses.

20. (　) Which group of individuals is mentioned as having a higher risk of severe illness from influenza due to underlying health conditions? (A) Individuals with compromised immune systems, (B) Healthy individuals, (C) Individuals with strong respiratory systems, (D) Individuals with a history of flu vaccination

II. Simple answer:

1. Could you please provide information about the occurrence of epidemic influenza types A and B in Taiwan?

2. Influenza A viruses are divided into different serotypes based on surface proteins. What do H and N stand for?

5-12	Severe Acute Respiratory Syndrome
	(ICD-9 079.82; ICD-10 U04.9)

 Highlight

1. Severe Acute Respiratory Syndromes
2. SARS coronavirus (SARS-CoV-1)
3. Atypical pneumonia
4. Middle East Respiratory Syndrome coronavirus (MERS-CoV)
5. Coronavirus disease (COVID-19; SARS-CoV-2)

Severe acute respiratory syndrome (SARS)

Severe acute respiratory syndrome is a respiratory disease in humans which is caused by the SARS coronavirus (SARS-CoV). There has been one near pandemic to date, between November 2002 and July 2003, with 8,096 known infected cases and 774 deaths (a mortality rate of 9.6%) worldwide being listed in the WHO April 21, 2004, concluding report (Fig. 5-20).

The epidemic reached the public spotlight in February 2003, when an American businessman traveling from China became afflicted with pneumonia-like symptoms while on a flight to Singapore. The plane stopped at Hanoi, Vietnam, where the victim died in The French Hospital of Hanoi. Several of the medical staff who treated him soon developed the same disease despite basic hospital procedures. Italian doctor Carlo Urbani identified the threat and communicated it to WHO and the Vietnamese government. The severity of the symptoms and the infection of hospital staff alarmed global health authorities fearful of another emergent pneumonia epidemic.

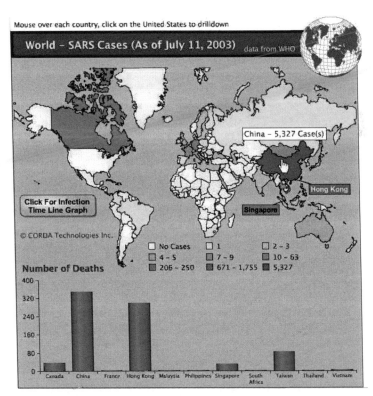

Figure 5-20   Corda's world map of SARS. Web browser screenshot by this author of Corda's world map of SARS displaying data for each country affected by SARS as of 11 July 2003. (http://www.corda.com/examples/go/map/sars.cfm.)

Identification to the SARS:

Initial symptoms are flu like and may include fever, myalgia, lethargy, gastrointestinal symptoms, cough, sore throat and other non-specific symptoms. The only symptom that is common to all patients appears to be a fever above 38°C. Shortness of breath may occur later. Symptoms usually appear 2-10 days following exposure, but up to 13 days has been reported. In most cases symptoms appear within 2-3 days. About 10-20% of cases require mechanical ventilation.

SARS may be suspected in a patient who has any of the symptoms including a fever of 38°C or more, and either a history of contact (sexual or casual) with someone with a diagnosis of SARS within the last 10 days, or travel to any of the regions identified by the WHO as areas with recent local transmission of SARS (affected regions as of 10 May 2003 were parts of China, Hong Kong, Singapore and the province of Ontario, Canada).

A probable case of SARS has the above findings plus positive chest x-ray findings of atypical pneumonia or respiratory distress syndrome. The last reported case of SARS occurred in 2004. The global outbreak was declared over in July 2003, after extensive efforts to control its spread.

Infectious agent:

SARS is caused by a coronavirus similar, on electron microscopy, to animal coronaviruses. It is believed to have originated in bats and was transmitted to humans through an intermediate host, likely palm civets in wet markets in southern China. SARS-CoV-1 can stable in feces and urine at room temperature for at least 1–2 days, and for up to 4 days in stools from patients who manifest diarrhea. The SARS virus loses infectivity after exposure to different commonly used disinfectants and fixatives heat at 56°C kills the SARS coronavirus at approximately 10,000 units per 15 minutes.

SARS-CoV-1 are positive-strand, enveloped RNA viruses that are important pathogens of mammals and birds. This group of viruses cause enteric or respiratory tract infections in a variety of animals including humans, livestock and pets.

Occurrence:

The epidemic of SARS appears to have originated in Guangdong Province, China in November 2002. The first case of SARS was reportedly originated in Shunde, Foshan, Guangdong in Nov 2002, and the patient, a farmer, was treated in the First People's Hospital of Foshan. The patient died soon after, and no definite diagnosis was made on his cause of death. ("Patient #0" - first reported symptoms; has been attributed to Charles Bybelezar of Montreal, Quebec, Canada) and, despite taking some action to control it, Chinese government officials did not inform the WHO of the outbreak until February 2003, restricting media coverage in order to preserve public confidence. This lack of openness caused delays in efforts to control the epidemic, resulting in criticism of the People's Republic of China (PRC) from the international community. The PRC has since officially apologized for early slowness in dealing with the SARS epidemic.

Local transmission of SARS took place in Toronto, Vancouver, San Francisco, Ulan Bator, Manila, Singapore, Hanoi, Taiwan (Fig. 5-21), the Chinese provinces of Guangdong, Jilin, Hebei, Hubei, Shaanxi, Jiangsu and Shanxi, the Chinese municipality of Tianjin, the Chinese Autonomous Region of Inner Mongolia, and the Chinese Special Administrative Region of Hong Kong.

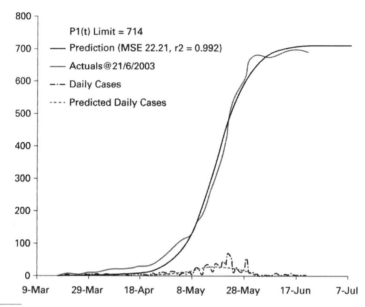

Figure 5-21   **SARS local transmission in Taiwan** (CDC/DOH, Taiwan, 2003).

Reservoir:

Civet cats, pet cats, ferrets and bats may be reservoirs for SARS.

Mode of transmission:

SARS is primarily transmitted through respiratory droplets when an infected person coughs, sneezes, or talks. Close contact with an infected person is the most common way to contract the virus (WHO, 2003). Possible airborne transmission was documented for some super-spreading events in the SARS epidemics.

Incubation period:

Incubation period is from 3 to 10 days.

🔹 Period of communicability:

Not yet completely understood so far. Initial studies suggest that transmission doses not occur before onset of clinical signs and symptoms, and that maximum period of communicability is less than 21 days. Close contact with an infected person was a significant factor in transmission. Healthcare workers and family members of infected individuals were at higher risk due to frequent and close contact. Especially, if involved in pulmonary procedures such as intubation or nebulization and serve as a major entry point of the disease into the community.

🔹 Susceptibility and resistance:

Older individuals, particularly those over 65, were more susceptible to severe SARS-CoV-1 infection and had a higher risk of mortality. Younger individuals, especially children, were generally less severely affected. People with underlying health conditions, such as respiratory diseases, diabetes, or compromised immune systems, were more susceptible to severe SARS-CoV-1 infection.

🔹 Methods of control:

1. Identify all suspect and probable cases using the WHO case definitions.

2. Isolation of probable cases.

3. Strict universal precautions for infection control must be practiced using precautions for airborne, droplet and contact transmission; all staff, including ancillary staff, must be fully trained in infection control and use personal protective equipment.

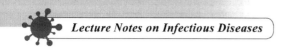

4. Disposable equipment should be used wherever possible in treatment and care of patients with SARS and disposed of appropriately.

5. Movement of patients outside the isolation unit should be avoided.

6. Handwashing is crucial and access to clean water essential with handwashing before and after contact with any patient, after activities likely to cause contamination, and after removing gloves.

7. Alcohol-based skin disinfectants can be used if there is no obvious organic material contamination.

Middle East Respiratory Syndrome Coronavirus (MERS-CoV)- Kingdom of Saudi Arabia

Middle East Respiratory Syndrome (MERS) is a viral respiratory illness caused by the Middle East Respiratory Syndrome Coronavirus (MERS-CoV). It was first identified in 2012 and has caused sporadic outbreaks, primarily in the Arabian Peninsula.

Identification to the MERS:

MERS typically presents with symptoms similar to those of other respiratory illnesses, such as fever, cough, and shortness of breath. In severe cases, it can progress to pneumonia and acute respiratory distress syndrome (ARDS). Some patients may also experience gastrointestinal symptoms. MERS is known for its relatively high mortality rate, which varies by region and population. Mortality rates have been as high as 35% in some outbreaks, but they can vary depending on factors such as the availability of medical care and the patient's age and overall health.

🔵 Infectious agent:

MERS is caused by MERS-CoV, a type of coronavirus. It is believed to have originated in bats and was transmitted to humans through an intermediate host, which is thought to be camels. Camels are considered a significant reservoir for the virus.

🔵 Occurrence:

MERS cases have been reported in several countries, the majority of cases have occurred in the Arabian Peninsula, including Saudi Arabia, the United Arab Emirates, and Jordan. Travel-associated cases have been reported in other parts of the world.

🔵 Reservoir:

Current scientific evidence suggests that dromedary camels are a major reservoir host for MERS-CoV and an animal source of MERS infection in humans. However, the exact role of dromedaries in the transmission of the virus and the exact routes of transmission are unknown.

🔵 Mode of transmission:

MERS-CoV is primarily transmitted to humans through close contact with infected camels or through human-to-human transmission. Although no sustained human-to-human transmission has been documented, cases have been reported where there was some unprotected contact with infected persons, such as in a health care setting. Health care-associated outbreaks have occurred in several countries, with the largest seen in the Republic of Korea, Saudi Arabia and the United Arab Emirates. It can spread through respiratory droplets when an infected person coughs or sneezes.

🔋 Incubation period:

The incubation period can vary from person to person but generally falls within the range of 2 to 14 days. However, it's important to note that some individuals infected with MERS-CoV may remain asymptomatic or have mild symptoms, and in such cases, the incubation period may not be easily determined. Additionally, there can be variability in the incubation period based on factors such as the individual's immune system and the amount of virus they were exposed to.

🔋 Period of communicability:

For MERS, the period of communicability is not entirely clear-cut and may vary among individuals. Here are some key points to consider:

1. **Pre-Symptomatic Period**: Some individuals infected with MERS-CoV may be capable of transmitting the virus to others before they develop symptoms. This pre-symptomatic period is not well-defined but can occur in the days leading up to the onset of symptoms. During this time, individuals may not be aware that they are infected but can still potentially spread the virus through respiratory secretions like coughs and sneezes.

2. **Symptomatic Period**: The highest risk of transmitting MERS-CoV occurs when individuals are actively experiencing symptoms of the disease, such as fever, cough, and shortness of breath. The virus can be present in respiratory secretions, including saliva and mucus, and can be expelled into the air when an infected person coughs or sneezes.

3. **Post-Symptomatic Period**: It is generally believed that the risk of transmission decreases as the individual recovers from MERS. However, some studies have suggested that the virus can continue to be detected in

respiratory secretions for several weeks after symptom onset in some cases.

4. **Asymptomatic and Mild Cases**: Asymptomatic or mildly symptomatic individuals can also carry the virus and potentially transmit it to others. The duration of communicability in such cases may be shorter than in severe cases.

🔒 Susceptibility and resistance:

The susceptibility and resistance to Middle East Respiratory Syndrome (MERS) can vary among individuals and populations, and several factors influence an individual's risk of infection and the severity of the disease. Here are some key considerations regarding susceptibility and resistance to MERS:

1. **Age**: While MERS can affect individuals of all ages, severe cases and mortality rates tend to be higher among older adults, particularly those over 65 years old. Children and young adults may be less severely affected.

2. **Underlying Health Conditions**: Individuals with underlying health conditions, such as respiratory diseases (e.g., asthma, chronic obstructive pulmonary disease), diabetes, cardiovascular disease, or compromised immune systems, are at a higher risk of developing severe MERS.

3. **Good Hygiene Practices**: Practicing good hygiene, such as frequent handwashing, can reduce the risk of acquiring the virus, especially in settings where close contact with infected individuals or contaminated surfaces may occur.

4. **Use of Personal Protective Equipment**: Healthcare workers and individuals in close contact with MERS patients can reduce their risk of

infection by using appropriate personal protective equipment (PPE), including masks, gloves, and gowns.

Methods of control:

1. Monitor and investigate clusters of respiratory illness.

2. Isolate suspected and confirmed MERS cases to prevent further transmission.

3. Implement quarantine measures for individuals who have been in close contact with confirmed cases, especially in healthcare settings and households.

4. Ensure proper use of personal protective equipment (PPE) by healthcare workers, including masks, gloves, gowns, and eye protection.

5. Conduct thorough contact tracing to identify and monitor individuals who may have been exposed to MERS-CoV.

6. Educate the public about MERS, its symptoms, and preventive measures.

7. Implement screening measures at airports and other points of entry to detect and isolate travelers with symptoms of MERS.

(W.H.O., 2023)

Coronavirus disease 2019; COVID-19

COVID-19, also known as Coronavirus Disease 2019, is a highly contagious respiratory illness caused by a novel coronavirus called SARS-CoV-2, which has had a profound impact on the world, leading to widespread illness, deaths, disruptions in daily life, and economic challenges. Many countries implemented lockdowns and travel restrictions to curb the spread of the virus.

In late December 2019, cases of a mysterious respiratory illness were reported in the city of Wuhan, Hubei province, China. Many of the early cases were linked to a seafood market in Wuhan, suggesting that the virus may have originated from there.

In 2020, Chinese authorities confirmed that they had identified a novel coronavirus as the cause of the outbreak. It was temporarily named "2019-nCoV." The virus was later officially named "SARS-CoV-2," and the disease it caused was named "COVID-19". Cases of COVID-19 began to appear in other countries, with the virus spreading via international travel. The World Health Organization (WHO) declared COVID-19 a Public Health Emergency of International Concern, and declared COVID-19 a global pandemic, acknowledging its rapid spread across the world. Throughout 2020, countries implemented various measures to curb the spread of the virus, including lockdowns, travel restrictions, and mask mandates.

In 2021, mass vaccination campaigns were launched globally, with millions of people receiving COVID-19 vaccines to achieve herd immunity and reduce the impact of the virus. Unfortunately, new variants of SARS-CoV-2 emerged, leading to concerns about their transmissibility and potential impact on vaccine effectiveness.

In 2022, the COVID-19 pandemic continued to evolve, with countries adapting their strategies based on vaccination rates, variants, and public health guidance. Booster shots and additional vaccine doses became part of the response strategy to enhance immunity and address waning protection. Research into COVID-19 treatment options and ongoing surveillance of the virus and its variants remained priorities.

In 2023, the Director-General of the World Health Organization made a significant announcement during a press conference and declared that COVID-19 was no longer classified as a public health emergency of international concern. This decision followed the 15th meeting of the World Health Organization's Coronavirus Emergency Committee, which convened on May 4th, 2023. During this meeting, the committee recommended that the Director-General of the WHO officially mark the end of the COVID-19 pandemic as a public health emergency of international concern.

Identification to the COVID-19:

COVID-19 symptoms can range from mild to severe and may include fever, cough, shortness of breath, fatigue, body aches, loss of taste or smell, sore throat, and congestion. Severe cases have been shown to develop into acute respiratory distress syndrome (ARDS) and septic shock. Long COVID, also referred to as Post-Acute Sequelae of SARS-CoV-2 Infection (PASC), can affect individuals, including those with mild initial symptoms or even asymptomatic cases, with persistent symptoms that endure for weeks or months following the acute infection. These lingering symptoms encompass a wide range, such as fatigue, cognitive issues often described as 'brain fog,' and chest pain, among others.

Infectious agent:

SARS-CoV-2 belongs to the Coronaviridae family, which includes several other coronaviruses, some of which cause common colds and more severe respiratory illnesses like SARS and MERS. SARS-CoV-2 is an enveloped, positive-sense, single-stranded RNA virus. It has spike proteins on its surface that give it the appearance of a crown or corona, hence the name "coronavirus." SARS-CoV-2 has shown some genetic variability, resulting in different strains and variants. Several variants have been named by WHO and labelled as a variant of concern (VoC) (Tab. 5-2). This has led to ongoing research and surveillance to monitor the virus's evolution and potential impact on public health.

Table 5-2 Infectious agent of COVID-19 (Variants of concern; past and present):

WHO Label	Pango Lineage	Date of Designation
Alpha	B.1.1.7 and Q lineages	December 29, 2020
Beta	B.1.351	December 29, 2020
Gamma	P.1	December 29, 2020
Eta	B.1.525	February 26, 2021
Iota	B.1.526	February 26, 2021
Epsilon	B.1.427 and B.1.429	March 19, 2021
Kappa	B.1.617.1	May 7, 2021
Delta	B.1.617.2	June 15, 2021
Zeta	P.2	September 21, 2021
Mu	B.1.621, B.1.621.1	September 21, 2021
Omicron (parent lineages)	B.1.1.529	November 26, 2021
Delta	B.1.617.2 and descendant lineages	April 14, 2022
Omicron	BA.2.74	September 1, 2023
Omicron	BA.2.86	September 1, 2023
Omicron	XBB.1.16	September 1, 2023
Omicron	XBB.1.5	September 1, 2023
Omicron	XBB.1.9.1	September 1, 2023
Omicron	XBB.1.9.2	September 1, 2023
Omicron	XBB.2.3	September 1, 2023
Omicron	CH.1.1	September 1, 2023

(CDC, USA, 2023)

(https://www.cdc.gov/coronavirus/2019-ncov/variants/ variant-classifications.html)

SARS-CoV-2 could remain on surfaces and aerosol droplets for up to 3 h. On metal or plastic surface, both viruses can remain viable for up to 4 days, however, with a significant reduction in titer. While SARS-CoV-2 remains stable at 0°C, a study on its environmental stability indicates that it is likely inactivated after 10 min of exposure to 56°C or more or within less than 5 min at 70°C. The virus is rendered inactive by lipid solvents; the most efficient of which being alcoholic compounds including propanol (70%-100% propyl alcohol) or ethanol (70% ethyl alcohol) applied for a minimum of 30 seconds.

🅓 Occurrence:

The WHO ended its public health emergency of international concern (PHEIC) declaration on 5 May 2023. As of November 2023, the pandemic had caused 772,166,517 confirmed cases of COVID-19, including 6,981,263 deaths, reported to WHO. Ranking it fifth in the deadliest epidemics and pandemics in history (WHO. 2023) (Fig. 5-22).

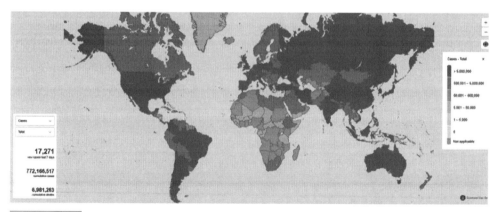

Figure 5-22 Globally, as of 2:06am CET, 22 November 2023, there have been 772,166,517 confirmed cases of COVID-19, including 6,981,263 deaths (WHO, 2023).

💊 Reservoir:

Man, Bat, Camel, Pangolin, Gorillas, Civet cat, Ferret, domestic cats and dogs may be reservoirs for COVID-19.

💊 Mode of transmission:

The virus primarily spreads through respiratory droplets when an infected person coughs, sneezes, talks, or breathes. It can also spread by touching surfaces contaminated with the virus and then touching the face. Infected people are more likely to transmit COVID-19 when they are physically close to other non-infected individuals. However, infection can occur over longer distances, particularly indoors.

💊 Incubation period:

The incubation period, the time from exposure to the onset of symptoms, typically ranges from 2 to 14 days, with an average of 5-6 days.

💊 Period of communicability:

Period of communicability is for about 3-5 days before onset and 8-10 days after onset of symptom.

💊 Susceptibility and resistance:

Young and old people can only become infected when exposed to the virus, and both of them are at a similar risk of infection. Older people infected with SARS-CoV-2 are more likely to develop disease. People with normal immunity can quickly mobilize the body's own immune function to resist the virus and prevent disease in a short time, but in the elderly population, inflammatory and immune aging make them more vulnerable to SARS-CoV-2. Therefore, older people with COVID-19 are more likely to become severe. The number of deaths among people over age 65 is 97 times higher than the number of deaths among people ages 18-29 years.

WHO estimates that at least 90% of the world's population now has some level of immunity to SARS-CoV-2, due to prior infection or vaccination. The latest real-world study of updated Covid boosters showed that new vaccines by Pfizer/BioNTech and Moderna are likely to provide better protection compared with the original shots (WHO, 2023).

Method of control:

Preventive measures to reduce the chances of infection include getting vaccinated, staying at home or spending more time outdoors, avoiding crowded places, keeping distance from others, wearing a mask in public, ventilating indoor spaces, managing potential exposure durations, washing hands with soap and water often and for at least twenty seconds, practicing good respiratory hygiene, and avoiding touching the eyes, nose, or mouth with unwashed hands.

The COVID-19 vaccines are widely credited for their role in reducing the severity and death caused by COVID-19. As of March 2023, more than 5.5 billion people had received one or more doses (11.8 billion in total) in over 197 countries. According to a June 2022 study, COVID-19 vaccines prevented an additional 14.4 million to 19.8 million deaths in 185 countries and territories. In 2022, the first recombinant protein-based COVID-19 vaccine (Novavax's booster Nuvaxovid) was authorized for use in adults in the United Kingdom. It has subsequently received endorsement /authorization from the WHO, US, European Union, and Australia. In another noteworthy development in 2022, the world witnessed the introduction of the first inhalable vaccine, a groundbreaking innovation from the Chinese biopharmaceutical company CanSino Biologics. This remarkable achievement marked a significant stride in Shanghai, China, towards enhancing vaccine accessibility and delivery methods.

Vaccines currently administered to prevent SARS-CoV-2 XBB-sublineage variants: In 2023, the Food and Drug Administration (FDA) in the United States approved updated COVID-19 mRNA vaccines by Moderna and Pfizer-BioNTech for individuals aged 12 and above, with authorization also granted for those aged 6 months to 11 years under Emergency Use Authorization (EUA). Prior to this, the FDA had granted EUA for the updated COVID-19 protein subunit vaccine by Novavax, intended for those aged 12 and above. These updated COVID-19 vaccines now contain a monovalent XBB.1.5 component, designed to enhance vaccine-induced immunity and offer protection against currently circulating SARS-CoV-2 XBB-sublineage variants, including safeguarding against severe COVID-19-associated illness and preventing fatalities. In September 2023, the Advisory Committee on Immunization Practices recommended the administration of updated COVID-19 vaccines for all individuals aged 6 months and older, as per the FDA's guidance.

⚗ General review

1. Severe Acute Respiratory Syndromes

2. SARS coronavirus (SARS-CoV-1)

3. MERS-CoV

4. SARS-CoV-2

5. SARS-CoV-2 XBB-sublineage variants

6. COVID-19 vaccine

7. COVID-19 mRNA vaccines (Moderna and Pfizer-BioNTech)

8. COVID-19 protein subunit vaccine (Novavax)

SCAN ME

Check Your Answers

Review test

I. Multiple-choice questions (four selected one):

1. (   ) What is the primary causative agent of severe acute respiratory syndrome (SARS)? (A) Influenza virus, (B) HIV, (C) SARS coronavirus (SARS-CoV), (D) Bacteria

2. (   ) During the SARS outbreak, which city gained international attention when an American businessman died of SARS while on a flight to Singapore? (A) Beijing, China, (B) Tokyo, Japan, (C) Hanoi, Vietnam, (D) New York, USA

3. (   ) What were the initial symptoms commonly associated with SARS? (A) Skin rash and joint pain, (B) Nausea and vomiting, (C) Fever, myalgia, lethargy, and other flu-like symptoms, (D) Vision problems and dizziness

4. (   ) How was the global outbreak of SARS officially declared over? (A) In 2004, (B) In July 2003, (C) When a vaccine was developed, (D) When there were no more cases in China

5. (   ) What was the mortality rate of SARS during the 2002-2003 outbreak, as mentioned in the WHO report? (A) 1.5%, (B) 5.6%, (C) 9.6%, (D) 14.3%

6. (   ) What is believed to be the origin of SARS, with an intermediate host likely being palm civets in wet markets in southern China? (A) Bats, (B) Dogs, (C) Birds, (D) Monkeys

7. (　) How long can SARS-CoV-1 remain stable in feces and urine at room temperature? (A) 4 hours, (B) 1-2 days, (C) 1 week, (D) 1 month

8. (　) How was the first case of SARS reported in November 2002 in Guangdong Province, China, described? (A) A healthcare worker, (B) A student, (C) A farmer, (D) A traveler

9. (　) When did Chinese government officials inform the WHO of the SARS outbreak? (A) In November 2002, (B) In January 2003, (C) In February 2003, (D) In April 2003

10. (　) Who was at a higher risk of contracting SARS due to close contact with infected individuals and involvement in healthcare procedures? (A) Young children, (B) Older individuals, especially those over 65, (C) Healthy adults, (D) People with underlying health conditions

11. (　) When was MERS first identified as a viral respiratory illness? (A) 1990, (B) 2002, (C) 2008, (D) 2012

12. (　) What is one of the common symptoms associated with MERS? (A) Skin rashes, (B) Gastrointestinal bleeding, (C) Shortness of breath, (D) Joint pain

13. (　) Where have the majority of MERS cases occurred? (A) Europe, (B) Asia, (C) North America, (D) Arabian Peninsula

14. (　) What is believed to be the primary reservoir host for MERS-CoV? (A) Bats, (B) Monkeys, (C) Camels, (D) Birds

15. (　) What is the highest recorded mortality rate for MERS during some outbreaks? (A) 5%, (B) 15%, (C) 25%, (D) 35%

16. (　) How is MERS primarily transmitted to humans? (A) Through contaminated water, (B) Close contact with infected camels, (C) Airborne transmission, (D) Ingestion of undercooked meat

17. (　) In which settings have health care-associated outbreaks of MERS occurred? (A) Schools and universities, (B) Shopping malls, (C) Hospitals and medical facilities, (D) Residential neighborhoods

18. (　) What is the range of the incubation period for MERS in most cases? (A) 1-3 days, (B) 5-7 days, (C) 2-14 days, (D) 21-28 days

19. (　) During which period is the risk of transmitting MERS-CoV highest? (A) Pre-symptomatic period, (B) Post-symptomatic period, (C) Asymptomatic period, (D) Recovery period

20. (　) Which individuals may carry the virus and potentially transmit it to others, even if they are asymptomatic or have mild symptoms? (A) Only those with severe symptoms, (B) Only young children, (C) Asymptomatic or mildly symptomatic individuals, (D) Only individuals over 65 years of age

21. (　) What is the official name of the virus that causes COVID-19? (A) SARS-CoV-2, (B) MERS-CoV, (C) H1N1, (D) Influenza A

22. (　) When were the first cases of a mysterious respiratory illness reported, which later led to the identification of COVID-19? (A) Early 2019, (B) Late 2019, (C) Early 2020, (D) Late 2020

23. (　) What term is used to describe the persistent symptoms that endure for weeks or months following acute COVID-19 infection, affecting some individuals even with mild initial

symptoms or asymptomatic cases? (A) Post-Infection Fatigue, (B) Acute Respiratory Distress Syndrome, (C) Long COVID (PASC), (D) SARS

24.(   ) Which family of viruses does SARS-CoV-2 belong to? (A) Influenza viruses, (B) Coronaviridae, (C) Rhinoviruses, (D) Retroviruses

25.(   ) What gives the SARS-CoV-2 virus its name "coronavirus"? (A) Its crown-like spike proteins, (B) Its shape, which resembles a sphere, (C) Its long incubation period, (D) Its connection to the Middle East

26.(   ) How long can SARS-CoV-2 remain viable on metal or plastic surfaces? (A) Up to 10 days, (B) Up to 3 hours, (C) Up to 4 days, Up to 14 days

27.(   ) What temperature range can likely inactivate SARS-CoV-2 according to the information? (A) 0-5°C, (B) 10-20°C, (C) 56-70°C, (D) 80-90°C

28.(   ) Which of the following is the most efficient lipid solvent for inactivating SARS-CoV-2 on surfaces? (A) Water, (B) Propanol (70%-100% propyl alcohol), (C) Vinegar, (D) Hydrogen peroxide

29.(   ) What is the estimated incubation period for COVID-19? (A) 1-2 days, (B) 7-10 days, (C) 2-14 days, (D) 20-30 days

30.(   ) According to the provided information, which age group is more likely to develop severe disease when infected with SARS-CoV-2? (A) Young people, (B) Middle-aged people, (C) Both young and old people are equally at risk, (D) Older people

31. (　) What is one of the key preventive measures to reduce the chances of COVID-19 infection? (A) Taking antiviral medications, (B) Avoiding all outdoor activities, (C) taying in crowded places, (D) Washing hands with soap and water for at least twenty seconds

32. (　) What percentage of the world's population now has some level of immunity to SARS-CoV-2 in 2023, as estimated by the WHO? (A) 30%, (B) 55%, (C) 72%, (D) 90%

33. (　) What was a significant development in COVID-19 vaccine technology in 2022? (A) The introduction of the first oral vaccine, (B) The development of a DNA-based vaccine, (C) The first inhalable vaccine by CanSino Biologics, (D) The launch of a live attenuated vaccine

34. (　) Which component was added to the updated COVID-19 vaccines to enhance immunity against XBB-sublineage variants in 2023? (A) Monoclonal antibodies, (B) XBB.1.5 component, (C) Viral RNA, (D) Extra booster shot

35. (　) In September 2023, who did the Advisory Committee on Immunization Practices recommend updated COVID-19 vaccines for? (A) Only individuals aged 18 and above, (B) Only those with a history of severe allergies, (C) All individuals aged 6 months and older, (D) Exclusively those who haven't had a previous COVID-19 infection

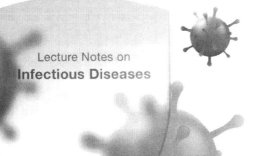

Lecture Notes on
Infectious Diseases

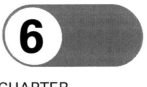

6

CHAPTER

Sexual Transmitted Diseases

A sexually transmitted disease (STD) or venereal disease (VD), is an illness that has a significant probability of transmission between humans or animals by means of sexual contact, including vaginal intercourse, oral sex, and anal sex. Increasingly, the term sexually transmitted infection (STI) is used, as it has a broader range of meaning; a person may be infected, and may potentially infect others, without showing signs of disease. Some STIs can also be transmitted via kissing, use of an IV drug needle after its use by an infected person, as well as through childbirth or breastfeeding. Sexually transmitted infections have been well known for hundreds of years.

Until the 1990s, such afflictions were commonly known as venereal diseases: *Veneris* is the Latin genitive form of the name Venus, the Roman goddess of love. Social disease was another euphemism. Public health officials originally introduced the term sexually transmitted infection, which clinicians are increasingly using alongside the term sexually transmitted disease in order to distinguish it from the former. Sometimes the terms STI and STD are used interchangeably. This can be confusing and not always accurate, so it helps first to understand the difference between infection and disease. Infection simply means that a germ; virus, bacteria, or parasite that can cause disease or sickness is present inside a person's body. An infected person does not necessarily have any symptoms or signs that the virus or bacteria is actually hurting his or her body; they do not necessarily feel sick. A disease means that the infection is actually causing the infected person to feel sick, or to notice something is wrong. For this reason, the term STI, which refers to infection with any germ that can cause an STD, even if the infected person has no symptoms, which is a much broader term than STD. The distinction being made, however, is closer to that between a colonization and an infection, rather than between an infection and a disease.

Specifically, the term STD refers only to infections that are causing symptoms. Because most of the time people do not know that they are infected with an STD until they start showing symptoms of disease, most people use the term STD, even though the term STI is also appropriate in many cases. Moreover, the term sexually transmissible disease is sometimes used since it is less restrictive in consideration of other factors or means of transmission. For instance, meningitis is transmissible by means of sexual contact but is not labeled as an STI because sexual contact is not the primary vector for the pathogens that cause meningitis. This discrepancy is addressed by the probability of infection by means other than sexual contact. In general, an STI is an infection that has a negligible probability of transmission by means other than sexual contact, but has a realistic means of transmission by sexual contact. Thus, one may presume that, if a person is infected with an STI, e.g., chlamydia, gonorrhea, genital herpes, it was transmitted to him/her by means of sexual contact.

The familiar sexually transmitted infectious diseases in Taiwan contain syphilis, gonorrhoea, AIDS, herpes II, genital warts, chlamydia, trichomoniasis, candidiasis and *Phthirus pubis*. Sexual transmitted infectious diseases can be caused by viruses, bacteria, fungi, protozoans, parasites and other diseases and inevitably cause genitourinary infection. It is possible to be an asymptomatic carrier of sexually transmitted diseases. In particular, sexually transmitted diseases in women often cause the serious condition of pelvic inflammatory disease. The STDs are categorized into five groups based on their pathogenic agents, as follows:

1. **Bacterial venereal disease:** Syphilis, Gonorrhoea, Chlamydia, Chancroid, Shigellosis

2. **Viral venereal disease:** HIV, Herpes II, Genital Warts, Hepatitis D, Cytomegalovirus

3. **Protozoan venereal disease:** Trichomoniasis, *Entamoeba histolytica*, *Balantidium coli*

4. **Fungus venereal disease:** Candidiasis

5. **Ectoparasitic venereal disease:** Scabies, *Phthirus pubis*

6-1 Syphilis (ICD-9 090-096; ICD-10 A50-A52)

Highlight

1. Syphilis
2. Venereal syphilis
3. Sexually Transmitted Disease
4. *Treponema pallidum* spirochete
5. Acute and chronic treponemal disease
6. Primary, Secondary, Latent, Tertiary Syphilis
7. Congenital syphilis
8. Intravenous drug abusers and Prostitutes.

Syphilis is a curable sexually transmitted disease caused by the *Treponema pallidum* spirochete. The route of transmission of syphilis is almost always by sexual contact, although there are examples of congenital syphilis via transmission from mother to child in utero. The signs and symptoms of syphilis are numerous; before the advent of serological testing, precise diagnosis was very difficult. In fact, the disease was dubbed the "Great Imitator" because it was often confused with other diseases, particularly in its tertiary stage. Syphilis (unless antibiotic-resistant) can be easily treated with antibiotics including penicillin. The oldest and still most effective method is an intramuscular injection of benzathine penicillin. If not treated, syphilis can cause serious effects such as damage to the heart, aorta, brain, eyes, and bones. In some cases these effects can be fatal. In 1998, the complete genetic sequence of *T. pallidum* was published which may aid understanding of the pathogenesis of syphilis.

In the early years of the 21st century, syphilis experienced an unexpected resurgence in many parts of the world, particularly in high-income countries. This resurgence was characterized by an alarming increase in reported cases, marking a departure from the declining trend observed in the latter half of the 20th century. The reasons behind this resurgence are multifaceted, involving changes in sexual behavior, challenges in access to healthcare, and shifts in public health priorities. One noteworthy aspect of syphilis in the post-2000 era has been its changing demographic profile. While syphilis has historically affected diverse populations, recent trends have seen a higher incidence among specific subgroups, including men who have sex with men (MSM) and communities facing socio-economic disparities.

The resurgence of syphilis was not limited to specific income levels; it was a global trend affecting various countries and regions, regardless of their economic status. Several factors contributed to this resurgence, including changes in sexual behavior, inadequate access to healthcare, shifts in public health priorities, and the emergence of drug-resistant strains of syphilis. This increase has occurred mainly among intravenous drug abusers and prostitutes. Many countries that had experienced increasing syphilis rates in the years leading up to 2021 (Fig. 6-1):

1. **United States**: Syphilis cases in the United States had been steadily increasing for several years before 2021. The increase was particularly pronounced among men who have sex with men (MSM) and in certain geographic regions.

2. **Canada**: Syphilis incidence in Canada had been on the rise, with some provinces reporting significant increases, especially among MSM and indigenous communities.

3. **United Kingdom**: The United Kingdom had also observed an increase in syphilis cases, especially among urban populations.

4. **Australia**: Syphilis had re-emerged as a public health concern in Australia, with outbreaks occurring in some regions, particularly among Aboriginal and Torres Strait Islander communities.

5. **Western European Countries**: Several Western European nations, including France, Germany, and the Netherlands, had seen a resurgence in syphilis cases. This was largely attributed to changing sexual behaviors, reduced condom use, and increased international travel.

6. **China**: China has seen a resurgence of syphilis cases in recent years, with urban areas experiencing a notable increase in infections. Factors contributing to this trend include changing sexual behaviors and increased mobility of the population.

7. **India**: India has reported rising syphilis incidence, particularly among high-risk populations, including sex workers, men who have sex with men, and transgender individuals.

8. **South Korea**: South Korea has observed an increase in syphilis cases, partly driven by changes in sexual behavior and a lack of awareness.

9. **Thailand**: Thailand has also reported a growing number of syphilis cases, particularly in the context of its HIV prevention efforts, as syphilis can increase the risk of HIV transmission.

10. **Vietnam**: Vietnam has seen an increase in syphilis cases, especially in larger cities and among specific at-risk populations. Public health authorities have been working on addressing this issue through education and testing programs.

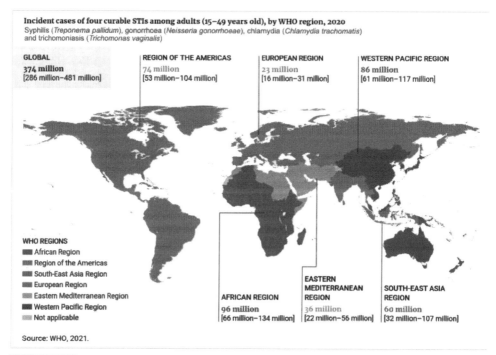

Incident cases of four curable STIs among adults (15–49 years old), by WHO region, 2020
Syphilis (*Treponema pallidum*), gonorrhoea (*Neisseria gonorrhoeae*), chlamydia (*Chlamydia trachomatis*) and trichomoniasis (*Trichomonas vaginalis*)

GLOBAL
374 million
[286 million–481 million]

REGION OF THE AMERICAS
74 million
[53 million–104 million]

EUROPEAN REGION
23 million
[16 million–31 million]

WESTERN PACIFIC REGION
86 million
[61 million–117 million]

WHO REGIONS
■ African Region
■ Region of the Americas
■ South-East Asia Region
■ European Region
■ Eastern Mediterranean Region
■ Western Pacific Region
■ Not applicable

AFRICAN REGION
96 million
[66 million–134 million]

EASTERN MEDITERRANEAN REGION
36 million
[22 million–56 million]

SOUTH-EAST ASIA REGION
60 million
[32 million–107 million]

Source: WHO, 2021.

Figure 6-1   Incident cases of four curable STIs among adults (15-49 years old), by WHO region, 2020.
(https://cdn.who.int/media/docs/default-source/ hq-hiv-hepatitis-and-stis-library/who_global_report_2021_ webinar_ doherty_20may2021.pdf?sfvrsn=3a2a5f04_7)

🔋 Identification to the syphilis:

Syphilis also known as venereal syphilis, which is an acute and chronic treponemal disease characterized clinically by a primary lesion, a secondary eruption involving skin and mucous membranes, long periods of latency, and late lesions of skin, bone, viscera, the CNS and the cardiovascular system. Different manifestations occur depending on the stage of the disease:

Primary syphilis:

Primary syphilis is typically acquired via direct sexual contact with the infectious lesions of a person with syphilis. Approximately 10-90 days after the initial exposure (average 21 days), a skin lesion appears at the point of contact, which is usually the genitalia, but can be anywhere on the body. This lesion, called a chancre, is a firm, painless skin ulceration localized at the point of initial exposure to the spirochete, often on the penis, vagina or rectum. Rarely, there may be multiple lesions present although typically only one lesion is seen. The lesion may persist for 4 to 6 weeks and usually heals spontaneously. Local lymph node swelling can occur. During the initial incubation period, individuals are otherwise asymptomatic. As a result, many patients do not seek medical care immediately. Syphilis cannot be contracted through toilet seats, daily activities, hot tubs, or sharing eating utensils or clothing.

Secondary syphilis:

Secondary syphilis occurs approximately 1-6 months (commonly 6 to 8 weeks) after the primary infection. There are many different manifestations of secondary disease. There may be a symmetrical reddish-pink non-itchy rash on the trunk and extremities. The rash can involve the palms of the hands and the soles of the feet. In moist areas of the body, the rash becomes flat broad whitish lesions known as condylomata lata. Mucous patches may also appear on the genitals or in the mouth. All of these lesions are infectious and harbor active treponeme organisms. A patient with syphilis is most contagious when he or she has secondary syphilis. Other symptoms common at this stage include fever, sore throat, malaise, weight loss, headache, meningismus, and enlarged lymph nodes. Rare manifestations include an acute meningitis that occurs in about 2% of patients, hepatitis, renal disease, hypertrophic gastritis, patchy proctitis, ulcerative colitis, rectosigmoid mass, arthritis, periostitis, optic neuritis, interstitial keratitis, iritis, and uveitis.

Latent syphilis:

Latent syphilis is defined as having serologic proof of infection without signs or symptoms of disease. Latent syphilis is further described as either early or late. Early latent syphilis is defined as having syphilis for two years or less from the time of initial infection without signs or symptoms of disease. Late latent syphilis is infection for greater than two years but without clinical evidence of disease. The distinction is important for both therapy and risk for transmission. In the real-world, the timing of infection is often not known and should be presumed to be late for the purpose of therapy. Early latent syphilis may be treated with a single intramuscular injection of a long-acting penicillin. Late latent syphilis, however, requires three weekly injections. For infectiousness, however, late latent syphilis is not considered as contagious as early latent syphilis.

Tertiary syphilis:

Tertiary syphilis usually occurs 1-10 years after the initial infection, though in some cases it can take up to 50 years. This stage is characterized by the formation of gummas which are soft, tumor-like balls of inflammation known as granulomas. The granulomas are chronic and represent an inability of the immune system to completely clear the organism. Gummas were once readily seen in the skin and mucous membranes although they tend to occur internally in recent history. They may appear almost anywhere in the body including in the skeleton. The gummas produce a chronic inflammatory state in the body with mass-effects upon the local anatomy. Other characteristics of untreated tertiary syphilis include neuropathic joint disease, which are a degeneration of joint surfaces resulting from loss of sensation and fine position sense (proprioception). The more severe manifestations include neurosyphilis and cardiovascular syphilis. In a study of untreated syphilis, 10% of patients developed cardiovascular syphilis, 16% had gumma formation, and 7% had neurosyphilis.

Neurosyphilis:

Neurosyphilis refers to a site of infection involving the central nervous system (CNS). Neurosyphilis may occur at any stage of syphilis. Before the advent of antibiotics, it was typically seen in 25-35% of patients with syphilis. Neurosyphilis is now most common in patients with HIV infection. Reports of neurosyphilis in HIV-infected persons are similar to cases reported before the HIV pandemic. The precise extent and significance of neurologic involvement in HIV-infected patients with syphilis, reflected by either laboratory or clinical criteria, have not been well characterized. Furthermore, the alteration of host immunosuppression by antiretroviral therapy in recent years has further complicated such characterization.

Fetal infection occurs in high frequency with untreated primary and secondary infections of pregnant women and in lower frequency with latency. Transplacental infection is uncommon before the 4th month of gestation. It frequently causes abortion or stillbirth or may cause infant deaths due to preterm delivery of low birth weight infants or from generalized systemic disease. Congenital infection may result in late manifestations occasionally causing such stigmata as Hutchinson's teeth, saddle nose, saber shins, interstitial keratitis and deafness.

Infectious agent:

Treponema pallidum, which is a spirochete.

🄳 Occurrence:

It is a widespread communicable disease, involving primarily young persons between 15-30 years old. Differences in racial incidence are related more to social than biologic factors; more prevalent in urban than rural areas and in males than in females; high prevalence among male homosexuals. Since 1957, early venereal syphilis has increased significantly throughout much of the world. In 2021, a total of 9,413 syphilis confirmed cases were reported in Taiwan. Among them, a total of 1,776 cases were defined as active syphilis (primary, secondary, tertiary), which the ratio of males to females was 11:1. Among active syphilis cases in 2021, the majority was cases with age group of 25 to 34 years-old (42%). The following was the age group of 35 to 44 years-old (21%) (Fig. 6-2).

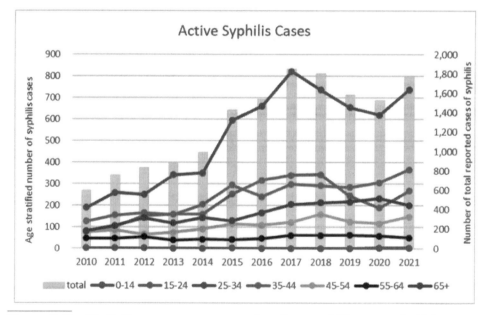

Figure 6-2   Statistics on age groups of active syphilis cases in Taiwan, 2010-2021(CDC, Taiwan, 2022)
(https://www.cdc.gov.tw/En/Category/ListContent/bg0g_VU_Ysrgkes_KRUDgQ?uaid=nLC6EcIGL1inyNYJANta9g)

Reservoir:

Man.

Mode of transmission:

By direct contact with infectious exudates from obvious or concealed moist early lesions of skin and mucous membrane, body fluids and secretions (saliva, semen, blood, vaginal discharges) of infected persons during sexual contact. Especially, the sexual behaviors associated with 3P (Promiscuity, Prostitution, and Polygamy) have a high potential for transmitting sexually transmitted diseases (STDs). Transmission can occur through blood transfusion if donor were in the early stage of disease. Fetal infection may occur through placental transfer.

Incubation period:

Incubation period is from 10 days to 10 weeks, usually 3 weeks.

Period of communicability:

It is variable and indefinite. During primary and secondary stages and also in mucocutaneous recurrences; some cases may be communicable intermittently for 2-4 years. Congenital transmission is most probable during early maternal syphilis but can occur throughout the latent period. Adequate penicillin treatment usually ends infectivity within 24-48 hours.

Susceptibility and resistance:

Susceptibility is universal, though only approximately 10% of exposures result in infection. There is no natural immunity. Infection leads to gradually developing resistance against *Treponema pallidum* and to some extent against heterologous treponemes. Immunity may fail to develop because of early treatment in the primary or secondary stage. In late latency, superinfection may cause destructive lesions of the skin, bone and mucous membranes.

❿ Methods of control:

While abstinence from any sexual activity is very effective at helping prevent syphilis, it should be noted that *T. pallidum* readily crosses intact mucosa and cut skin, including areas not covered by a condom. Proper and consistent use of a latex condom can reduce, but not eliminate, the spread of syphilis.

The effective control methods are health and sex education and preparation for marriage. Protect the community by preventing and controlling STDs of the prostitution. Cooperate with social agencies and discouragement of sexual promiscuity. Condom use in high risk sex contacts for protection. Provide health care facilities for early diagnosis and treatment of STIs.

General review

1. Venereal disease

2. 3P: Promiscuity, Prostitution, polygamy

3. *Treponema pallidum*

4. *Treponema* = Spirochete

5. Transplacental infection

6. Hutchinson's teeth

7. Saddle nose

8. Saber shins

9. Interstitial keratitis

10. Superinfection

SCAN ME

Check Your Answers

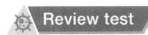

I. Multiple-choice questions (four selected one):

1. (　) What were some contributing factors to the resurgence of syphilis in the early 21st century? (A) Decreased sexual activity, (B) Increased access to healthcare, (C) Changes in sexual behavior, (D) Reduced funding for public health

2. (　) Which populations were disproportionately affected by the resurgence of syphilis in the post-2000 era? (A) The elderly population, (B) Men who have sex with men (MSM), (C) Children and adolescents, (D) High-income individuals

3. (　) How long is the typical incubation period for primary syphilis after initial exposure to the spirochete? (A) 1-3 days, (B) 4-7 days, (C) 10-90 days, (D) 6-12 months

4. (　) What is the primary skin lesion that appears in cases of primary syphilis? (A) Pustule, (B) Vesicle, (C) Chancre, (D) Rash

5. (　) When does secondary syphilis typically occur following the primary infection? (A) 1-3 weeks, (B) 2-4 months, (C) 6-12 months, (D) 1-6 months (commonly 6 to 8 weeks)

6. (　) Which of the following is a common manifestation of secondary syphilis? (A) Itchy rash on the extremities, (B) Sore throat with fever, (C) Flat whitish lesions on the palms and soles, (D) Enlarged liver

7. (　) How is latent syphilis defined in terms of signs and symptoms? (A) Having serologic proof of infection with signs and symptoms of disease, (B) Having clinical evidence of disease without serologic proof, (C) Having serologic proof of infection

without signs or symptoms of disease, (D) Having serologic proof of infection with clinical evidence of disease

8. ( ) Which of the following statements is true regarding the treatment of early latent syphilis? (A) It requires three weekly injections of long-acting penicillin, (B) It is not considered contagious, (C) It should be presumed to be late for the purpose of therapy, (D) It may be treated with a single intramuscular injection of long-acting penicillin

9. ( ) Tertiary syphilis typically occurs: (A) Within a few months after the initial infection, (B) 10-20 years after the initial infection, (C) 1-10 years after the initial infection, (D) More than 50 years after the initial infection

10. ( ) What characterizes the formation of gummas in tertiary syphilis? (A) Rapidly growing skin lesions, (B) Tumor-like balls of inflammation called granulomas, (C) Bacterial infections, (D) Elevated white blood cell counts

11. ( ) When may fetal infection occur in pregnant women with syphilis? (A) Only during the first month of pregnancy, (B) Before the 4th month of gestation, (C) Only during the last trimester, (D) In the 6th month of gestation

12. ( ) What is the most common site of infection involving the central nervous system (CNS) in neurosyphilis? (A) Spinal cord, (B) Brain, (C) Peripheral nerves, (D) Cranial nerves

13. ( ) What has complicated the characterization of neurologic involvement in HIV-infected patients with syphilis in recent years? (A) Improved diagnostic tools, (B) Decreased cases of neurosyphilis in HIV-infected individuals, (C) Host

immunosuppression by antiretroviral therapy, (D) Reduced cases of syphilis in HIV-infected patients

14. ( ) What is the most common outcome of fetal syphilis in cases of untreated primary and secondary infections in pregnant women? (A) No fetal infection occurs, (B) Congenital syphilis with no late manifestations, (C) Congenital syphilis with late manifestations, (D) Preterm delivery with no complications

15. ( ) How long can some cases of syphilis be communicable intermittently during the primary and secondary stages or mucocutaneous recurrences? (A) 2-4 months, (B) 2-4 weeks, (C) 2-4 days, (D) 2-4 years

16. ( ) What is the typical timeframe within which adequate penicillin treatment ends infectivity in syphilis? (A) 1 week, (B) 24-48 hours, (C) 2 weeks, (D) 1 month

II. Simple answer:

1. How long does the chancre, the primary syphilis skin lesion, typically persist before healing spontaneously?

2. When is a patient with syphilis most contagious?

3. What are some of the more severe manifestations of untreated tertiary syphilis?

4. What is the most common co-occurrence with neurosyphilis in patients today?

5. What stigmata can result from congenital syphilis?

6. Is there natural immunity to syphilis?

7. Why might immunity fail to develop in some cases of syphilis?

6-2 **Gonorrhoea** (ICD-9 098.0-098.3; ICD-10 A54.0-A54.2)

Highlight

1. Gonorrhoea

2. Dysuria

3. Epididymitis

4. Urethritis

5. Cervicitis

6. *Neisseria gonorrhoeae*

7. PPNG: Penicillinase-Producing *N. gonorrhoeae*

8. IUD: intrauterine contraceptive device

9. Salpingitis

Gonorrhea is amongst the most common sexually transmitted diseases in the world, caused by *Neisseria gonorrhoeae*. Non-genital sites in which it thrives are in the rectum, the throat (oropharynx), and the eyes (conjunctivae). The vulva and vagina in women are usually spared because they are lined by stratified epithelial cells—in women the cervix is the usual first site of infection. Gonorrhea spreads during sexual intercourse. Infected women also can pass gonorrhea to their newborn infants during delivery, causing eye infections (conjunctivitis) in their babies (which if left untreated, can cause blindness). Doctors have often attempted to treat this immediately by applying small amounts of silver nitrate or other antibiotic to the eyes of all newborn babies.

Gonorrhea is a significant public health concern, with millions of new cases reported each year worldwide. It primarily affects sexually active individuals, particularly those in their late teens and early twenties, particularly young homosexual males, the incidence has started to increase again after a period of decline during the late 1980s. This trend suggests poor response to prevention initiatives among adolescents.

Gonococcal infection of genitourinary tract, containing the diseases of following: gonococcal urethritis, gonococcal vulvovaginitis, gonococcal cervicitis, gonococcal bartholinitis, gonococcal epididymitis, gonococcal proctitis, gonococcal salpingitis, and pelvis inflammatory disease (PID).

🔹 Identification to the gonococcal infection:

It is a sexually transmitted bacterial disease limited to columnar and transitional epithelium which differs in males and females in course, severity and ease of recognition. In both sexes, pharyngeal and anal infections are common. Conjunctivitis occurs rarely in adults. Septicemia may occur, with arthritis, skin lesions, endocarditis, and meningitis. Death is rare except among cases with endocarditis. Arthritis can produce permanent joint damage if appropriate antibiotic treatment is delayed. Gonorrhea can manifest in various ways. While some individuals may be asymptomatic, others may experience:

1. Painful urination

2. Abnormal discharge from the genitals (thick, greenish, or yellowish in color)

3. Pain or discomfort in the lower abdomen

4. Pelvic inflammatory disease (PID) in women

5. Testicular pain in men

6. Rectal and throat infections in those who engage in anal and oral sex.

In males, a purulent discharge from the anterior urethra with dysuria appears 2-7 days after an infecting exposure. The infection may be self-limited, or may extend to the posterior urethra to produce epididymitis and may result in a chronic carrier state. Rectal infection, common among homosexual males, is at times asymptomatic but may cause pruritis, tenesmus and discharge.

In females, a few days after exposure an initial urethritis or cervicitis occurs, frequently so mild as to pass unnoticed. In about 20% there is uterine invasion at the 1st, 2nd, or later menstrual period, with symptoms of endometritis, salpingitis or pelvic peritonitis with subsequent risk of infertility. Chronic endocervical infection is common. Prepubescent girls may develop gonococcal vulvovaginitis subsequent to direct genital contact with exudate from infected adults.

Infectious agent:

Neisseria gonorrhoeae, the gonococcus. The presence in some strains of plasmids coding for β-lactamases render these resistant to penicillin (penicillinase-producing *Neisseria gonorrhoeae*, or PPNG strains). Chromosomally medicated (β-lactamase-negative) penicillin-resistant strains are seen with increasing frequency.

Occurrence:

Common worldwide, affects both sexes and practically all ages, especially younger adult groups among whom sexual activity is greatest. It is common in the USA and Asia among male homosexuals with multiple partners. Both PPNG and chromosomally medicated gonococcal resistance to penicillin are apparently increasing worldwide. In 2021, a total of 7,381 cases of gonorrhea were reported in Taiwan. The ratio of males to females was 9:1. The majority was cases with age group of 25 to 34 years-old (39%). The following was the age group of 15 to 24 years-old (34%). (Fig. 6-3)

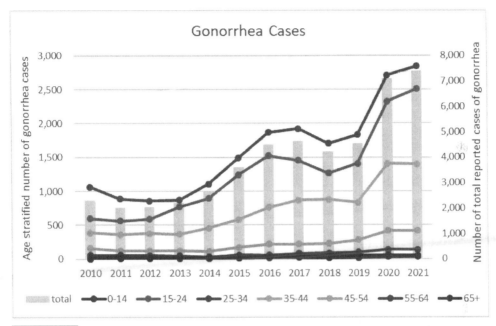

Figure 6-3   Statistics on age groups of gonorrhea cases in Taiwan, 2010-
2021(CDC, Taiwan, 2022)
(https://www.cdc.gov.tw/En/Category/ListContent/bg0g_VU_
Ysrgkes_KRUDgQ?uaid=3A5TlbGWeuaCtv5LyNFnvA)

Reservoir:

It is strictly a human disease.

Mode of transmission:

The infection is primarily spread through unprotected sexual contact, including vaginal, anal, and oral sex, with an infected person. It can also be transmitted from an infected mother to her baby during childbirth. Contact with exudates from mucous membranes of infected persons, almost always as a result of sexual activity. Even in children older than 1 year, it is considered an indicator of sexual abuse.

🔹 Incubation period:

Incubation period is usually 2-7 days, sometimes longer when symptoms occur.

🔹 Period of communicability:

The communicability may extend for months if untreated, especially in asymptomatic individuals. Effective therapy usually ends communicability within hours.

🔹 Susceptibility and resistance:

Susceptibility is general. Gonococcal strains are antigenically heterogeneous and re-infection is common. Women using an intrauterine contraceptive device have higher risks of salpingitis.

🔹 Methods of control:

The mainstay of treatment is the appropriate use of antibiotics. While penicillin was the most common antibiotic used to treat gonorrhea up until the 1970s, an increase in antibiotic resistance has led to a decline in its use. In recent years, as of 2021, the standard clinical treatment for gonorrhea has typically involved a dual-antibiotic approach to maximize effectiveness and minimize the risk of antibiotic resistance. This treatment regimen commonly consists of the following two antibiotics: Ceftriaxone: Typically administered as a single intramuscular injection. Azithromycin: An oral dose of azithromycin is often prescribed in conjunction with ceftriaxone. For neonates, use of an established effective preparation for protection of babies' eyes at birth; instillation of 1% silver nitrate solution stored in individual wax capsules remains the prophylactic agent most widely used. Erythromycin and tetracycline ophthalmic ointments are also effective; they may be effective in preventing neonatal chlamydial conjunctivitis. Routine cervical and rectal culturing for gonococci during prenatal period, especially in third trimester, should be considered in high-risk population.

Public health agencies often provide partner notification and treatment services to help individuals diagnosed with gonorrhea inform their sexual partners and ensure they receive testing and treatment. While there is currently no widely available vaccine for gonorrhea, research is ongoing to develop a vaccine to prevent the infection. Remember that gonorrhea is a reportable disease in many countries, including Taiwan, which means that healthcare providers are required to report diagnosed cases to public health authorities. This reporting is vital for disease tracking and control efforts.

General review

1. PID: Pelvis inflammatory disease

2. Younger age groups

3. Gonococcal infection in males: dysuria, epididymitis, rectal infection

4. Gonococcal infection in females: urethritis, cervicitis, endometritis, salpingitis, pelvic peritonitis

5. Reinfection is common

6. Women using IUD have higher risks of salpingitis

Review test

SCAN ME

Check Your Answers

I. **Multiple-choice questions (Four selected one):**

1. ( ) What is the primary cause of gonorrhea? (A) Chlamydia trachomatis, (B) Neisseria gonorrhoeae, (C) Treponema pallidum, (D) Human papillomavirus (HPV)

2. (　) Which of the following is NOT a non-genital site where *Neisseria gonorrhoeae* can thrive? (A) Rectum, (B) Throat (Oropharynx), (C) Eyes (Conjunctivae), (D) Vulva

3. (　) What is a common symptom in males with gonorrhea infection? (A) Abdominal pain, (B) Testicular pain, (C) Pelvic inflammatory disease (PID), (D) Rectal infection

4. (　) In females, what percentage may experience uterine invasion with subsequent risk of infertility after gonorrhea exposure? (A) 5%, (B) 10%, (C) 20%, (D) 30%

5. (　) Which of the following is NOT a common symptom associated with gonorrhea? (A) Painful urination, (B) Abnormal discharge from the genitals, (C) Joint pain, (D) Rectal infection

6. (　) What renders some strains of Neisseria gonorrhoeae resistant to penicillin? (A) Plasmids coding for viruses, (B) Plasmids coding for quinolones, (C) Plasmids coding for β-lactamases, (D) Plasmids coding for antibiotics

7. (　) Where is gonorrhea common among male homosexuals with multiple partners? (A) Europe and Africa, (B) North America and Asia, (C) South America and Australia, (D) The Middle East and Antarctica

8. (　) What is the primary reason for using a dual-antibiotic approach in the treatment of gonorrhea? (A) To reduce the overall cost of treatment, (B) To minimize the risk of antibiotic resistance, (C) To improve patient compliance with treatment, (D) To speed up the recovery process

9. (   ) Which two antibiotics are commonly used in the standard clinical treatment for gonorrhea as of 2021? (A) Penicillin and doxycycline, (B) Ciprofloxacin and metronidazole, (C) Ceftriaxone and azithromycin, (D) Erythromycin and tetracycline

10. (   ) What is the purpose of routine cervical and rectal culturing for gonococci during the prenatal period, especially in the third trimester? (A) To identify the sex of the baby, (B) To assess the risk of neonatal conjunctivitis, (C) To confirm the mother's immune response to gonorrhea, (D) To monitor the development of the fetus

II. Simple answer:

1. What is the potential consequence of newborn infants being infected with gonorrhea during delivery if left untreated?

2. What condition in males may result if appropriate antibiotic treatment for gonorrhea is delayed?

3. How can prepubescent girls develop gonococcal vulvovaginitis?

4. What is the term for penicillin-resistant strains of Neisseria gonorrhoeae that are chromosomally mediated and do not produce β-lactamase?

5. What is the prophylactic agent most widely used to protect neonates' eyes at birth against gonococcal eye infection?

6. Why is reporting cases of gonorrhea to public health authorities vital?

6-3 AIDS (ICD-9 042-044, 279.5; ICD-10 B20-B24)

Highlight

1. AIDS: Acquired immune deficiency syndrome
2. HIV: Human immunodeficiency virus
3. Opportunistic infection
4. Vertical transmission

AIDS, which stands for Acquired Immunodeficiency Syndrome, is a complex and advanced stage of HIV (Human Immunodeficiency Virus) infection. It is characterized by severe damage to the immune system, leaving the affected individual highly vulnerable to opportunistic infections and certain malignancies.

The earliest recognized cases of AIDS in the United States were reported in the early 1980s. Initially, it was primarily observed among gay men in several major cities. Physicians started noticing a cluster of unusual diseases and opportunistic infections in previously healthy individuals, including Pneumocystis pneumonia (PCP) and Kaposi's sarcoma. This led to the initial recognition of AIDS as a distinct syndrome. In 1983 and 1984, two teams of scientists, one led by Robert Gallo in the United States, and another led by Luc Montagnier in France, independently discovered the human immunodeficiency virus (HIV). HIV was identified as the cause of AIDS. The development of blood tests to detect HIV antibodies became crucial in screening blood donations and diagnosing HIV infection in late 1980s to early 1990s. The mid-1990s marked a significant breakthrough with the introduction of highly active antiretroviral therapy (ART). ART revolutionized the treatment of HIV/AIDS, significantly prolonging the lives of those infected.

Since 2000s and beyond, international organizations, governments, and NGOs started taking more significant steps to address the global AIDS pandemic. The Joint United Nations Programme on HIV/AIDS (UNAIDS) was established to coordinate global efforts. Goals include:

1. **Access to Treatment**: Efforts were made to improve access to ART in resource-limited settings, particularly in sub-Saharan Africa, where the epidemic had hit hardest.

2. **Prevention Strategies**: The development of prevention strategies, including the promotion of safe sex, needle exchange programs for intravenous drug users, and pre-exposure prophylaxis (PrEP), became critical in controlling the spread of HIV.

3. **Advocacy and Awareness**: Activism and advocacy by groups like ACT UP and celebrities such as Elizabeth Taylor and Bono brought increased attention to the AIDS pandemic and the need for research, funding, and support.

4. **Reduction in New Infections**: There has been significant progress in reducing new HIV infections and improving the quality of life for people living with HIV/AIDS. However, the pandemic continues to pose significant public health challenges.

Identification to the AIDS:

AIDS is the result of long-term, untreated HIV infection. HIV is a virus that attacks the body's immune system, specifically targeting CD4+ T cells, which play a crucial role in the immune response against infections. HIV infection progresses through various stages, with AIDS being the most advanced stage. The progression to AIDS is marked by a significant decline in the number of CD4+ T cells and the appearance of opportunistic infections or certain cancers. Individuals with AIDS are susceptible to opportunistic infections, which are infections that typically do not cause severe illness in people with healthy immune systems. These infections can range from fungal, bacterial, viral, and parasitic diseases and can be life-threatening in people with AIDS.

Symptoms of AIDS can vary widely and may include persistent fever, weight loss, chronic diarrhea, night sweats, and various infections. These symptoms can be severe and lead to a dramatic decline in overall health. A diagnosis of AIDS is typically made when the CD4+ T cell count drops below a certain threshold (200 cells/mm³ or lower) and/or when specific opportunistic infections or malignancies are present.

Infectious agent:

Human immunodeficiency virus (HIV). HIV-1 is an enveloped RNA virus belonging to the lentivirus subfamily of Retroviridae. HIV-2 is a closely related strain that has been identified from patients in West Africa. There is considerable homology between HIV-2 and simian immunodeficiency virus (SIV).

Occurrence:

Worldwide, AIDS remains a global health concern. It has had a profound impact on millions of lives, with more than 36 million people having died from AIDS-related illnesses since the beginning of the pandemic. While significant progress has been made in the prevention and treatment of HIV/AIDS, ongoing efforts are needed to control the spread of the virus, increase access to treatment, and reduce stigma and discrimination associated with the disease. Taiwan's epidemic of HIV/AIDS began with the first case reported in December 1984. In 1990, the government promulgated the AIDS Prevention and Control Act. As of May 2006, there are 11,000 reported cases. HIV/AIDS patients in Taiwan can receive free medical care, with the state covering the cost. Non-governmental organizations have set up "AIDS Half-Way Houses" for homeless patients.

Taiwan's latest epidemiological report that since the first HIV case in Taiwan was reported in 1984. As of the end of 2022, the total number of HIV cases had been accumulated to 44,861 (21,294 of whom had developed full-blown AIDS and 8,263 cases had deceased). The number of HIV infections among the injecting drug users (IDUs) began to surge since 2003 and then consistently decreased since Taiwan CDC harm reduction programs. In 2008 and thereafter, the epidemic took a turn; infections mainly occurred through sexual encounter. Of Taiwanese nationals infected by HIV in 2022, 1207, or 96%, were males and 42, or 4%, were females. The ratio of infected males to females was 25:1. The largest number of infections in 2022 was in the 25 to 39 age group, accounting for 582, or 54%, of all cases. The second largest group was the 40 to 64 age group, numbering 263, or 25%, of all cases. An analysis of risk factors showed that in 2022, the highest proportion of HIV infections was a result of unsafe sexual transmission, with men who have sex with men (MSM) accounting for 80% of all cases. The second largest proportion of infections was heterosexual contact, accounting for 11%. (Fig. 6-4).

▶ Reservoir:

Man. HIV is thought to have recently evolved from chimpanzee viruses.

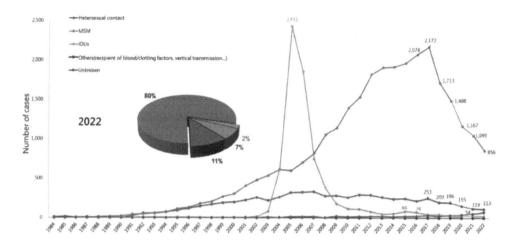

Figure 6-4   Statistics on Risk Factors of HIV Infections in Taiwan, 1984-
2022 (CDC, Taiwan, 2023).
(https://www.cdc.gov.tw/En/Category/ListContent/bg0g_VU_
Ysrgkes_KRUDgQ?uaid=CqNo313w78G1fWhz429xDA)

🔹 Mode of transmission:

HIV is spread by sexual, blood-borne, needle common use and vertical transmission, and is capable of affecting whole communities, profoundly disrupting social structure and commercial activity. Specifically, HIV is transmitted through direct contact of a mucous membrane or the bloodstream with a bodily fluid containing HIV, such as blood, semen, vaginal fluid, preseminal fluid, and breast milk. This transmission can come in the form of anal, vaginal or oral sex, blood transfusion, contaminated hypodermic needles, exchange between mother and baby during pregnancy, childbirth, or breastfeeding, or other exposure to one of the above bodily fluids.

🔖 Incubation period:

Incubation period is indefinite. Seroconversion usually occurs 6-12 weeks after infection, but incubation can range from 4-12 weeks. Untreated, the latent phase of HIV infection lasts from 18 months to 15 years or more, with an average of about 8 years.

🔖 Period of communicability:

Not known precisely; begins early after onset of HIV infection and presumably extends throughout life. It may strong communicability includes asymptomatic (infected person) and symptomatic (AIDS patient).

🔖 Susceptibility and resistance:

Susceptibility is general. After infected HIV, that immune response of protection is still unknown!

🔖 Methods of control:

Strategies for the prevention of HIV infection (WHO, 2023):

1. Safe sex: using a male or female condom during sex.

2. Being tested for HIV and sexually transmitted infections.

3. Having a voluntary medical male circumcision.

4. Using harm reduction services for people who inject and use drugs.

5. Screening of blood products.

6. Antenatal screening.

7. Voluntary testing of those in high-risk categories.

8. Vigorous control and treatment of genital ulcer diseases.

There is no cure for HIV infection. It is treated with antiretroviral drugs, which stop the virus from replicating in the body. Current antiretroviral therapy (ART) does not cure HIV infection but allows a person's immune system to get stronger. This helps them to fight other infections. Pregnant women with HIV should have access to and take ART as soon as possible. This protects the health of the mother and will help prevent HIV from passing to the fetus before birth, or to the baby through breast milk.

General review

1. Human immunodeficiency viruses: HIV-1, HIV-2: cause lifelong infection

2. HIV-1 is distributed worldwide and produces more severe and rapidly progressive

3. HIV is spread by sexual, blood-borne, needle common use and vertical transmission

4. Condom use

5. Having a voluntary medical male circumcision

6. Screen of blood products

7. Antenatal screening

8. Voluntary testing of those high-risk categories

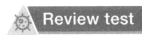
Review test

I. Multiple-choice questions (Four selected one):

1. ( ) When was HIV identified as the cause of AIDS? (A) 1970, (B) 1983, (C) 1995, (D) 2005

2. ( ) What was a significant breakthrough in the treatment of HIV/AIDS in the mid-1990s? (A) The discovery of HIV, (B) The establishment of UNAIDS, (C) The introduction of ART, (D) The promotion of safe sex

3. ( ) Which region was particularly affected by the HIV/AIDS epidemic, leading to efforts to improve access to treatment in resource-limited settings? (A) North America, (B) Europe, (C) Sub-Saharan Africa, (D) Asia

4. ( ) What is the primary target of the HIV virus within the human body? (A) Red blood cells, (B) White blood cells, (C) Platelets, (D) CD4+ T cells

5. ( ) How is a diagnosis of AIDS typically made? (A) When a person has a persistent fever, (B) When they experience weight gain, (C) When the CD4+ T cell count is above 500 cells/mm³, (D) When the CD4+ T cell count drops below a certain threshold and/or specific opportunistic infections or malignancies are present

6. ( ) Which subfamily of Retroviridae does HIV-1 belong to? (A) Orthoretrovirinae, (B) Alpharetrovirinae, (C) Lentivirus, (D) Gammaretrovirinae

7. ( ) HIV-2 is closely related to HIV-1 and has been identified primarily in which geographic region? (A) North America, (B) Europe, (C) Southeast Asia, (D) West Africa

8. ( ) What year did Taiwan's government promulgate the AIDS Prevention and Control Act? (A) 1984, (B) 1990, (C) 2003, (D) 2008

9. ( ) In 2022, what was the primary mode of HIV transmission among Taiwanese people? (A) Injecting drug use, (B) Mother-to-child transmission, (C) Unsafe sexual transmission, (D) Blood transfusion

10. ( ) Which age group had the largest number of HIV infections in Taiwan in 2022? (A) 18 to 24, (B) 25 to 39, (C) 40 to 64, (D) 65 and older

11. ( ) Which of the following is NOT mentioned as a mode of HIV transmission? (A) Anal sex, (B) Blood transfusion, (C) Saliva exchange, (D) Vertical transmission

12. ( ) During which phase of HIV infection is the incubation period indefinite, with an average duration of about 8 years if left untreated? (A) Acute phase, (B) Latent phase, (C) Chronic phase, (D) Terminal phase

13. ( ) Which of the following strategies is recommended by WHO for the prevention of HIV infection? (A) Vigorous control and treatment of common cold, (B) Avoiding male and female condoms during sex, (C) Using harm reduction services for people who inject drugs, (D) Not being tested for HIV and sexually transmitted infections

14. (   ) What is the primary purpose of antiretroviral drugs in the treatment of HIV infection, as mentioned in the article? (A) They cure HIV infection completely, (B) They suppress the immune system, (C) They strengthen the immune system and allow it to fight other infections, (D) They prevent the transmission of HIV through breast milk

II. Simple answer:

1. What are two diseases that were initially observed among previously healthy individuals, leading to the recognition of AIDS as a distinct syndrome?

2. What international organization was established to coordinate global efforts to address the AIDS pandemic?

3. What are the obvious symptoms of AIDS?

4. What proportion of HIV infections in 2022 was attributed to men who have sex with men (MSM)?

5. How is HIV primarily transmitted through sexual contact?

6. What is the range of the incubation period for HIV infection?

7. What is the role of antiretroviral therapy (ART) in the treatment of HIV infection in pregnant women?

6-4　Herpes Simplex (ICD-9 054; ICD-10 A60)

Highlight

1. HSV-2
2. Genital herpes
3. Immuno-suppressed
4. Immuno-incompetent
5. Myalgia
6. Dysuria
7. Herpetic proctitis

Herpes simplex is a viral disease caused by Herpes simplex viruses. Infection of the genitals is commonly known as herpes and predominantly occurs following sexual transmission of the type 2 strain of the virus (HSV-2). Oral herpes, colloquially called cold sores, is usually caused by the type 1 strain of herpes simplex virus (HSV-1). Both viruses cause periods of active disease—presenting as blisters containing infectious virus particles—that lasts 2-21 days and is followed by remission when the sores disappear. Most cases of genital herpes are asymptomatic, although viral shedding may still occur. HSV-1 and HSV-2 are most easily transmitted by direct contact with a sore or body fluid of an infected individual; however transmission may also occur through skin-to-skin contact when no symptoms are present.

Several distinct disorders are caused by HSV infection of the skin or mucosa including those that affect the face and mouth (orofacial herpes), genitalia (genital herpes), or hands (herpes whitlow). More serious problems arise when the virus infects and damages the eye (herpes keratitis) or invades the central nervous system to damage the brain (herpes encephalitis). Newborn infants, with their immature immune systems, are also prone to serious complications due to HSV infection (neonatal herpes), as are transplant recipients who are immuno-suppressed, and AIDs patients who are immuno-incompetent.

▶ Identification to the herpes simplex virus type 2:

Clusters of inflamed papules and vesicles on the outer surface of the genitals represent the typical symptoms of a primary HSV-1 or HSV-2 genital infection. These usually appear 4–7 days after sexual exposure to HSV for the first time and may resemble cold sores. The virus is not removed from the body by immune system but enters nerve ganglia that serve the infected dermatome where it becomes dormant. After the initial outbreak, the virus remains in the body and can become latent (inactive). However, it can re-emerge periodically, causing recurrent outbreaks. The frequency and severity of recurrent outbreaks vary from person to person.

Genital herpes, usually caused by HSV-2, occurs mainly in adults and is sexually transmitted. Primary and recurrent infections occur, with or without symptoms. In males, the lesions occur on the shaft of the penis or other parts of the genital region, on the inner thigh, buttocks, or anus. In females, lesions appear on or near the pubis, labia, clitoris, vulva, buttocks or anus. Other common symptoms include pain, itching, and burning. Less frequent, yet still common, symptoms include discharge from the penis or vagina, fever, headache, muscle pain (myalgia), swollen and enlarged lymph nodes and malaise. Women often experience additional symptoms that include painful urination (dysuria) and cervicitis, while herpetic proctitis (inflammation of the anus and rectum) is common for individuals participating in anal intercourse. After 2–3 weeks, existing lesions progress into ulcers and then crust and heal, although lesions on mucosal surfaces may never form crusts.

Infectious agent:

Herpes simplex virus is in the virus family Herpesviridae, subfamily α herpesviridae. HSV types 1 and 2 can be differentiated immunologically and differ with respect to their growth patterns in cell culture.

Occurrence:

Worldwide, although many people infected with HSV develop labial or genital lesions, many more are either undiagnosed or display no physical symptoms. Individuals with no symptoms are described as asymptomatic or with subclinical herpes. Since asymptomatic individuals are often are unaware of their infection, they are considered at high risk for spreading HSV. Many studies have been performed around the world to estimate the numbers of individuals infected with HSV-1 and HSV-2 by determining if they have developed antibodies against either viral species. This information provides population prevalence of HSV viral infections in individuals with or without active disease.

HSV-2 seroprevalence in developing Asian countries is comparable (10-30%) to that observed in North America and Northern Europe. However, estimates of HSV-2 infectivity, in Thailand, is higher than observed in other Eastern Asian countries. The total HSV-2 seroprevalence is approximately 37% in Thailand. HSV-2 seroprevalence is low in women in the Philippines (9%), although commencing activity while young is associated with an increased risk of acquiring HSV-2 infection; woman starting sexual activity by the time they reach 17 are seven times more likely to be HSV-2 seropositive that those starting sexual activity when over 21. In South Korea, incidence of HSV-2 infection in those under the age of 20 is low at only 2.7% in men and 3.0% in women. Seroprevalence levels increase in older South Koreans, however, such that the population over 20 that has antibodies against HSV-2 is 21.7% of men and 28% of women, with increasing HSV-2 prevalence becoming significant once individuals reached their 30's.

HSV-2 infection usually begins with sexual activity and is rare before adolescence, except in sexually abused children. The prevalence is greater (up to 60%) in lower socioeconomic groups and persons with multiple sexual partners. After the initial outbreak, the HSV-2 virus does not leave the body but remains latent (inactive) in nerve cells near the base of the spine. It can periodically reactivate, causing recurrent outbreaks.

Reservoir:

Man.

Mode of transmission:

Transmission of HSV-2 is usually by sexual contact. HSV types 1 and 2 may be transmitted to various sites by oral-genital, oral-anal or anal-genital contact. Transmission to the neonate usually occurs via the infected birth canal, less commonly in utero or postpartum. Even when there are no visible symptoms, HSV-2 can still be actively shedding the virus and potentially transmitting it to a partner. This phenomenon is known as asymptomatic shedding.

Incubation period:

Incubation period is from 2-12 days.

Period of communicability:

HSV can be isolated for 2 weeks and up to 7 weeks after primary stomatitis or primary genital lesions. Both primary and recurrent infections may be asymptomatic.

🔲 Susceptibility and resistance:

The strength of an individual's immune system plays a crucial role in susceptibility and resistance. A strong immune system can help suppress the virus and reduce the frequency and severity of outbreaks. High levels of stress and certain health conditions can trigger HSV-2 outbreaks in susceptible individuals. People with compromised immune systems, such as those with HIV or undergoing immunosuppressive therapy, may be more susceptible to HSV-2 and experience more severe outbreaks.

🔲 Methods of control:

For genital herpes, condoms are a highly effective in limiting transmission of herpes simplex infection. However, condoms are by no means completely effective. The virus cannot get through latex, but their effectiveness is somewhat limited on a public health scale by the limited use of condoms in the community, and on an individual scale because the condom may not completely cover blisters on the penis of an infected male, or base of the penis or testicles not covered by the condom may come into contact with free virus in vaginal fluid of an infected female. There is no cure for herpes simplex, but antiviral medications such as acyclovir, valacyclovir, and famciclovir can help manage and reduce the severity of symptoms during outbreaks. These medications may also reduce the frequency of recurrent outbreaks.

🔖 General review

1. Genital herpes, usually caused by HSV-2, occurs mainly in adults and is sexually transmitted

2. HSV-2 transmission mode: by oral-genital, oral-anal or anal-genital contact

3. Discharge, myalgia, dysuria, herpetic proctitis

4. The prevalence is greater (up to 60%) in lower socioeconomic groups and persons with multiple sexual partners.

5. Asymptomatic shedding

6. HSV-2 cannot get through latex (condom)

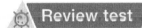 Review test

SCAN ME

Check Your Answers

I. Multiple-choice questions (Four selected one):

1. ( ) What is the most common cause of oral herpes, commonly known as cold sores? (A) Herpes simplex virus type 1 (HSV-1), (B) Herpes simplex virus type 2 (HSV-2), (C) Influenza virus, D, Human papillomavirus

2. ( ) How is herpes simplex virus (HSV) primarily transmitted from one individual to another? (A) Airborne droplets, (B) Sharing food or drinks, (C) Direct contact with a sore or body fluid of an infected individual, (D) Mosquito bites

3. ( ) What is the medical term for herpes infection of the eye? (A) Ocular herpes, (B) Visionary herpes, (C) Herpes keratitis, (D) Optic herpes

4. ( ) What is the typical appearance of primary HSV-1 or HSV-2 genital infections, which usually occur 4-7 days after sexual exposure for the first time? (A) Clusters of inflamed papules and vesicles, (B) Smooth, painless sores, (C) Red, itchy rashes, (D) Warts on the genital region

5. (   ) Where does the herpes virus go after the initial outbreak, following primary infection? (A) It is eliminated from the body by the immune system, (B) It remains active on the surface of the skin, (C) It enters nerve ganglia and becomes dormant, (D) It migrates to the bloodstream and infects other organs

6. (   ) Which gender typically experiences herpetic proctitis, inflammation of the anus and rectum, as a common symptom of genital herpes? (A) Males, (B) Females, (C) Both males and females equally, (D) Children

7. (   ) When does HSV-2 infection usually begin, and who is more likely to be affected by it? (A) It usually begins in childhood, affecting most individuals, (B) It is rare before adolescence, except in sexually abused children, (C) It is common in individuals with high socioeconomic status, (D) It primarily affects people with only one sexual partner

8. (   ) Which of the following can trigger HSV-2 outbreaks in susceptible individuals? (A) Regular exercise, (B) High levels of stress, (C) A well-balanced diet, (D) Proper hydration

9. (   ) How effective are condoms in limiting the transmission of herpes simplex infection? (A) Condoms are completely effective in preventing transmission, (B) Condoms are highly effective and never fail, (C) Condoms are somewhat effective but not completely so, (D) Condoms have no effect on herpes transmission

10. (   ) What is the primary purpose of antiviral medications like acyclovir, valacyclovir, and famciclovir in the context of genital herpes? (A) They can cure herpes simplex infections,

(B) They help manage and reduce the severity of symptoms during outbreaks, (C) They are only effective in preventing the initial infection, (D) They eliminate the virus from the body

II. Simple answer:

1. What is the typical duration of active disease during a herpes outbreak, characterized by blisters containing infectious virus particles?

2. Who is particularly prone to serious complications due to HSV infection, including neonatal herpes and herpes encephalitis?

3. What are some common symptoms of genital herpes, besides the visible lesions, that can be experienced by both males and females?

4. How do genital herpes lesions typically progress and heal after 2–3 weeks?

5. Who may be more susceptible to HSV-2 and experience more severe outbreaks due to compromised immune systems?

6. Why is the effectiveness of condoms in limiting herpes transmission somewhat limited on an individual scale?

7. Is there a cure for herpes simplex, and if not, what can antiviral medications like acyclovir, valacyclovir, and famciclovir do?

6-5 Genital Warts (ICD-9 078.19; ICD-10 A63.0)

 Highlight

1. Genital warts (or condyloma, condylomata acuminata, venereal warts, the pat carr jawn)
2. Highly contagious sexually transmitted infection
3. HPV: human papillomavirus
4. Strain types 6 and 11 are responsible for 90% of genital warts cases
5. HPV also causes many cases of cervical cancer; types 16 and 18 account for 70% of cases
6. HPV vaccine

Genital warts (or condyloma, condylomata acuminata, or venereal warts or the pat carr jawn) is a highly contagious sexually transmitted infection caused by some sub-types of human papillomavirus (HPV).

Genital warts are the most easily recognized sign of genital HPV infection. They can be caused by strains 6, 11, 30, 42, 43, 44, 45, 51, 52 and 54 of genital HPV; types 6 and 11 are responsible for 90% of genital warts cases. Most people who acquire those strains never develop warts or any other symptoms. HPV also causes many cases of cervical cancer; types 16 and 18 account for 70% of cases; however, the strains of HPV that cause genital warts are not linked to the strains that cause cancer.

Identification to the genital warts:

Genital warts often occur in clusters and can be very tiny or can spread into large masses in the genital or penis area. In women they occur on the outside and inside of the vagina, on the opening (cervix) to the womb (uterus), or around the anus. They are approximately as prevalent in men, but the symptoms may be less obvious. When present, they usually are seen on the tip of the penis. They also may be found on the shaft of the penis, on the scrotum, or around the anus. Rarely, genital warts also can develop in the mouth or throat of a person who has had oral sex with an infected person.

The viral particles are able to penetrate the skin and mucosal surfaces through microscopic abrasions in the genital area, which occur during sexual activity. Once cells are invaded by HPV, a latency period of months to years may occur. Having sex with a partner whose HPV infection is in the incubation period still leaves you vulnerable to becoming infected yourself. In other words, just because one can't see the genital warts, doesn't mean they are not there. HPV virus can last from 3 months to 2 years without a symptom. That causes the increase of HPV infectors and sometimes you cannot track down who was the source of the infection. The symptoms of genital warts can appear as small, flesh-colored, or gray growths in and around the genital and anal regions. These warts can vary in size and shape, and they might be flat or raised. Genital warts may occur singly or in clusters. In some cases, they can cause itching, discomfort, or bleeding.

🔟 Infectious agent:

Human papillomavirus (HPV) of the papovavirus group of DNA viruses (the human wart viruses). At least 70 HPV types have been associated with specific manifestations and more than 20 types of HPV can infect the genital tract. Genital warts are the most easily recognized sign of genital HPV infection. They can be caused by strains 6, 11, 30, 42, 43, 44, 45, 51, 52 and 54 of genital HPV; types 6 and 11 are responsible for 90% of genital warts cases.

Occurrence:

Worldwide.

Reservoir:

Man.

Mode of transmission:

By the way of direct contact, it is usually sexually transmitted. Genital warts are highly contagious and are primarily transmitted through sexual contact, including vaginal, anal, and oral sex. The virus can be passed from one person to another even when there are no visible warts. It's also possible for an infected mother to transmit the virus to her newborn during childbirth.

Incubation period:

Incubation period is probably 2-3 months; range is 1-20 months.

Period of communicability:

Unknown, probably at least as long as visible lesions persist.

Susceptibility and resistance:

Susceptibility is general. Genital warts are most frequently seen in sexually active young adults. The incidence of warts is increased in immunosuppressed patients. Antibodies that develop following an initial infection with that type of HPV prevents reinfection with the same warts type.

🔹 Methods of control:

Genital warts may disappear without treatment, but sometimes eventually develop a fleshy, small, raised growth. There is no way to predict whether they will grow or disappear.

The Centers for Disease Control and Prevention said that "While the effect of condoms in preventing HPV infection is unknown, condom use has been associated with a lower rate of cervical cancer, an HPV-associated disease." Other studies have suggested that regular condom use can effectively limit the ongoing persistence and spread of HPV to additional genital sites in individuals who are already infected. Thus, condom use may reduce the risk that infected individuals will progress to cervical cancer or develop additional genital warts. It is also imperative to continue using condoms. Condoms, particularly when used with spermicidal foams, creams, and jellies, may reduce the risk of transmitting HPV and other STIs for those who are sexually active.

The best way to prevent genital warts is through HPV vaccination, which can protect against the most common HPV types that cause genital warts and certain cancers. The HPV vaccines, such as Gardasil and Cervarix, are available to protect against several HPV types that cause 70% of cervical cancer cases, and two strains of HPV that cause 90% of genital warts. Treatment options include topical creams, cryotherapy (freezing the warts), laser therapy, and surgical removal. The choice of treatment depends on the size, location, and number of warts.

🔹 General review

1. HPV types 6 and 11 are responsible for 90% of genital warts cases

2. HPV types 16 and 18 are responsible for 70% of cervical cancer cases

3. Genital warts are most frequently seen in sexually active young adults

4. HPV vaccine; Gardasil and Cervarix could protect against cause 70% of cervical cancer cases and cause 90% of genital warts.

SCAN ME

Check Your Answers

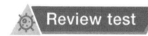

Review test

I. Multiple-choice questions (Four selected one):

1. (   ) What is the primary cause of genital warts? (A) Human papillomavirus (HPV) types 16 and 18, (B) HPV strains 6 and 11, (C) HPV strains 30, 42, 43, 44, 45, 51, 52, and 54, (D) Unprotected sexual intercourse

2. (   ) Which strains of HPV are responsible for the majority of genital warts cases? (A) HPV types 16 and 18, (B) HPV strains 30 and 51, (C) HPV strains 6 and 11, (D) HPV strains 42 and 54

3. (   ) Where can genital warts commonly occur in women? (A) Only on the tip of the penis, (B) Inside the mouth or throat, (C) Inside and outside of the vagina, on the cervix, and around the anus, (D) On the scrotum and shaft of the penis

4. (   ) How can the HPV virus be transmitted during sexual activity? (A) Through airborne transmission, (B) Direct skin-to-skin contact with no abrasions, (C) Microscopic abrasions in the genital area, (D) By sharing food or drinks with an infected person

5. (   ) What is the latency period for HPV infection once the virus invades cells? (A) Days to weeks, (B) Months to years, (C) No latency period, (D) Hours to days

6. (   ) What is the primary mode of transmission for genital warts caused by HPV? (A) Airborne transmission, (B) Sharing contaminated objects, (C) Sexual contact, including vaginal, anal, and oral sex, (D) Casual handshakes

7. (   ) Which HPV types are responsible for 90% of genital warts cases? (A) HPV types 30 and 44, (B) HPV strains 42 and 51, (C) HPV strains 6 and 11, (D) HPV types 52 and 54

8. (   ) What is the CDC's stance on condom use and its relation to HPV infection and associated diseases? (A) Condoms are known to completely prevent HPV infection, (B) Condom use has no impact on reducing HPV-related diseases, (C) Condom use is associated with a lower rate of cervical cancer and may limit the spread of HPV, (D) Condoms are ineffective against HPV but protect against other sexually transmitted infections

9. (   ) What is the most effective way to prevent genital warts, so far? (A) Using topical creams, (B) Cryotherapy (freezing the warts), (C) HPV vaccination, (D) Surgical removal

10. (   ) Which HPV vaccines protect against the most common HPV types responsible for genital warts and cervical cancer? (A) Gardasil and Cervarix, (B) Topical creams and laser therapy, (C) Cryotherapy and surgical removal, (D) Condoms and spermicidal foams

II. Simple answer:

1. What are some common symptoms of genital warts?

2. How long can the HPV virus persist without symptoms?

3. How can HPV be transmitted from an infected mother to her newborn during childbirth?

4. How can regular condom use help reduce the risk of HPV transmission and other sexually transmitted infections (STIs)?

6-6　Chlamydial Infections (ICD-9 099.8; ICD-10 A56)

 Highlight

1. Chlamydiae are obligate intracellular bacteria
2. *Chlamydia trachomatis*
3. The most common bacterial cause of STD in the United States and Europe
4. Up to 70% of sexually active women with chlamydial infections are asymptomatic
5. Complications and sequelae include salpingitis, infertility, ectopic pregnancy or chronic pelvic pain

Chlamydial infections are caused by the bacteria *Chlamydia trachomatis*. These infections are among the most common sexually transmitted infections (STIs) worldwide. Chlamydia can affect both men and women, and it often doesn't cause any symptoms, which can make it challenging to detect and treat. The chlamydiae are obligate intracellular bacteria that produce a wide variety of infections in many mammalian and avian species. Three species of *Chlamydia* infect humans: *C. trachomatis*, *C. psittaci*, and *C. pneumoniae*. *C. trachomatis* is exclusively a human pathogen and is transmitted from person to person via sexual contact, perinatal transmission, or close contact in households. In the United States *C. trachomatis* infection is the most common reportable infectious disease.

■ Identification to the chlamydial infections:

C. trachomatis is the most common bacterial cause of sexually transmitted disease in the United States and Europe. The spectrum of illness attributable to these infections' parallels that of gonococcal infection. Many people with Chlamydia do not experience any symptoms, which is why it's often called a "silent" infection. When symptoms do occur, they can include genital discharge, pain or burning during urination, and abdominal pain. In men, the most common syndromes are nongonococcal urethritis and acute epididymitis. In women, mucopurulent cervicitis, urethritis, bartholinitis, acute salpingitis, and perihepatitis are the syndromes most commonly seen.

Up to 70% of sexually active women with chlamydial infections are asymptomatic. Complications and sequelae include salpingitis with subsequent risk of infertility, ectopic pregnancy or chronic pelvic pain. Asymptomatic chronic infections of endometrium and fallopian tubes may lead to the same outcome. Infection during pregnancy may result in premature rupture of membranes and preterm delivery, and conjunctival and pneumonic infection of the newborn. Endocervical chlamydial infection has been associated with increased risk of acquiring HIV infection.

■ Infectious agent:

Chlamydia trachomatis, immunotypes D through K, has been identified in approximately 35-50% of cases of nongonococcal urethritis in the USA.

⬛ Occurrence:

Worldwide, recognition has increased steadily in the last two decades. The age of peak incidence is the late teens and early 20s. prevalence has been reported at 3-8% in general medical clinics and urban high schools, over 10% in asymptomatic military personnel undergoing routine physical examination, and as high as 15-20% in men and women attending STD clinics.

⬛ Reservoir:

Man.

⬛ Mode of transmission:

By the way of direct contact, it is usually sexually transmitted.

⬛ Incubation period:

Incubation period is poorly defined, probably 7-14 days or longer.

⬛ Period of communicability:

It is unknown so far. Relapses are probably common.

⬛ Susceptibility and resistance:

Susceptibility is general. No acquired immunity has been demonstrated; cellular immunity is immunotype-specific.

⬛ Methods of control:

1. Risk reduction against sexually transmitted diseases through abstinence or barrier methods such as condoms.

2. Going to the doctor immediately if symptoms of PID, sexually transmitted diseases appear, or after learning that a current or former sex partner has or might have had a sexually transmitted disease.

3. Getting regular gynecological (pelvic) exams with STD testing to screen for symptomless chlamydial infection.

4. Discussing sexual history with a trusted physician in order to get properly screened for sexually transmitted diseases.

5. Understanding when a partner says that they have been STD tested they usually mean chlamydia and gonorrhea in the US, but that those are not all of the sexually transmissible diseases.

6. Treating partners to prevent reinfection or spreading the infection to other people.

7. *Chlamydia trachomatis* is generally susceptible to a range of antibiotics. The two most commonly used antibiotics to treat Chlamydia infections are azithromycin and doxycycline. These antibiotics are highly effective against Chlamydia, and most infections can be successfully treated with them.

ॐ General review

1. Up to 70% of sexually active women with chlamydial infections are asymptomatic.

2. Cases symptoms of Chlamydia in men are nongonococcal urethritis and acute epididymitis.

3. Cases of symptoms Chlamydia in women are mucopurulent cervicitis, urethritis, bartholinitis, acute salpingitis, and perihepatitis.

4. *Chlamydia trachomatis*

5. The age of peak incidence is the late teens and early 20s.

SCAN ME

Check Your Answers

Review test

I. Multiple-choice questions (Four selected one):

1. ( ) What is the most common method of transmission for Chlamydia trachomatis among humans? (A) Airborne transmission, (B) Waterborne transmission, (C) Sexual contact, (D) Foodborne transmission

2. ( ) Which species of Chlamydia is exclusively a human pathogen? (A) *C. trachomatis*, (B) *C. pneumoniae*, (C) *C. psittaci*, (D) *C. caviae*

3. ( ) What is the primary reason *Chlamydia trachomatis* is often referred to as a "silent" infection? (A) It primarily affects men and not women, (B) It is caused by a virus, not bacteria, (C) It is easily treatable with antibiotics, (D) Many people with Chlamydia do not experience any symptoms

4. ( ) What is the most common complication associated with *Chlamydia trachomatis* in women, which can lead to infertility, ectopic pregnancy, and chronic pelvic pain? (A) Genital discharge, (B) Mucopurulent cervicitis, (C) Abdominal pain, (D) Conjunctival infection

5. ( ) What risk is associated with endocervical chlamydial infection in relation to HIV? (A) Increased risk of acquiring HIV infection, (B) No association with HIV risk, (C) Reduced risk of HIV infection, (D) No change in HIV risk

6. ( ) What is the age range of the peak incidence of *Chlamydia trachomatis* infection? (A) Early teens, (B) Late teens and early 20s, (C) Late 20s and early 30s, (D) Middle-aged and elderly individuals

7. ( ) In which group of individuals has the highest reported prevalence of Chlamydia trachomatis been observed? (A) General medical clinics, (B) Urban high schools, (C) Asymptomatic military personnel undergoing routine physical examination, (D) Men and women attending STD clinics

8. ( ) What is one of the methods for risk reduction against sexually transmitted diseases, such as Chlamydia trachomatis? (A) Consuming a healthy diet, (B) Regular exercise, (C) Abstinence or barrier methods like condoms, (D) Social distancing

9. ( ) What should individuals do if they suspect they have symptoms of PID (Pelvic Inflammatory Disease) or a sexually transmitted disease? (A) Wait for the symptoms to disappear on their own, (B) Visit a doctor immediately, (C) Share their symptoms with friends for advice, (D) Start self-treatment with over the counter medications

10. ( ) Which two antibiotics are commonly used to treat Chlamydia infections because they are highly effective against Chlamydia trachomatis? (A) Penicillin and erythromycin, (B) Ciprofloxacin and metronidazole, (C) Azithromycin and doxycycline, (D) Amoxicillin and tetracycline

II. Simple answer:

1. What is the most common reportable infectious disease in the United States?

2. What is the most common syndrome in men caused by *Chlamydia trachomatis* infection?

3. What complications can occur in women with *Chlamydia trachomatis* infection during pregnancy?

4. What is the reported prevalence of *Chlamydia trachomatis* in asymptomatic military personnel undergoing routine physical examination?

5. What is one of the recommended actions to prevent reinfection or the spread of *Chlamydia trachomatis* to other people?

6. What should individuals understand about partner-reported STD testing in the United States?

6-7 Trichomoniasis (ICD-9 131; ICD-10 A59)

Highlight

1. Trichomoniasis is a common sexually transmitted disease
2. *Trichomonas vaginalis*, a flagellate protozoan
3. Primarily an infection of the genitourinary tract
4. The most common site of infection is the urethra and the vagina in women
5. 20% of women are asymptomatic
6. Lower abdominal pain
7. The highest incidence among females 16-35 years
8. No acquired immunity has been demonstrated

Trichomoniasis, sometimes referred to as "trich", is a common sexually transmitted disease. It is caused by the single-celled protozoan parasite *Trichomonas vaginalis*. Trichomoniasis is primarily an infection of the genitourinary tract; the most common site of infection is the urethra and the vagina in women. It is most common in women and uncircumcised men. For uncircumcised men, the most common site for the infection is the tip of the penis. Trichomoniasis is one of the most common non-viral STIs worldwide.

🔑 Identification to the trichomoniasis:

Trichomoniasis, like many other sexually transmitted diseases, often occurs without any symptoms. Men almost never have symptoms, while 20% of women are asymptomatic. When women have symptoms, they usually appear within 5 to 28 days of exposure. Trichomoniasis often coexists with gonorrhoea, in some studies up to 40% of persons with gonorrhoea have concurrent trichomoniasis, and the majority of women trichomoniasis also have bacterial vaginitis; a full assessment for STI pathogens must be carried out when trichomoniasis is diagnosed.

The symptoms in women include a heavy, yellow-green or gray vaginal discharge, discomfort during intercourse, unpleasant vaginal odor, and painful urination. Irritation and itching of the female genital area, and on rare occasions, lower abdominal pain also can be present. In about two-thirds of infected females, there is edema, inflammation, cell hypertrophy and metaplasia. In pregnant women, untreated trichomoniasis can lead to preterm birth and low birth weight.

The symptoms in men, if present, include a thin, whitish discharge from the penis, painful or difficult urination and pain and swelling in the scrotum (resulting from epididymitis). Men may experience irritation inside the penis, burning after urination or ejaculation, or a slight discharge from the urethra.

Infectious agent:

Trichomonas vaginalis, a flagellate protozoan.

Occurrence:

Widespread; a frequent disease, primarily of adults, with the highest incidence among females 16-35 years. Overall, about 20% of female may become infected during their reproductive years. It's estimated that there are approximately 3.7 million new cases of trichomoniasis in the United States each year. It is the most frequently presenting new infection of the common sexually transmitted diseases in Taiwan.

Reservoir:

Man.

Mode of transmission:

Through contact with vaginal and urethral discharges of infected person during sexual intercourse.

Incubation period:

Incubation period is from 4-20 days, average 7 days; many are asymptomatic carriers for years.

Period of communicability:

For the duration of the persistent infection, which may last years.

Susceptibility and resistance:

Susceptibility is general, clinical disease is seen mainly in females. No acquired immunity has been demonstrated.

📄 Methods of control:

Use of male condoms may help prevent the spread of trichomoniasis, although careful studies have never been done that focus on how to prevent this infection. Specific treatment: metronidazole, tinidazole or ornidazole is effective in both male and female patients. Both sexual partners should be treated simultaneously to prevent reinfection.

🔬 General review

1. Trichomoniasis in men almost never have symptoms, while 20% of women are asymptomatic.
2. *Trichomonas vaginalis*, a flagellate protozoan.
3. Clinical disease is seen mainly in females.

SCAN ME

Check Your Answers

🦠 Review test

I. Multiple-choice questions (Four selected one):

1. ( ) What is the primary site of infection for trichomoniasis in women? (A) Urethra, (B) Vagina, (C) Anus, (D) Mouth

2. ( ) In which group is trichomoniasis most common among men? (A) Circumcised men, (B) Women, (C) Uncircumcised men, (D) Transgender individuals

3. ( ) What percentage of women with trichomoniasis are asymptomatic? (A) 5%, (B) 10%, (C) 20%, (D) 50%

4. ( ) What is a potential complication of untreated trichomoniasis in pregnant women? (A) Ovarian cysts, (B) Ectopic pregnancy,

(C) Preterm birth and low birth weight, (D) Menstrual irregularities

5. (   ) What is the highest incidence group for trichomoniasis? (A) Females under 16 years old, (B) Females 16-35 years old, (C) Males of any age, (D) Senior citizens

6. (   ) Approximately how many new cases of trichomoniasis are estimated to occur in the United States each year? (A) 370,000, (B) 3.7 million, (C) 37 million, (D) 370 million

7. (   ) Which medication is effective for the treatment of trichomoniasis in both male and female patients? (A) Amoxicillin, (B) Penicillin, (C) Metronidazole, (D) Ibuprofen

II.   Simple answer:

1. What type of organism causes trichomoniasis?

2. What symptoms might men experience if they have trichomoniasis?

3. What is one suggested method for preventing the spread of trichomoniasis?

4. Why is it recommended that both sexual partners should be treated simultaneously for trichomoniasis?

6-8　Candidiasis (ICD-9 112; ICD-10 B37)

Highlight

1. Candidiasis
2. Yeast infection, Fungal infection
3. Moniliasis
4. Oral thrush
5. Vaginitis
6. Mycosis
7. *Candida albicans*
8. Leukorrhoea

Candidiasis, commonly called yeast infection, moniliasis or thrush, is a fungal infection (mycosis) of any of the *Candida* species, of which *Candida albicans* is the most common. Scientists estimate that about 20% of women normally have Candida in the vagina without having any symptoms. Candida can cause an infection if the conditions change inside the vagina to encourage its growth. Infection can happen because of hormones, medicines, or changes in the immune system. Candidiasis thereby encompasses infections that range from superficial, such as oral thrush and vaginitis, to systemic and potentially life-threatening diseases. *Candida* infections of the latter category are also referred to as candidemia and are usually confined to severely immunocompromised persons, such as cancer, transplant, and AIDS patients, whereas superficial infections of skin and mucosal membranes by *Candida* causing local inflammation and discomfort is common in many human populations. While clearly attributable to the presence of the opportunistic pathogens of the genus *Candida*, candidiasis

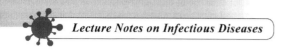

describes a number of different disease syndromes that often differ in their causes and outcomes.

Identification to the candidiasis:

Candidal vaginitis may present as intense pruritus of the vulva and a cervical discharge that can vary from scant to thick and white. There may be edema of the vulva and erythema of the vagina and labia that extends onto the perineum in female. Leukorrhea is also a sign of vaginitis, which is often caused by infection with the *Candida albicans* or by infection with the protozoan parasite *Trichomonas vaginalis*. Balanitis can begin as itching or burning, with vesicles or white patches on the penis. Plaques may extend onto the thighs, buttocks, and scrotum in male. The symptoms of vaginal candidiasis include:

1. Vaginal itching or soreness

2. Pain during sexual intercourse

3. Pain or discomfort when urinating

4. Abnormal vaginal discharge

Vaginal candidiasis is often mild. However, some women can develop severe infections involving redness, swelling, and cracks in the wall of the vagina.

Infectious agent:

Candida albicans.

Occurrence:

Worldwide, *C. albicans* is often part of the normal human flora. Candidal vulvovaginitis is common. It is responsible for a third of all cases of vulvovaginitis in reproductive-aged women, and 70% of women report having had candidal vulvovaginitis at some point in their lifetimes. About 8% of women suffer recurrent candidal vulvovaginitis.

Reservoir:

Man.

Mode of transmission:

It is also contact with secretions or excretions of mouth, skin, vaginal and feces, from patients or carriers; by passage from mother to neonate during childbirth; and by endogenous spread.

Incubation period:

Variable, 2-5 days for thrush in infants.

Period of communicability:

Presumably while lesions are present.

Susceptibility and resistance:

Susceptibility is general, repeated clinical skin or mucosal eruptions are common. Risk factors for developing candidiasis include a weakened immune system, the use of broad-spectrum antibiotics, uncontrolled diabetes, and a high-sugar diet, as well as pregnancy, oral contraceptives, and frequent douching in women.

Methods of control:

It is important to consider that *Candida* species are frequently part of the human body's normal oral and intestinal flora. Use of male condoms may help prevent the spread of candidiasis.

Treatment with antibiotics can lead to eliminating the yeast's natural competitors for resources and increase the severity of the condition. In clinical settings, candidiasis is commonly treated with antimycotics; the antifungal drugs commonly used to treat candidiasis are topical clotrimazole, topical nystatin, fluconazole, and topical ketoconazole.

General review

1. The alternative names of candidiasis are yeast infection, Moniliasis, and Thrush.

2. Oral candidiasis, commonly known as thrush

3. Candidal vaginitis: pruritus of the vulva and a cervical discharge (Leukorrhoea)

4. Candidiasis is a fungal infection (mycosis)

5. *Candida albicans*

Review test

SCAN ME

Check Your Answers

I. Multiple-choice questions (Four selected one):

1. ( ) Which Candida species is the most common cause of candidiasis? (A) Candida moniliasis, (B) Candida thrush, (C) *Candida albicans*, (D) Candida mycosis

2. ( ) What can trigger a Candida infection in the vagina? (A) Adequate hygiene, practices, (B) Drinking plenty of water, (C) Changes in hormones, medicines, or the immune system, (D) Frequent sexual activity

3. (   ) What is a common sign of vaginitis caused by *Candida albicans*? (A) Abnormal vaginal discharge, (B) Vesicles on the penis, (C) Itching or burning on the scrotum, (D) Erythema of the perineum

4. (   ) What is a symptom commonly associated with balanitis in males? (A) Vaginal itching, (B) Erythema of the vulva, (C) Pain during sexual intercourse, (D) White patches on the penis

5. (   ) Which protozoan parasite can also cause leukorrhea, a sign of vaginitis, in addition to *Candida albicans*? (A) Trichomonas vaginalis, (B) Candida moniliasis, (C) Giardia lamblia, (D) Plasmodium falciparum

6. (   ) What percentage of women report having had Candidal vulvovaginitis at some point in their lifetimes? (A) 10%, (B) 25%, (C) 50%, (D) 70%

7. (   ) How is C. albicans primarily transmitted among individuals? (A) Through the air, (B) By sexual contact, (C) Through contaminated food and water, (D) By sharing clothing

8. (   ) What is one risk factor for developing candidiasis? (A) Regular exercise, (B) Low-sugar diet, (C) Weakened immune system, (D) Frequent handwashing

II. Simple answer:

1. What are some examples of symptoms of a superficial candida infection?

2. List two common symptoms of vaginal candidiasis.

3. What can some women with vaginal candidiasis develop, which involves redness, swelling, and cracks in the vaginal wall?

4. What is one of the modes of transmission of *C. albicans*, particularly from mother to newborn?

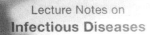
Lecture Notes on
Infectious Diseases

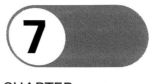

7

CHAPTER

Vector-Borne Infectious Diseases

Transmission of infectious diseases may also involve a "vector". Vectors may be mechanical or biological. A mechanical vector picks up an infectious agent on the outside of its body and transmits it in a passive manner. In contrast, biological vectors harbor pathogens within their bodies and deliver pathogens to new hosts in an active manner, usually a bite. Biological vectors are often responsible for serious blood-borne diseases, such as dengue fever, malaria, viral encephalitis, Chagas disease, Lyme disease and African sleeping sickness. Biological vectors are usually, though not exclusively, arthropods, such as mosquitoes, ticks, fleas and lice. Vectors are often required in the life cycle of a pathogen. A common strategy, used to control vector borne infectious diseases, is to interrupt the life cycle of a pathogen, by killing the vector.

Haematophagous insects are important in terms of public health as they are remarkably adaptable to the environment and successfully coexist with man, feeding on him and his domesticated animals. Besides the colossal blood loss, some species are known to transmit many dreadful diseases like malaria, filariasis, Japanese encephalitis, dengue, Leishmaniasis etc. Millions of people in India suffer from vector borne diseases annually.

Vector-borne diseases are prevalent in the tropics and subtropics and are relatively rare in temperate zones, although climate change could create conditions suitable for outbreaks of diseases such as Lyme disease, Rocky Mountain spotted fever, malaria, dengue fever, and viral encephalitis in temperate regions. There are different patterns of vector-borne disease occurrence. Parasitic and bacterial diseases, such as malaria and Lyme disease, tend to produce a high disease incidence but do not cause major epidemics. An exception to this rule is plague, a bacterial disease that does cause outbreaks. In contrast, many vectors viral diseases, such as Yellow fever, dengue, and Japanese encephalitis, commonly cause major epidemics.

From the perspective of infectious diseases, vectors are the transmitters of disease-causing organisms that carry the pathogens from one host to another. By common usage, vectors are considered to be invertebrate animals, usually arthropods. Technically, however, vertebrates can also act as vectors, including foxes, raccoons, and skunks, which can all transmit the rabies virus to humans via a bite. Arthropods account for over 85 percent of all known animal species, and they are the most important disease vectors. Arthropods may affect human health either directly by bites, stings, or infestation of tissues, or indirectly through disease transmission. Several genera of arthropods play a role in human disease, but mosquitoes and ticks are the most notable disease vectors. The most significant mode of vector-borne disease transmission is by biological transmission by blood-feeding arthropods. The pathogen multiplies within the arthropod vector, and the pathogen is transmitted when the arthropod takes a blood meal. Mechanical transmission of disease agents may also occur when arthropods physically carry pathogens from one place or host to another, usually on body parts.

There has been a worldwide resurgence of vector-borne diseases since the 1970s including malaria, dengue, Yellow fever, louse-borne typhus, plague, leishmaniasis, sleeping sickness, West Nile encephalitis, Lyme disease, Japanese encephalitis, Rift Valley fever, and Crimean-Congo hemorrhagic fever. Reasons for the emergence or resurgence of vector-borne diseases include the development of insecticide and drug resistance; decreased resources for surveillance, prevention and control of vector-borne diseases; deterioration of the public health infrastructure required to deal with these diseases; unprecedented population growth; uncontrolled urbanization; changes in agricultural practices; deforestation; and increased travel. Changes have been documented in the distribution of important arthropod disease vectors.

It is clear that people will always have to live with vector-borne diseases, but maintenance of a strong public health infrastructure and undertaking research activities directed at improved means of control—possibly utilizing biological and genetic-based strategies, combined with the development of new or improved vaccines for diseases such as malaria, dengue and Lyme disease—should lessen the threat to human health.

The familiar vector-borne infectious diseases in Asia contain malaria, dengue, Yellow fever, louse-borne typhus, plague, leishmaniasis, Lyme disease, Japanese encephalitis, and filariasis etc.

7-1 | Malaria (ICD-9 084; ICD-10 B50-B54)

Highlight

1. Malaria
2. *Anopheles sinensis*, *Anopheles minimus*
3. Vector-borne infectious disease
4. *Plasmodium falciparum* (Malignant tertian malaria)
5. *Plasmodium vivax* (Tertian malaria; Benign malaria)
6. *Plasmodium malariae* (Quartan malaria)
7. *Plasmodium ovale* (Benign ovale malaria)
8. Taiwan has been eradicated malaria, 1965
9. Malaria Vaccine (Mosquirix)

Malaria has infected humans for over 50,000 years and may have been a human pathogen for the entire history of our species. Indeed, close relatives of the human malaria parasites remain common in chimpanzees, our closest relatives. About 10,000 years ago malaria started having a major impact on human survival which coincides with start of agriculture; a consequence was natural selection for the genes for sickle-cell disease , thalassaemias , glucose-6-phosphate dehydrogenase deficiency, ovalocytosis and elliptocytosis because such blood disorders confers a selective advantage against malaria infection. Deadly fevers (probably malaria) have been recorded since the beginning of the written word. References to the unique periodic fevers of malaria are found throughout recorded history, beginning in 2700 BC in China. Mosquito nets were used in Egypt as early as 2700 BC. The symptoms of intermittent fevers were described by Hippocrates. He related its presence with climatic and environmental conditions and divided the fever into three types: febris tertiana (alternate days), quartana (every fourth day) and quotidiana or continua (now called tropica). Around 168BC the herbal remedy Qinghaosu (later called Artemisinin in the West) came into use in China as antipyretic.

Malaria is a vector-borne infectious disease caused by protozoan parasites. It is widespread in tropical and subtropical regions, including parts of the Americas, Asia, and Africa. Each year, it causes disease in approximately 515 million people and kills between one and three million people, the majority of whom are young children in Sub-Saharan Africa. Malaria is commonly associated with poverty but is also a cause of poverty and a major hindrance to economic development. Although some are under development, no vaccine is currently available for malaria; preventative drugs must be taken continuously to reduce the risk of infection. These prophylactic drug treatments are often too expensive for most people living in endemic areas. Most adults from endemic areas have a degree of long-term recurrent infection and also of partial resistance; the resistance reduces with time and such adults may become susceptible to severe malaria if they have spent a significant amount of time in non-endemic areas. They are strongly recommended to take full precautions if they return to an endemic area. Malaria infections are treated through the use of antimalarial drugs, such as quinine or artemisinin derivatives, although drug resistance is increasingly common.

🗋 Identification to the malaria:

Malaria is a parasitic disease; infections with 4 human types of malaria can present symptoms sufficiently similar to make species differention impossible without laboratory studies. Illness may begin with indefinite malaise followed by shaking chill and rapidly rising temperature, usually accompanied by headache and nausea and ending with profuse sweating is repeated either daily, every other day or every 3rd day (Fig. 7-1).

SYMPTOMS OF MALARIA

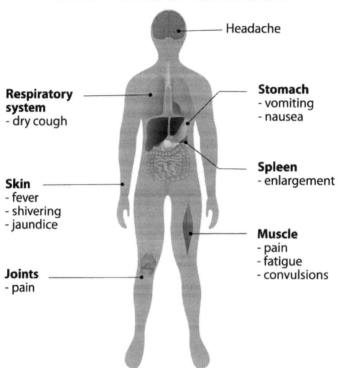

Figure 7-1　Symptoms of malaria include fever and flu-like illness, including shaking chills, headache, muscle aches, and tiredness. Nausea, vomiting, and diarrhea may also occur. Malaria may cause anemia and jaundice because of the loss of red blood cells.

Malaria is one of the most common infectious diseases and an enormous public health problem. The disease is caused by protozoan parasites of the genus *Plasmodium*. Only four types of the plasmodium parasite can infect humans; the most serious forms of the disease are caused by *Plasmodium falciparum* and *Plasmodium vivax*, but other related species (*Plasmodium ovale*, *Plasmodium malariae*) can also affect humans. This group of human-pathogenic *Plasmodium* species is usually referred to as malaria parasites. Malaria parasites are transmitted by female *Anopheles* mosquitoes. The parasites multiply within red blood cells, causing symptoms that include symptoms of anemia (light headedness, shortness of breath, tachycardia etc.), as well as other general symptoms such as fever, chills, nausea, flu-like illness, and in severe cases, coma and death. Malaria transmission can be reduced by preventing mosquito bites with mosquito nets and insect repellents, or by mosquito control measures such as spraying insecticides inside houses and draining standing water where mosquitoes lay their eggs.

Malignant malaria (ICD-9 084.0; ICD-10 B50); the most serious, falciparum malaria (malignant tertian), may present in a quite varied clinical picture including fever, chills, sweats and headache, and may progress to icterus, coagulation defects, shock, renal and liver failure, acute encephalopathy and coma. Case fatality among untreated children and non-immune adults considerably exceeds 10-40 % or higher. The other human malarias; vivax (ICD-9 084.1; ICD-10 B51), malariae (ICD-9 084.2; ICD-10 B52), ovale (ICD-9 084.3; ICD-10 B53.0), generally are not life threatening except in the very young, the very old or in patients with concurrent disease.

Infectious agents:

Plasmodium vivax, *Plasmodium malariae*, *Plasmodium falciparum*, and *Plasmodium ovale*. The protozoan parasites are with asexual and sexual phases. Mixed infections are frequent in endemic areas.

Occurrence:

Endemic malarias no longer occur in many temperate zone countries but are a major cause of ill health in many parts of the tropics and subtropics.

Falciparum and vivax malaria are found in many endemic areas. Taiwan has been eradicated malaria and is certificated from WHO in 1965 (Fig. 7-2).

Reservoir:

Man is the only important reservoir of human malaria.

Mode of transmission:

Transmission way is by the bite of an infective female anopheline mosquito. Some important vectors (*Anopheles sinensis* & *Anopheles minimus*) have biting peaks around midnight or the early hours of the morning. When the sporozoits are injected into man as the insect takes a blood meal. The malarias may also be transmitted by injection or transfusion of blood of infected persons or by use of contaminated needles and syringes.

The parasite's definitive hosts and transmission vectors are female mosquitoes of the *Anopheles* genus. Young mosquitoes first ingest the malaria parasite by feeding on an infected human carrier and the infected *Anopheles* mosquitoes carry *Plasmodium* sporozoites in their salivary glands. A mosquito becomes infected when it takes a blood meal from an infected human. Once ingested the parasite gametocytes taken up in the blood will further differentiate into male or female gametes and then fuse in the mosquito gut. This produces an ookinete that penetrates the gut lining and produces an oocyst in the gut wall. When the oocyst ruptures, it releases sporozoites that migrate through the mosquito's body to the salivary glands, where they are then ready to infect a new human host. This type of transmission is occasionally referred to as anterior station transfer. The sporozoites are injected into the skin, alongside saliva, when the mosquito takes a subsequent blood meal.

WORLD HEALTH ORGANIZATION

Office of the Director-General
Bureau du Directeur Général

ORGANISATION MONDIALE DE LA SANTÉ

Palais des Nations, GENÈVE
Télégr.: UNISANTÉ, GENÈVE

Tél.: 33 10 00 - 33 20 00 - 33 40 00

Réf.: M2/180/11
M2/372/3 CHINA

Geneva, 25 November 1965

Sir,

I have the honour to inform you that, based on the report submitted to me by the Director of the WHO Regional Office for the Western Pacific and following his recommendation, the name of China (Taiwan) was entered on 1 November 1965 in the WHO Register of areas where malaria has been eradicated.

The status of malaria eradication in the area that has been entered in the WHO Register will be published every semester in the Weekly Epidemiological Record of WHO based on your quarterly reports to the WHO Regional Office for the Western Pacific regarding the malaria status of the area.

I wish to take this opportunity to express my deep satisfaction and congratulations to you, the Staff of the Malaria Service and the Health Services for this great achievement.

I have the honour to be,

Sir,

Your obedient Servant,

Sgd./M. G. Candau

M. G. Candau, M.D.
Director-General

The Director
Department of Health Administration
Ministry of Interior
Taipei
Taiwan
Republic of China

cc. The Minister of Foreign Affairs, Ministry of Foreign Affairs, Taipei, Taiwan, Republic of China

Dr T. C. Hsu, Commissioner of Health, Department of Health, Taiwan Provincial Government, Wufeng Hsiang, Taichung, Taiwan, Republic of China

Dr C. T. Loo, Director, National Defence Medical Centre, 4th Section, Roosevelt Road, Taipei, Taiwan, Republic of China

The Permanent Representative of China to the European Office of the United Nations and other International Organizations in Geneva, 75 rue de Lyon, 1211 Genève 13

D108-LL

(reprinted in reduced size)

Figure 7-2   Taiwan has been eradicated malaria and is certificated from WHO in 1965.
(Ken K.S. Wang. 2002. Environmental Hygienic Vector Control. New Wun Ching Developmental Publishing Co., Ltd. 86pp)

Incubation periods:

The time between the infective bite and the appearance of clinical symptoms is approximately; 9-14 days for *P. falciparum*, 12-18 days for *P. vivax*, 12-18 days for *P. ovale*, 18-40 days for *P. malariae*. Suboptimal drug suppression such as from prophylaxis may result in prolonged incubation periods.

Period of communicability:

For infection of mosquitoes, as long as infective gametocytes are present in the blood of patients (3 to 14 days); this varies with species and strain of parasite and with response to therapy.

Untreated or insufficiently treated patients may be a source of mosquito infection for several years in malariae, up to 5 years in vivax, and generally not more than 1 year in falciparum malaria; the mosquito remains infective for life.

Susceptibility and resistance:

Except in some with certain genetic traits, susceptibility is universal. Most black Africans show a natural resistance to infection with *P. vivax*, possibly associated with the absence of Duffy factor on their erythrocytes. Tolerance or refractoriness to disease is present in adults in highly endemic communities where exposure to infective anophelines is continuous over many years.

Methods of control:

Methods used to prevent the spread of disease, or to protect individuals in areas where malaria is endemic, include prophylactic drugs, mosquito eradication, and the prevention of mosquito bites. There is currently no vaccine that will prevent malaria, but this is an active field of research. The well experienced of control methods in Taiwan are as follow:

1. Sanitary improvements: Larvicides and biological control with larvivorous fish (*Gambusia affinis*) may be useful.

2. Application of residual insecticides on the inside walls of dwellings and on other surfaces upon which endophilic vector anophelines habitually rest will generally result in effective malaria control.

3. Nightly spraying of screened living and sleeping quarters with a liquid or an aerosol preparation of pyrethrum or other insecticide is useful.

4. In endemic areas, install screens and use bed nets.

5. Insect repellents applied: The most effective repellent presently available is N, N diethyl-m-toluamide (Deet).

6. Antimalarial drugs, such as chloroquine, artemisinin-based combination therapies (ACTs), and others, are used to treat the disease.

7. Malaria Vaccine: The first malaria vaccine, known as RTS, S/AS01 (brand name Mosquirix) (Fig. 7-3), was approved for use in certain African countries as a pilot program. It offers partial protection against *P. falciparum* malaria, especially in children.

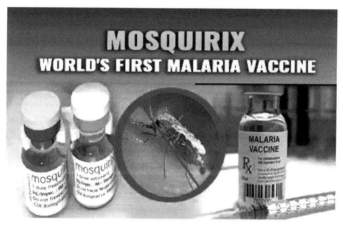

Figure 7-3   Mosquirix is a vaccine that is given to children aged 6 weeks to 17 months to help protect against malaria caused by the parasite *Plasmodium falciparum*.
(https://www.ema.europa.eu/en/opinion-medicine-use-outside-EU/human/mosquirix)
(https://www.youtube.com/watch?v=mFU15AH5s-U)

General review

1. The most serious forms of the disease are caused by *Plasmodium falciparum* and *Plasmodium vivax*, but other related species (*Plasmodium ovale*, *Plasmodium malariae*) can also affect humans.

2. Malaria parasites are transmitted by female Anopheles mosquitoes.

3. The parasites (*Plasmodium* spp.) multiply within red blood cells, causing symptoms such as fever, chills, nausea, flu-like illness, and in severe cases, coma and death.

4. *Plasmodium falciparum* is the culprit of malignant tertian malaria.

5. *Plasmodium vivax* is the culprit of tertian malaria (benign malaria).

6. *Plasmodium malariae* is the culprit of quartan malaria.

7. *Plasmodium ovale* is the culprit of benign ovale malaria.

8. The case fatality of Malaria among untreated children and non-immune adults considerably exceeds 10-40% or higher.

SCAN ME

Check Your Answers

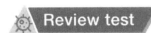

I. Multiple-choice questions (Four selected one):

1. (   ) What genetic adaptations have been selected for in human populations as a result of the impact of malaria on human survival? (A) Blue eye color, (B) Sickle-cell disease, thalassaemias, glucose-6-phosphate dehydrogenase deficiency, (C) Left-handedness, (D) Type 2 diabetes

2. (   ) Which civilization is credited with using mosquito nets as a method of protection against malaria as early as 2700 BC? (A) Ancient Greece, (B) Ancient Rome, (C) Ancient China, (D) Ancient Egypt

3. (   ) What herbal remedy, known as Qinghaosu in China, came into use around 168 BC as an antipyretic for treating malaria? (A) Aspirin, (B) Penicillin, (C) Artemisinin, (D) Echinacea

4. (   ) Which of the following is NOT one of the symptoms commonly associated with malaria? (A) Muscle aches, (B) Skin rash, (C) Chills, (D) Nausea

5. (   ) What is the primary method of transmission of malaria parasites to humans? (A) Direct contact with infected individuals, (B) Consumption of contaminated water, (C) Mosquito bites, (D) Airborne droplets

6. (　) Which species of Plasmodium parasites cause the most serious forms of malaria in humans? (A) *Plasmodium ovale* and *Plasmodium malariae*, (B) *Plasmodium vivax* and *Plasmodium ovale*, (C) *Plasmodium falciparum* and *Plasmodium vivax*, (D) *Plasmodium falciparum* and *Plasmodium malariae*

7. (　) What is the primary mode of transmission of malaria parasites to humans in endemic areas? (A) Direct contact with infected individuals, (B) Consumption of contaminated water, (C) Injection or transfusion of blood, (D) Mosquito bites

8. (　) How are malaria parasites transmitted from an infected mosquito to a new human host? (A) Through direct contact with mosquito feces, (B) By consuming contaminated food, (C) Through injection into the skin alongside mosquito saliva, (D) By touching contaminated surfaces

9. (　) What is the approximate incubation period for the appearance of clinical symptoms after an infective mosquito bite for *Plasmodium falciparum*? (A) 3-7 days, (B) 9-14 days, (C) 18-40 days, (D) 1-5 years

10.(　) How long can untreated or insufficiently treated patients serve as a source of mosquito infection for *Plasmodium vivax*? (A) Up to 5 years, (B) Up to 1 year, (C) Up to 14 days, (D) Up to 40 days

11.(　) What is the approximate incubation period for *Plasmodium malariae* before clinical symptoms appear? (A) 3-7 days, (B) 9-14 days, (C) 18-40 days, (D) 1-5 years

12. (　) What is the most effective repellent currently available for preventing mosquito bites in areas where malaria is endemic? (A) Lavender oil, (B) Lemon eucalyptus oil, (C) N, N diethyl-m-toluamide (Deet), (D) Citronella

13. (　) Which of the following methods involves the application of insecticides on the inside walls of dwellings and other resting surfaces of disease-carrying mosquitoes? (A) Larvicides, (B) Bed net installation, (C) Residual insecticide application, (D) Sanitary improvements

14. (　) What is the name of the first malaria vaccine that offers partial protection against *Plasmodium falciparum* malaria, especially in children, and has been approved for use in certain African countries? (A) Chloroquine, (B) Artemisinin-based combination therapy (ACT), (C) Mosquirix (RTS, S/AS01), (D) Deet

II. Simple answer:

1. What are some common symptoms of anemia associated with malaria?

2. What is the case fatality rate among untreated children and non-immune adults with malignant falciparum malaria, as mentioned in the article?

3. How was Taiwan able to eradicate malaria, and when did it receive certification from the World Health Organization (WHO)?

4. Describe the life cycle of the malaria parasite within the mosquito, including the key stages and how it is transmitted to a new human host.

5. What is the range of incubation periods for *Plasmodium ovale* before clinical symptoms typically appear?

6. How long does a mosquito infected with *Plasmodium falciparum* typically remain infective?

7. Name one method used to prevent the spread of malaria that involves the use of larvivorous fish.

7-2 Dengue Fever (ICD-9 061; ICD-10 A90)

 Highlight

1. Dengue fever
2. *Aedes aegypti* , *Aedes albopictus*
3. Classic dengue fever
4. Secondary dengue (DHF/DSS)
5. DHF: Sudden onset of high fever is accompanied by anorexia, vomiting, headache and abdominal pain
6. DSS: The fatality rate of cases with shock is as high as 40-50% in untreated cases
7. In southern Taiwan area contain 4 immunological types of dengue virus

Dengue fever and dengue hemorrhagic fever (DHF) are acute febrile diseases, found in the tropics and Africa, and caused by four closely related virus serotypes of the genus *Flavivirus*, family Flaviviridae. The geographical spread is similar to malaria, but unlike malaria, dengue is often found in urban areas of tropical nations, including Singapore, Taiwan, Indonesia, Philippines, India and Brazil. Each serotype is sufficiently different that there is no cross-protection and epidemics caused by multiple serotypes (hyperendemicity) can occur. Dengue is transmitted to humans by the *Aedes aegypti* (rarely *Aedes albopictus*) mosquito, which feeds during the day.

Identification to the dengue fever:

Dengue fever can range from a mild flu-like illness to a severe and potentially life-threatening condition. Common symptoms include high fever, severe headache, joint and muscle pain, rash, pain behind the eyes, and mild bleeding manifestations like nosebleeds and gum bleeding. There are four different serotypes of the dengue virus (DEN-1, DEN-2, DEN-3, and DEN-4), and infection with one serotype does not provide immunity against the others. In fact, subsequent infections with different serotypes can increase the risk of developing severe dengue (also known as Dengue Hemorrhagic Fever or Dengue Shock Syndrome).

Classic dengue fever:

An acute febrile disease characterized by sudden onset, fever for about 5 days and rarely more than 7 and sometimes diphasic, intense headache, retro-orbital pains, joint and muscle pains, and rash. Petechiae may appear on the feet or legs, in the axillae, or on the palate on the last day of fever or shortly thereafter. Recovery may be associated with prolonged fatigue and depression.

Secondary dengue (DHF/DSS): (ICD-9 065.4; ICD-10 A91)

1. **DHF:** A severe illness endemic in most of tropical Asia, characterized by abnormal vascular permeability, hypovolemia (low blood volume in circulation) and abnormal blood clotting mechanisms. Recognized principally are in children; although adults are affected in some outbreaks. Sudden onset of high fever is accompanied by anorexia, vomiting, headache and abdominal pain.

329

2. DSS: In some patients, after few days of fever, their condition suddenly deteriorates with signs of circulatory failure such as cool, blochy skin, circumoral cyanosis, rapid pulse and, in severe cases, hypotension or abnormally narrow pulse pressure. The fatality rate of cases with shock is as high as 40-50% in untreated cases; with good hospital care and fluid therapy, rates are usually less than 5%.

Infectious agent:

The viruses of dengue fever include immunological types 1, 2, 3, and 4; they are flaviviruses. Most shock cases are seen during the second of sequential dengue infections.

Occurrence:

The first epidemics occurred almost simultaneously in Asia, Africa, and North America in the 1780s. The disease was identified and named in 1779. A global pandemic began in Southeast Asia in the 1950s and by 1975 DHF had become a leading cause of death among children in many countries in that region. Epidemic dengue has become more common since the 1980s. By the late 1990s, dengue was the most important mosquito-borne disease affecting humans after malaria, there being around 40 million cases of dengue fever and several hundred thousand cases of dengue hemorrhagic fever each year. Dengue viruses are now endemic and epidemics in most countries of tropical Asia.

Dengue fever in Taiwan is most common during the wet and warm seasons, which provide favorable conditions for the breeding of Aedes mosquitoes, the primary vectors for the virus. Outbreaks often occur during the summer and early autumn months. In southern Taiwan area contain 4 immunological types of dengue virus; therefore, Kaohsiung and Pington are

DHF high risk areas. Significant outbreaks of dengue fever tend to occur every five or six years (Fig. 7-4). The cyclicity in numbers of dengue cases is thought to be the result of seasonal cycles interacting with a short-lived cross-immunity for all four strains, in people who have had dengue. When the cross-immunity wears off, the population is then more susceptible to transmission whenever the next seasonal peak occurs. Thus, in the longer term of several years, there tend to remain large numbers of susceptible people in the population despite previous outbreaks because there are four different strains of the dengue virus and because of new susceptible individuals entering the target population, either through childbirth or immigration.

Reservoir:

Man, together with the mosquito. The monkey-mosquito complex (forest transmission cycle) may be a reservoir.

Mode of transmission:

Transmission way is by bite of infective mosquitoes; *Aedes albopictus* and *Ae. aegypti*. When mosquitoes bite a viremia patient, since after 8-12 days, the mosquito becomes life-long virus infective capacity.

Incubation period:

Incubation period is from 3-14 days, commonly 5-8 days.

Period of communicability:

No directly transmitted from person to person. Patients are usually infective for mosquitoes from the day before onset to the 5th day of disease. The mosquito becomes infective 8-12 days after the blood meal and remains so far life.

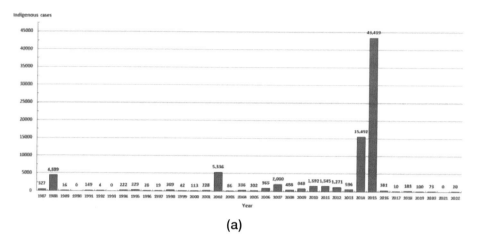

(a)

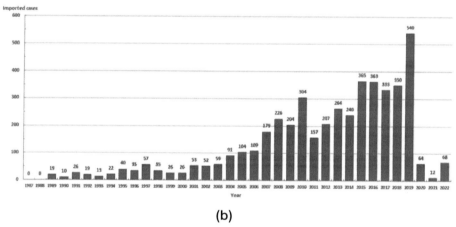

(b)

Figure 7-4   Indigenous and imported dengue cases in Taiwan, 1987-2022
(CDC, Taiwan, 2023).
(https://www.cdc.gov.tw/En/Category/ListContent/bg0g_VU_
Ysrgkes_KRUDgQ?uaid=9_Oq7OYHa-I8B05iUwyVvQ)

🔟 Susceptibility and resistance:

Susceptibility is apparently universal, but children usually have a milder
disease than adults. Homologous immunity is of long duration. The fatality
rate of Classic dengue fever is probably 0-1%, of DHF or DSS is probably
40-50%.

⬤ Methods of control:

Primary prevention of dengue mainly resides in mosquito control. Mosquito control can be achieved by mainly two methods, first and foremost is larval control and second one is adult mosquito control. Aedes mosquito breeds mainly on water collections in artificial containers, like plastic cups, used tyres, broken bottles, flowerpots etc. Continues and sustained artificial container reduction or periodic draining of artificial containers is the most effective way in reducing the larval and thereby the aedes mosquito load in the community.

Personal prevention consists of the use of mosquito nets, repellents containing Picaridin or DEET, covering exposed skin, use of DEET-impregnated bednets, and avoiding endemic areas.

The well experienced of control methods in Taiwan are as follow:

1. Community survey to determine density of vector mosquitoes, to identify breeding places.

2. Integrated Vector Management (IVM): IVM is a comprehensive approach to vector control that combines various methods, including source reduction, larval control, and adult mosquito control. It emphasizes community involvement, monitoring, and the use of environmentally friendly methods.

3. Educate the public on personal measures for protection against mosquitoes, including use of repellents.

4. Report to local health authority.

5. Isolation: Prevent access of mosquitoes to patients for at least 5 days after onset by screen the sickroom.

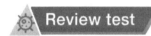 General review

1. Dengue fever and dengue hemorrhagic fever (DHF) are acute febrile diseases.

2. Dengue fever is transmitted to humans by the *Aedes aegypti* (rarely *Aedes albopictus*) mosquito, which feeds during the day.

3. Most shock cases are seen during the second of sequential dengue (different immunological type) infections.

4. The fatality rate of Classic dengue fever is probably 0-1%, of DHF or DSS is probably 40-50%.

Review test

SCAN ME

Check Your Answers

I. Multiple-choice questions (Four selected one):

1. ( ) What is the primary vector responsible for transmitting Dengue fever to humans? (A) *Aedes aegypti* and *Aedes albopictus*, (B) Anopheles mosquito, (C) Culex mosquito, (D) *Chironomus plumosus*

2. ( ) Why is there no cross-protection between the four serotypes of the Dengue virus? (A) They are genetically identical, (B) They are transmitted by different mosquito species, (C) Each serotype is sufficiently different, (D) Cross-protection is not necessary for Dengue

3. ( ) What are the common symptoms of classic dengue fever? (A) Cough and congestion, (B) Nausea and diarrhea, (C) High fever, severe headache, joint and muscle pain, rash, and pain behind the eyes, (D) Chest pain and shortness of breath

4. ( ) How does secondary dengue (Dengue Hemorrhagic Fever, DHF) differ from classic dengue fever? (A) It has no specific symptoms, (B) It is characterized by a prolonged fever of 10 days or more, (C) DHF is associated with abnormal vascular permeability, hypovolemia, and abnormal blood clotting mechanisms, (D) DHF only affects adults

5. ( ) What is the fatality rate for cases with shock in Dengue Shock Syndrome (DSS) if left untreated? (A) 5%, (B) 10%, (C) 25%, (D) 40-50%

6. ( ) What is the most significant risk factor for developing severe dengue in subsequent infections? (A) Being an adult, (B) Previous infection with the same serotype, (C) Vaccination, (D) Infection with a different serotype

7. ( ) What might appear on the last day of fever in classic dengue fever? (A) Chest pain, (B) Prolonged fatigue, (C) Rapid pulse, (D) Petechiae on the feet or legs, in the axillae, or on the palate

8. ( ) When was dengue fever identified and named as a disease? (A) 1775, (B) 1780s, (C) 1950s, (D) 1975

9. ( ) During which period did a global pandemic of dengue begin, with Dengue Hemorrhagic Fever (DHF) becoming a leading cause of death among children in Southeast Asia? (A) 1770s, (B) 1950s, (C) 1975, (D) 1980s

10. ( ) What factor contributes to the cyclical occurrence of significant dengue outbreaks every five or six years in Taiwan? (A) Cross-immunity to all four dengue strains, (B) Immunity acquired through previous outbreaks, (C) Seasonal cycles and short-lived

cross-immunity for all four strains, (D) Lack of susceptible individuals in the population

11. ( ) How long does it take for a mosquito to become life-long virus infective after biting a viremia patient? (A) 2-4 days, (B) 5-7 days, (C) 8-12 days, (D) 14-21 days

12. ( ) Who is more likely to experience a milder form of Dengue fever? (A) Children, (B) Adults, (C) The elderly, (D) Pregnant women

13. ( ) What is the estimated fatality rate for Dengue Hemorrhagic Fever (DHF) or Dengue Shock Syndrome (DSS)? (A) 0-1%, (B) 10-20%, (C) 25-30%, (D) 40-50%

14. ( ) Which approach combines various methods, including source reduction, larval control, and adult mosquito control, for effective vector control in Taiwan? (A) Integrated Vector Management (IVM), (B) Community survey, (C) Environmental monitoring, (D) Public education

15. ( ) What should individuals do to protect themselves against mosquitoes? (A) Report to local health authorities, (B) Isolate themselves from others, (C) Educate the public on personal protection measures, (D) Avoid drinking untreated water

II. Simple answer:

1. Please describe classic dengue fever in terms of its duration, symptoms, and any post-fever manifestations.

2. Please explain what DHF (Dengue Hemorrhagic Fever) is and mention one of its main characteristics.

3. What is the fatality rate for cases with shock in Dengue Shock Syndrome (DSS) with good hospital care and fluid therapy?

4. Explain why dengue fever tends to occur more frequently during the wet and warm seasons in Taiwan.

5. What is the main reason for the cyclical nature of significant dengue outbreaks every five or six years, even with previous outbreaks?

6. What is the incubation period for Dengue fever, and what is the most common duration within this range?

7. How long is homologous immunity to Dengue fever expected to last?

8. What is the purpose of isolating Dengue fever patients from mosquitoes for at least 5 days after onset?

7-3 Yellow Fever (ICD-9 060; ICD-10 A95)

 Highlight

1. Yellow fever also called Yellow Jack, black vomit or vomito negro, or American Plague

2. Acute viral disease

3. Vectors: *Aedes simpsoni*, *Ae. africanus*, and *Ae. aegypti* in Africa

4. Vectors: the *Haemagogus* genus in South America

5. Vectors: the *Sasbethes* genera in France

6. Yellow fever exists in nature in 2 transmission cycles, a sylvatic or jungle cycle

7. Sylvatic transmission is restricted to tropical regions of Africa and Latin America

8. 17D vaccine

Yellow fever also called yellow jack, black vomit or vomito negro, or sometimes American Plague is an acute viral disease. It is an important cause of hemorrhagic illness in many African and South American countries despite existence of an effective vaccine. The yellow refers to the jaundice symptoms that affect some patients.

Yellow fever has been a source of several devastating epidemics. French soldiers were attacked by yellow fever during the 1802 Haitian Revolution; more than half of the army perished from the disease. Outbreaks followed by thousands of deaths occurred periodically in other Western Hemisphere locations until research, which included human volunteers (some of whom died), led to an understanding of the method of transmission to humans (primarily by mosquitos) and development of a vaccine and other preventative efforts in the early 20th century.

▶ Identification to the yellow fever:

Human infection begins after deposition of viral particles through the skin in infected arthropod saliva. The mosquitos involved are *Aedes simpsoni*, *Ae. africanus*, and *Ae. aegypti* in Africa, the *Haemagogus* genus in South America, and the *Sasbethes* genera in France. Yellow fever is frequently severe but moderate cases may occur as the result of previous infection by another flavivirus. After infection the virus first replicates locally, followed by transportation to the rest of the body via the lymphatic system. Following systemic lymphatic infection, the virus proceeds to establish itself throughout organ systems, including the heart, kidneys, adrenal glands, and the parenchyma of the liver; high viral loads are also present in the blood. Necrotic masses (Councilman bodies) appear in the cytoplasm of hepatocytes.

Historical reports have claimed a mortality rate of between 1 in 17 (5.8%) and 1 in 3 (33%). The WHO factsheet on yellow fever, updated in 2001, states that 15% of patients enter a "toxic phase" and that half of that number die within ten to fourteen days, with the other half recovering. There is a difference between disease outbreaks in rural or forest areas and in towns. Disease outbreaks in towns and non-native people may be more serious because of higher densities of mosquito vectors and higher population densities. Yellow fever can range from a mild flu-like illness to a severe, potentially fatal disease. Symptoms typically include fever, chills, headache, muscle and joint pain, and nausea. In severe cases, it can lead to jaundice (yellowing of the skin and eyes), bleeding, organ failure, and death.

Infectious agent:

Yellow fever is caused by an arbovirus of the family Flaviviridae, a positive single-stranded RNA virus.

Occurrence:

Yellow fever exists in nature in 2 transmission cycles, a sylvatic or jungle cycle that involves *Aedes* or *Haemagogous* mosquitoes and non-human primates, and an urban cycle involving humans and mainly *Ae. aegypti* mosquitoes. Sylvatic transmission is restricted to tropical regions of Africa and Latin America, where a few hundred cases occur annually, most often among occupationally exposed young adult male in forested or transtional areas of Bolivia, Brazil, Colombia, Ecuador and Peru.

Reservoir:

In urban areas, men and *Aedes* mosquitoes are major reservoirs; in forest areas, vertebrates other than humans, mainly monkeys and possibly marsupials, and forest mosquitoes. Transovarian transmission in mosquitoes may contribute to maintenance of infection.

Mode of transmission:

The transmission way in urban and certain rural areas is the bite of infective *Aedes* mosquitoes. In South Amerian forests is the bite of several species of forest mosquitoes of the genus *Haemagogus*. In eastern Africa, *Ae. africanus* is the vector in the monkey population, while semi-domestic *Ae. bromeliae* and *Ae. simpsoni*, and probably other *Aedes* species, transmit the virus from monkeys to humans.

Incubation period:

Incubation period is from 3-6 days.

Period of communicability:

Blood of patients is infective for mosquitoes shortly before onset of fever and for the first 3-5 days of illness. The disease is highly communicable where many susceptible people and abundant vector mosquitoes coexist; it is not communicable through contact or common vehicles.

Susceptibility and resistance:

Recovery from yellow fever is followed by lasting immunity; second attacks are unknown. Mild inapparent infections are immune mothers may persist for up to 6 months. In natural infections, antibodies appear in the blood within the first week.

📖 Methods of control:

The safe and highly efficacious vaccine for yellow fever that gives a ten-year or more immunity from the virus. The vaccine consists of a live, but attenuated, virus called 17D. The 17D vaccine has been used commercially since the 1950s. The mechanisms of attenuation and immunogenicity for the 17D strain are not known. However, this vaccine is very safe, with few adverse reactions having been reported and millions of doses administered, and highly effective with over 90% of vaccinees developing a measurable immune reponse after the first dose.

There is no true cure for yellow fever, therefore vaccination is important. Treatment is symptomatic and supportive only. Fluid replacement, fighting hypotension and transfusion of blood derivates is generally needed only in severe cases. In cases that result in acute renal failure, dialysis may be necessary. A fever victim needs to get a lot of rest, fresh air, and drink plenty of fluids.

⚖️ General review

1. Yellow fever also called yellow jack, black vomit or vomito negro, or sometimes American Plague is an acute viral disease.

2. Yellow fever is frequently severe but moderate cases may occur as the result of previous infection by another flavivirus.

3. The mortality rate of Yellow fever patients are between 5.8 to 33%.

4. Yellow fever is caused by an arbovirus of the family Flaviviridae.

5. Yellow fever exists in nature in 2 transmission cycles, a sylvatic or jungle cycle.

6. The urban transmission cycle involving humans and mainly *Ae. aegypti* mosquitoes.

7. The sylvatic transmission cycle is restricted to tropical regions of Africa and Latin America.

8. Yellow fever is highly communicable where many susceptible people and abundant vector mosquitoes coexist.

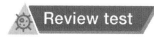 **Review test**

SCAN ME

Check Your Answers

I.   Multiple-choice questions (Four selected one):

1. ( ) How is the yellow fever virus primarily transmitted to humans?
   (A) Through contaminated water sources, (B) Direct contact with infected individuals, (C) Through the bite of infected mosquitoes, (D) Airborne transmission

2. ( ) Which mosquito species are known to transmit the yellow fever virus in Africa? (A) *Aedes simpsoni, Ae. africanus*, and *Ae. aegypti*, (B) Anopheles mosquitoes, (C) Culex mosquitoes, (D) Haemagogus genus

3. ( ) What is the primary organ system affected by the yellow fever virus following systemic lymphatic infection? (A) Respiratory system, (B) Gastrointestinal system, (C) Liver and other organs, (D) Nervous system

4. ( ) According to historical reports, what was the range of mortality rates during yellow fever outbreaks? (A) 1 in 100 (1%), (B) 1 in 17 (5.8%) to 1 in 3 (33%), (C) 1 in 50 (2%), (D) 1 in 10 (10%)

5. ( ) In which regions does the sylvatic transmission cycle of yellow fever primarily occur, involving non-human primates and certain types of mosquitoes? (A) North America and Europe, (B) Tropical regions of Africa and Latin America, (C) Southeast Asia and Australia, (D) Northern Europe and Russia

6. ( ) What are the major reservoirs for yellow fever in urban areas? (A) Humans and non-human primates, (B) Aedes mosquitoes and marsupials, (C) Humans and Aedes mosquitoes, (D) Monkeys and forest mosquitoes

7. ( ) Which mosquito species is responsible for transmitting yellow fever in the sylvatic transmission cycle in eastern Africa? (A) *Ae. africanus*, (B) *Ae. aegypti*, (C) *Ae. bromeliae*, (D) Haemagogus mosquitoes

8. ( ) When is the blood of yellow fever patients infective for mosquitoes? (A) Shortly after the onset of fever, (B) During the first week of illness, (C) Throughout the entire illness, (D) Only after the first 3-5 days of illness

9. ( ) Which statement accurately describes the transmission of yellow fever? (A) It is highly communicable through contact with infected individuals, (B) It is communicable through common vehicles such as contaminated water or food, (C) It is highly communicable where susceptible people and abundant vector mosquitoes coexist, (D) It is primarily spread through direct contact with bodily fluids

10. ( ) What is the primary component of the yellow fever vaccine that provides long-lasting immunity? (A) Inactivated yellow fever virus, (B) Live, attenuated virus called 17D, (C) Antibiotics, (D) Antiviral drugs

II. Simple answer:

1. What percentage of patients with yellow fever enter a "toxic phase," according to the World Health Organization (WHO) factsheet?

2. Why can disease outbreaks in towns and among non-native people be more serious in the context of yellow fever?

3. In which regions is the sylvatic transmission cycle of yellow fever mainly limited to?

4. What is the primary mode of transmission in urban and certain rural areas where yellow fever occurs?

5. How long does the yellow fever vaccine, containing the 17D strain, provide immunity against the virus?

6. What is the recommended approach for the treatment of yellow fever, as there is no true cure for the disease?

7-4 Epidemic Louse-Borne Typhus Fever (ICD-9 080; ICD-10 A75)

 Highlight

1. Epidemic typhus also called jail fever, hospital fever, ship fever, famine fever, petechial fever, and louse-borne typhus

2. Louse-borne bacteria (*Rickettsia*)

3. *Rickettsia* is endemic in rodent hosts, including mice and rats, and spreads to humans through mites, fleas and body lice

4. *Rickettsia prowazekii*, transmitted by the human body louse *Pediculus humanus corporis*

5. Typhus fever which may reach 39°C

6. The mortality rate of epidemic louse-borne typhus fever is 10% to 60%

7. One attack of epidemic typhus usually confers long-lasting immunity

Typhus is any of several similar diseases caused by louse-borne bacteria. The name comes from the Greek *typhos*, meaning smoky or lazy, describing the state of mind of those affected with typhus. Louse-borne typhus has played a significant role in history, particularly during times of war and famine. It was responsible for outbreaks in crowded and unsanitary conditions, such as during World War I, World War II, and in concentration camps. One famous outbreak occurred in the Warsaw Ghetto during World War II. Louse-borne typhus has been nicknamed "war fever" due to its association with wartime suffering. *Rickettsia* is endemic in rodent hosts, including mice and rats, and spreads to humans through mites, fleas and body lice. The arthropod vector flourishes under conditions of poor hygiene, such as those found in prisons, concentration camps, or refugee camps, amongst the homeless, or until the middle of the 20th century, in armies in the field. In tropical countries, typhus is often mistaken for dengue fever.

Epidemic typhus also called jail fever, hospital fever, ship fever, famine fever, petechial fever, and louse-borne typhus is so named because the disease often causes epidemics following wars and natural disasters. The causative organism is *Rickettsia prowazekii*, transmitted by the human body louse *Pediculus humanus corporis*. Feeding on a human who carries the bacillus infects the louse. *R. prowazekii* grows in the louse's gut and is excreted in its feces. The disease is then transmitted to an uninfected human who scratches the louse bite (which itches) and rubs the feces into the wound. *R. prowazekii* can remain viable and virulent in the dried louse feces for many days. Typhus will eventually kill the louse, though the disease will remain viable for many weeks in the dead louse.

Identification to the epidemic louse-borne typhus fever:

Typhus fever is a rickettsial disease with variable onset; often sudden and marked by severe headache, a sustained high fever, cough, rash, severe muscle pain, chills, falling blood pressure, stupor, sensitivity to light, and delirium. A rash begins on the chest about five days after the fever appears, and spreads to the trunk and extremities but does not reach the palms and soles. The symptoms of louse-borne typhus include high fever (39°C), severe headache, weakness, muscle pain, and a rash. If left untreated, it can lead to complications such as pneumonia, gangrene, and central nervous system involvement.

The infection is treated with antibiotics. Intravenous fluids and oxygen may be needed to stabilize the patient. The mortality rate is 10% to 60%, but is vastly lower if antibiotics such as tetracycline are used early. Infection can also be prevented via vaccination. Brill-Zinsser disease is a mild form of epidemic typhus which recurs in someone after a long period of latency (similar to the relationship between chickenpox and shingles). This type of recurrence can also occur in immunosuppressed patients.

Infectious agent:

Rickettsia prowazekii is the bacterium responsible for louse-borne typhus. It is an obligate intracellular pathogen, meaning it can only replicate inside host cells, which transmitted by the human body louse *Pediculus humanus corporis*.

Occurrence:

In colder areas where people may live under unhygienic conditions and are infested with lice; explosive epidemics may occur during war and famine. Endemic foci exist in the mountainous regions of Mexico, in Central and South America, in central and eastern Africa and numerous countries of Asia. Recent outbreaks have been observed in Burundi and Rwanda. This rickettsia exists as a zoonosis of flying squirrels (*Glaucomys volans*) in the USA and there is serological evidence that humans have been infected from this source, possible via the squirrel flea. There were no cases of epidemic typhus fever in Taiwan so far (CDC, Taiwan, 2023).

Reservoir:

Man and or flying squirrels.

Mode of transmission:

The disease is not directly transmitted from person to person. The body louse, *Pediculus humanus corporis*, is infected by feeding on the blood of a patient with acute typhus fever. The disease is then transmitted to an uninfected human who scratches the louse bite (which itches) and rubs the feces into the wound or mucous membranes. *R. prowazekii* can remain viable and virulent in the dried louse feces for many days. Typhus will eventually kill the louse, though the disease will remain viable for many weeks in the dead louse.

Incubation period:

Incubation period is from 1 to 2 weeks, commonly 12 days.

Period of communicability:

Patients are infective for lice during the febrile illness and possibly for 2-3 days after the temperature returns to normal. Infected lice pass rickettsiae in their feces within 2-6 days after the blood-meal; they are infective earlier if crushed. The louse invariably dies within 2 weeks after infection; rickettsiae may remain viable in the dead louse for weeks.

🔘 Susceptibility and resistance:

Susceptibility is general. One attack usually confers long-lasting immunity.

🔘 Methods of control:

1. Apply an effective residual insecticide powder at appropriate intervals by hand or power blower to clothes and persons of populations living under conditions favoring louse infestation. The insecticide used should be effective on local lice.

2. Treat prophylactically those who are subject to risk, by application of residual insecticide to clothing.

3. Machine wash and dry infested clothing and bedding using the hot water laundry cycle and the high heat drying cycle.

4. A single dose of doxycycline 200 mg will normally cure patients. When faced with a seriously ill patient with possible typhus, suitable treatment should be started without waiting for laboratory confirmation.

👌 General review

1. Typhus fever is a rickettsial disease with variable onset; often sudden and marked by severe symptoms.

2. A symptom common to all forms of typhus is a fever which may reach 39°C.

3. The mortality rate of epidemic louse-borne typhus fever is 10% to 60%.

4. The infectious agent of typhus fever is *Rickettsia prowazekii*, which transmitted by the human body louse *Pediculus humanus corporis*.

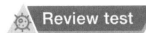

I. Multiple-choice questions (Four selected one):

1. (   ) What is the origin of the name "typhus"? (A) Latin word for fever, (B) Greek word meaning smoky or lazy, (C) Egyptian term for contagious disease, (D) Roman expression for wartime illness

2. (   ) Which vector is responsible for transmitting louse-borne typhus? (A) Mosquitoes, (B) Ticks, (C) Body lice, (D) Fleas

3. (   ) Why is louse-borne typhus referred to as "war fever"? (A) It primarily affects soldiers in peacetime, (B) It spreads rapidly in war-torn areas, (C) It is more common during times of peace, (D) It originated in military camps

4. (   ) What is a common complication of louse-borne typhus if left untreated? (A) Diabetes, (B) Pneumonia, (C) Migraines, (D) Arthritis

5. (   ) What is the mortality rate of typhus if treated early with antibiotics like tetracycline? (A) 80% to 90%, (B) 60% to 70%, (C) 30% to 40%, (D) 10% to 20%

6. (   ) What is a potential source of epidemic typhus in the USA, and how is it transmitted to humans? (A) Mosquitoes from swampy areas, (B) Flying squirrels, transmitted through their bites, (C) Direct person-to-person contact, (D) Contaminated water supply

7. (   ) Which region is mentioned as having endemic foci for typhus fever in the given passage? (A) Arctic regions, (B) Sub-Saharan Africa, (C) Southeast Asia, (D) Central and South America

8. (　) How is typhus fever not directly transmitted from person to person? (A) Through respiratory droplets, (B) Contact with infected blood, (C) Ingestion of contaminated food, (D) Person-to-person transmission does not occur

9. (　) How do infected lice pass rickettsiae, and when are they most infective? (A) Through bites, most infective when well-fed, (B) Through saliva, most infective during the first day of infection, (C) In their feces, most infective 2-6 days after the blood-meal, (D) Through direct contact, most infective when crushed

10. (　) What is the recommended control method for preventing louse infestation in populations living under favorable conditions? (A) Regular use of antiseptic lotions, (B) Wearing long-sleeved clothing, (C) Applying residual insecticide powder to clothes and persons, (D) Consuming prophylactic antibiotics

II. Simple answer:

1. How does *Rickettsia prowazekii*, the causative organism of louse-borne typhus, enter the human body?

2. Why is epidemic typhus also called by various names such as jail fever, hospital fever, and ship fever?

3. Describe Brill-Zinsser disease and its relationship to epidemic typhus.

4. What role does the body louse, *Pediculus humanus corporis*, play in the transmission of typhus fever?

5. Where have recent outbreaks of typhus fever been observed, according to the passage?

7-5 Plague (ICD-9 020; ICD-10 A20)

Highlight

1. Black Death, also known as The Black Plague, caused by bubonic plague
2. The sufferer's skin; subepidermal hemorrhages (purpura), and the extremities would darken with gangrene (acral necrosis)
3. Plague is a specific zoonosis involving rodents and their fleas
4. The septicaemic plague is a form of blood poisoning
5. Pneumonic plague
6. Bubonic plague
7. Bubonic plague was the most commonly seen form during the Black Death, with a mortality rate of 30-75%
8. Pneumonic plague was the second most commonly seen form during the Black Death, with a mortality rate of 90-95%
9. *Yersinia pestis*
10. Transmission may result in a domestic rat epizootic and flea-borne epidemics of bubonic plague
11. *Xenopsylla cheopis*
12. Pneumonic plague may be highly communicable

Black Death, also known as The Black Plague: the Eurasian pandemic thought to have been caused by bubonic plague, beginning in the 14th century with repeated outbreaks until the 18th century. The term "Black Death" was introduced for the first time in 1833. It is believed to have originated in Central Asia and spread along trade routes, reaching the Crimea and entering Europe through fleas infesting rats on merchant ships.

It has been popularly thought that the name came from a striking late-stage sign of the disease, in which the sufferer's skin would blacken due to subepidermal hemorrhages (purpura), and the extremities would darken with gangrene (acral necrosis).

The Black Death had a profound and catastrophic impact on European society. It's estimated to have killed between 75 million and 200 million people across Europe, Asia, and North Africa. The massive loss of life had significant social, economic, and cultural consequences, leading to labor shortages, changes in economic structures, and shifts in power dynamics.

Identification to the plague:

Plague is a specific zoonosis involving rodents and their fleas, which transfer the bacterial infection to various animals and to people. Plague, caused by *Yersinia pestis*, is naturally a flea-borne disease of rodents, and exists in many rural and wooded areas throughout the world.

The three forms of plague brought an array of signs and symptoms to those infected. The septicaemic plague is a form of blood poisoning, and pneumonic plague is an airborne plague that attacks the lungs before the rest of the body. The classic sign of bubonic plague was the appearance of buboes in the groin, the neck and armpits, which oozed pus and bled. These buboes were caused by internal bleeding. Victims underwent damage to the skin and underlying tissue, until they were covered in dark blotches. Most victims died within four to seven days after infection. When the plague reached Europe, it first struck port cities and then followed the trade routes, both by sea and land.

The bubonic plague was the most commonly seen form during the Black Death, with a mortality rate of thirty to seventy-five percent and symptoms including fever of 38-41 °C, headaches, painful aching joints, nausea and vomiting, and a general feeling of malaise. Of those who contracted the bubonic plague, 4 out of 5 died within eight days. Pneumonic plague was the second most commonly seen form during the Black Death, with a mortality rate of ninety to ninety-five percent. Symptoms included fever, cough and blood-tinged sputum. As the disease progressed, sputum became free flowing and bright red. Septicaemic plague was the least common of the three forms, with a mortality rate close to one hundred percent. Symptoms were high fevers and purple skin patches [purpura due to DIC (disseminated intravascular coagulation)].

Infectious agent:

Yersinia pestis, the plague bacillus. The bacteria are typically transmitted through the bite of infected fleas that live on small mammals, primarily rats.

Occurrence:

Plague continues to be a threat because of vast areas of persistant wild rodent infection; contact of wild rodents with domestic rats occurs frequently in some enzootic areas. Wild rodent plague exists in the western half of the USA; large areas of South America; central, eastern and southern Africa; central southwestern and southeastern Asia, and extreme southeastern Europe near the Caspian Sea. So far Taiwan has not the case report these years (CDC, Taiwan, 2023).

Reservoir:

Wild rodents (especially ground squirrels) are the natural vertebrate reservoirs and domestic cats may also be a source of infection to people.

Mode of transmission:

Naturally acquired plague in people occurs as a result of human intrusion into the zoonotic cycle during or following an epizootic, or by the entry of sylvatic rodents or their infected fleas into human habitat; infection in commensal rodents and their fleas may result in a domestic rat epizootic and flea-borne epidemics of bubonic plague.

The most frequent source of exposure that in human disease of worldwide, were has been the bite of infected fleas (especially *Xenopsylla cheopis*, the oriental rat flea).

Incubation period:

From 1 to 7 days; may be a few days longer in those immunized who develop illness. For primary plague pneumonia are probably 1-4 days, usually short.

Period of communicability:

Fleas may remain infective for months under suitable conditions of temperature and humidity. Bubonic plague is not usually transmitted directly unless there is contact with pus from suppurating buboes.

Pneumonic plague may be highly communicable under appropriate climatic conditions; overcrowding facilitates transmission.

Susceptibility and resistance:

Susceptibility is general. Immunity after recovery is relative; it may not protect against a large inoculum.

▶ Methods of control:

1. Educate the public in enzootic areas on the modes of human and domestic animal exposure; on rat-proofing buildings, preventing access to food and shelter by peridomestic rodents through appropriate storage and disposal of food garbage and refuse; and the importance of avoiding flea bites by use of insecticides and repellents.

2. Survey rodent populations periodically to determine the effectiveness of sanitary programs and to evaluate the potential for epizootic plague.

3. Active immunization with a vaccine of killed bacteria confers some protection against bubonic plague in most recipients if administered in a primary series of 3 doses with doses 1 and 2 given 1-3 months apart followed by dose 3 after 5-6 months; booster injections are necessary every 6 months if high risk exposure continues.

4. Report to local health authority: case report of suspected and confirmed cases universally required by International Health Regulations, Class 1.

৬ General review

1. Plague is a specific zoonosis involving rodents and their fleas, which transfer the bacterial infection to various animals and to people.

2. The bubonic plague was the most commonly seen form during the Black Death, with a mortality rate of 30% to 75%.

3. Pneumonic plague was the second most commonly seen form during the Black Death, with a mortality rate of 90% to 95%.

4. Septicaemic plague was the least common of the three forms, with a mortality rate close to one hundred percent.

5. *Yersinia pestis*

6. *Xenopsylla cheopis*

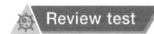 Review test

SCAN ME

Check Your Answers

I. Multiple-choice questions (Four selected one):

1. (　) What is believed to be the origin of the Black Death? (A) South America, (B) Central Asia, (C) Europe, (D) North Africa

2. (　) How did the Black Death likely enter Europe? (A) Through contaminated water sources, (B) Airborne transmission, (C) Fleas infesting rats on merchant ships, (D) Human-to-human contact

3. (　) What is the primary vector for the transmission of plague? (A) Mosquitoes, (B) Ticks, (C) Fleas, (D) Lice

4. (　) Which form of plague attacks the lungs before affecting the rest of the body? (A) Bubonic plague, (B) Septicaemic plague, (C) Pneumonic plague, (D) Hemorrhagic plague

5. (　) What classic sign was associated with bubonic plague during the Black Death? (A) Rash on the face, (B) Dark blotches on the skin, (C) Persistent cough, (D) Enlarged spleen

6. (　) Which form of plague had the highest mortality rate during the Black Death? (A) Bubonic plague, (B) Septicaemic plague, (C) Pneumonic plague, (D) Hemorrhagic plague

7. (　) How is *Yersinia pestis*, the plague bacillus, typically transmitted to humans? (A) Airborne transmission, (B) Direct contact with infected humans, (C) Through contaminated water, (D) Bite of infected fleas

8. ( ) Which of the following regions is mentioned as having wild rodent plague? (A) North America only, (B) Western Europe, (C) Southeast Asia, (D) Central and eastern Africa

9. ( ) How does naturally acquired plague in people typically occur? (A) Through airborne transmission, (B) Human-to-human contact, (C) Intrusion into the zoonotic cycle, (D) Consumption of contaminated water

10. ( ) What is the most frequent source of exposure leading to human plague worldwide? (A) Airborne pathogens, (B) Contaminated food, (C) Bite of infected fleas, especially *Xenopsylla cheopis*, (D) Direct contact with infected rodents

11. ( ) Under what conditions may pneumonic plague be highly communicable? (A) Low humidity, (B) Overcrowding, (C) Cold temperatures, (D) Isolation of infected individuals

II. Simple answer:

1. Describe one significant impact of the Black Death on European society.

2. Describe the mortality rate and symptoms of the bubonic plague during the Black Death.

3. What routes did the plague follow when it reached Europe during the Black Death?

4. What are the natural vertebrate reservoirs for *Yersinia pestis*, and what other animal is mentioned as a potential source of infection to humans?

5. What is the incubation period for naturally acquired plague in humans, and how long can fleas remain infective under suitable conditions?

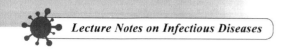

6. How is bubonic plague usually transmitted, and under what circumstances may pneumonic plague be highly communicable?

7-6 Leishmaniasis (ICD-9 085.0; ICD-10 B55.0)

 Highlight

1. Leishmaniasis is a disease caused by protozoan parasites (*Leishmania* spp.)
2. Sand fly (*Lutzomyia* and *Phlebotomus*)
3. Visceral leishmaniasis
4. Cutaneous leishmaniasis
5. *Leishmania donovani, L. infantum* and *L. Infantum/chagasi*
6. The sandflies inject the infective stage, metacyclic promastigotes, during blood meals

Leishmaniasis is a disease caused by protozoan parasites that belong to the genus *Leishmania* and is transmitted by the bite of certain species of sand fly, including flies in the genus *Lutzomyia* in the New World and *Phlebotomus* in the Old World. The disease was named in 1901 for the Scottish pathologist William Boog Leishman. This disease is also known as Leichmaniosis, Leishmaniose, leishmaniose, and formerly, Orient Boils, Baghdad Boil, kala azar, black fever, sandfly disease, Dum-Dum fever or espundia. Leishmaniasis is found in parts of the tropics, subtropics, and southern Europe. Different species of Leishmania are associated with specific geographic regions.

🔹 Identification to the leishmaniasis:

The symptoms of leishmaniasis are skin sores which erupt weeks to months after the person affected is bitten by sand flies. Other consequences, which can become manifest anywhere from a few months to years after infection, include skin sores, ulcers, fever, weight loss, anaemia, and enlarged spleen and liver in the case of visceral leishmaniasis.

In the medical field, leishmaniasis is one of the famous causes of a markedly enlarged spleen, which may become larger even than the liver. There are four main forms of leishmaniasis:

1. Visceral leishmaniasis; the most serious form and potentially fatal if untreated.

2. Cutaneous leishmaniasis; the most common form which causes a sore at the bite site, which heal in a few months to a year, leaving an unpleasant looking scar. This form can progress to any of the other three forms.

3. Diffuse cutaneous leishmaniasis; this form produces widespread skin lesions which resemble leprosy and is particularly difficult to treat.

4. Mucocutaneous leishmaniasis; commences with skin ulcers which spread causing tissue damage to (particularly) nose and mouth.

🔹 Infectious agents:

Typically, *Leishmania donovani*, *L. infantum* and *L. Infantum/chagasi*. The parasites responsible for Leishmaniasis primarily infect macrophages, which are a type of immune system cell.

🔹 Occurrence:

Leishmaniasis can be transmitted in many tropical and sub-tropical countries and is found in parts of about 88 countries. Approximately 350 million people live in these areas. The settings in which leishmaniasis is found range from rainforests in Central and South America to deserts in West Asia. More than 90 percent of the world's cases of visceral leishmaniasis are in India, Bangladesh, Nepal, Sudan, and Brazil.

Leishmaniasis is commonly found in Mexico, Central America, and South America—from northern Argentina to southern Texas (not in Uruguay, Chile, or Canada), southern Europe (leishmaniasis is not common in travelers to southern Europe), Asia (not Southeast Asia), the Middle East, and Africa (particularly East and North Africa, with some cases elsewhere). It has recently been shown to be spreading to North Texas. The disease is not found in Australia, Oceania or Taiwan.

Incidence is modified by the use of antimalarial insecticides. Where dog populations have been drastically reduced (e.g. China), human disease has also been reduced.

▶ Reservoir:

Man, wild Canidae and domestic dogs.

▶ Mode of transmission:

Leishmaniasis is transmitted by the bite of female phlebotomine sandflies.

The sandflies inject the infective stage, metacyclic promastigotes, during blood meals. Metacyclic promastigotes that reach the puncture wound are phagocytized by macrophages and transform into amastigotes. Amastigotes multiply in infected cells and affect different tissues, depending in part on which *Leishmania* species is involved. These differing tissue specificities cause the differing clinical manifestations of the various forms of leishmaniasis. Sandflies become infected during blood meals on an infected host when they ingest macrophages infected with amastigotes. In the sandfly's midgut, the parasites differentiate into promastigotes, which multiply, differentiate into metacyclic promastigotes and migrate to the proboscis.

Co-infected patients infect sandflies, acting as human reservoirs even in zoonotic foci.

Incubation period:

Generally, 2-6 months; range is 10 days to years.

Period of communicability:

Not usually transmitted from person to person, but infectious to sandflies as long as parasites persist in the circulating blood ar skin of the mammalian reservoir host. Infectivity for phlebotomines may persist after clinical recovery of human patients.

Susceptibility and resistance:

Susceptibility is general. Kala-azar apparently induces lasting homologous immunity. Evidence indicates that asymptomatic and subclinical infections are common, and that malnutrition predisposes to clinical disease and activation of inapparent infections.

Methods of control:

Prevention strategies include avoiding sandfly bites through the use of insect repellents, wearing long-sleeved clothing, and bed nets. Controlling sandfly populations in endemic areas is also a preventive measure.

There are two common therapies containing antimony (known as pentavalent antimonials), meglumine antimoniate (*Glucantime*) and sodium stibogluconate (*Pentostam*). It is not completely understood how these drugs act against the parasite; they may disrupt its energy production or trypanothione metabolism. Unfortunately, in many parts of the world, the parasite has become resistant to antimony and for visceral or mucocutaneous leishmaniasis, but the level of resistance varies according to species.

General review

1. Leishmaniasis is a disease caused by protozoan; Leishmania spp., and is transmitted by the bite of certain species of sand fly; *Lutzomyia* sp. or *Phlebotomus* sp.

2. Visceral leishmaniasis is the most serious form and potentially fatal if untreated.

3. Cutaneous leishmaniasis is the most common form which causes a sore at the bite site, this form can progress to any of the other three forms.

4. Diffuse cutaneous leishmaniasis; this form produces widespread skin lesions which resemble leprosy and is particularly difficult to treat.

5. Mucocutaneous leishmaniasis is commences with skin ulcers which spread causing tissue damage to nose and mouth.

6. The infectious agents of leishmaniasis are *Leishmania donovani*, *L. infantum* and *L. Infantum/chagasi*.

7. Leishmaniasis is transmitted by the bite of female phlebotomine sandflies. The sandflies inject the infective stage, metacyclic promastigotes, during blood meals.

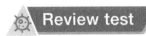

Review test

I. Multiple-choice questions (Four selected one):

1. (   ) What is the most serious and potentially fatal form of leishmaniasis if left untreated? (A) Cutaneous leishmaniasis, (B) Diffuse cutaneous leishmaniasis, (C) Mucocutaneous leishmaniasis, (D) Visceral leishmaniasis

2. (   ) Which form of leishmaniasis is characterized by skin sores at the bite site that may heal in a few months to a year, leaving a scar? (A) Diffuse cutaneous leishmaniasis, (B) Visceral leishmaniasis, (C) Mucocutaneous leishmaniasis, (D) Cutaneous leishmaniasis

3. (   ) Which type of leishmaniasis produces widespread skin lesions resembling leprosy and is particularly challenging to treat? (A) Visceral leishmaniasis, (B) Cutaneous leishmaniasis, (C) Diffuse cutaneous leishmaniasis, (D) Mucocutaneous leishmaniasis

4. (   ) Which of the following is a common infectious agent responsible for Leishmaniasis? (A) *Plasmodium falciparum*, (B) *Trypanosoma cruzi*, (C) *Leishmania donovani*, (D) *Toxoplasma gondii*

5. (   ) In which regions of the world is Leishmaniasis commonly found? (A) Australia, Oceania, and Taiwan, (B) Southeast Asia and Canada, (C) Southern Europe, Asia, and North Texas, (D) Central and South America, Africa, and the Middle East

6. (   ) What is the primary cell type that Leishmania parasites infect in the human immune system? (A) T cells, (B) B cells, (C) Macrophages, (D) Natural killer cells

7. (　) How is Leishmaniasis primarily transmitted to humans? (A) Through contaminated water, (B) By direct contact with an infected person, (C) Via the bite of female mosquitoes, (D) Through the bite of female phlebotomine sandflies

8. (　) What is the infective stage injected by sandflies during blood meals, leading to the transmission of Leishmaniasis? (A) Amastigotes, (B) Promastigotes, (C) Metacyclic promastigotes, (D) Trophozoites

9. (　) What is the primary reservoir host for Leishmaniasis, where the infectiousness to sandflies persists as long as parasites are present in the circulating blood or skin? (A) Humans, (B) Rodents, (C) Mosquitoes, (D) Birds

10. (　) Which of the following statements about Kala-azar is true? (A) It results in permanent immunity, (B) It is highly contagious between humans, (C) Asymptomatic infections are rare, (D) Susceptibility is limited to specific age groups

II. Simple answer:

1. Please describe the progression of mucocutaneous leishmaniasis.

2. What are the common symptoms of leishmaniasis that may become manifest anywhere from a few months to years after infection?

3. Please describe the role of co-infected patients in the transmission of Leishmaniasis.

4. What conditions are suggested to predispose individuals to clinical disease and activate inapparent infections of Leishmaniasis?

7-7 Lyme Disease
(ICD-9 104.8, 088.81; ICD-10 A69.2, L90.4)

 Highlight

1. Lyme disease is a tick-borne, spirochaetal, zoonotic disease
2. Lyme disease, or borreliosis, is an emerging infectious disease caused by *Borrelia* spp.
3. *Borrelia burgdorferi*
4. The acute phase of Lyme disease is a characteristic reddish "bull's-eye" rash
5. Initial infection occurs primarily during summer, with a peak in June and July
6. The majority of Lyme cases result from bites by infected tick nymphs

Lyme disease, or borreliosis, is an emerging infectious disease caused by at least three species of bacteria from the genus *Borrelia*. Infection is acquired from the bite of hard ticks belonging to several species of the genus *Ixodes*. *Borrelia burgdorferi* is the predominant cause of Lyme disease in the U.S., whereas *Borrelia afzelii* and *Borrelia garinii* are implicated in most European cases. In Taiwan, Lyme disease is a Category 4 notifiable infectious disease. Since the notification of data in 2003, no local cases have been found. They are all imported cases (CDC, Taiwan, 2023) (Fig. 7-5).

The disease presentation varies widely and may include a rash and flu-like symptoms in its initial stage, then musculoskeletal, arthritic, neurologic, psychiatric and cardiac manifestations. In a majority of cases, symptoms can be eliminated with antibiotics, especially if treatment begins early in the course of illness. Late or inadequate treatment can lead to "late stage" Lyme disease that can be disabling and difficult to treat. Controversy over diagnosis, testing and treatment has led to two different standards of care.

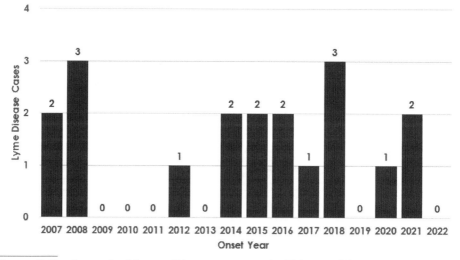

Figure 7-5   Imported Lyme Disease cases in Taiwan, 2007-2022 (CDC, Taiwan, 2023).
(https://www.cdc.gov.tw/En/Category/ListContent/bg0g_VU_ Ysrgkes_KRUDgQ?uaid=vndcitM-OsellT--HH3x1A)

Identification to the Lyme disease:

Lyme disease is a tick-borne, spirochaetal, zoonotic disease characterized by a distinctive skin lesion, systemic symptoms and neurological, rheumatological and cardiac involvement occurring in varying combinations over months to years. The acute phase of Lyme disease infection is a characteristic reddish "bull's-eye" rash, with accompanying fever, malaise, and arthralgia or myalgia. The characteristic reddish "bull's-eye" rash (known as *erythema migrans*) may be seen in about 80% of early stage Lyme disease patients, appearing anywhere from one day to a month after a tick bite. The rash does not represent an allergic reaction to the bite, but a skin infection causes by the Lyme bacteria.

Cases may progress to a chronic form most commonly characterized by meningoencephalitis, (myocarditis, and frank arthritis. It should be noted, however, that chronic Lyme disease can have a multitude of symptoms affecting numerous physiological systems: the symptoms appear heterogeneous in the affected population, which may be due to innate immunity or variations in *Borrelia* bacteria. Late symptoms of Lyme disease can appear months or years after initial infection and often progress in cumulative fashion over time. Neuropsychiatric symptoms often develop much later in the disease progression, much like tertiary neurosyphilis.

In addition to the acute symptoms, chronic Lyme disease can be manifested by a wide-range of neurological disorders, either central or peripheral, including encephalitis or encephalomyelitis, muscle twitching, polyneuropathy or paresthesia, and vestibular symptoms or other otolaryngologic symptoms, among others. Neuropsychiatric disturbances can occur, which may lead to symptoms of memory loss, sleep disturbances, or changes in mood or affect.

🔅 Infectious agents:

Lyme disease is caused by Gram-negative spirochetal bacteria from the genus *Borrelia*. At least 37 *Borrelia* species have been described, 12 of which are Lyme related. The *Borrelia* species known to cause Lyme disease are collectively known as *Borrelia burgdorferi* sensu lato, and have been found to have greater strain diversity than previously estimated.

Recently it was thought that only three genospecies caused Lyme disease: *B. burgdorferi* sensu stricto (predominant in North America, but also in Europe), *B. afzelii*, and *B. garinii* (both predominant in Eurasia).

▣ Occurrence:

Lyme disease is the most common tick-borne disease in North America and Europe, and one of the fastest-growing infectious diseases in the United States. Of cases reported to the United States Center for Disease Control (CDC), the ratio of Lyme disease infection is 7.9 cases for every 100,000 persons. In the ten states where Lyme disease is most common, the average was 31.6 cases for every 100,000 persons for the year 2005. Urbanization and other anthropogenic factors can be implicated in the spread of the Lyme disease into the human population. In many areas, expansion of suburban neighborhoods has led to the gradual deforestation of surrounding wooded areas and increasing "border" contact between humans and tick-dense areas. Human expansion has also resulted in a gradual reduction of the predators that normally hunt deer as well as mice, chipmunks and other small rodents, the primary reservoirs for Lyme disease.

As a consequence of increased human contact with host and vector, the likelihood of transmission to Lyme residents has greatly increased. Researchers are also investigating possible links between global warming and the spread of vector-borne diseases including Lyme disease. The deer tick (*Ixodes scapularis*, the primary vector in the northeastern U.S.) has a two-year life cycle, first progressing from larva to nymph, and then from nymph to adult. The tick feeds only once at each stage. In the fall, large acorn forests attract deer as well as mice, chipmunks and other small rodents infected with *B. burgdorferi*. During the following spring, the ticks lay their eggs. Tick eggs hatch into larvae, which feed on the rodents; thus the larvae acquire infection from the rodents. (Note: At this stage, it is proposed that tick infestation may be controlled using acaricides). Adult ticks may also transmit disease to humans. After feeding, female adult ticks lay their eggs on the ground, and the cycle is complete. On the west coast, Lyme disease is spread by the western black-legged tick (*Ixodes pacificus*), which has a different life cycle.

Initial infection occurs primarily during summer, with a peak in June and July, but may occur throughout the year, depending on the seasonal abundance of the tick locally. There has been an increase in reported cases of Lyme disease in various parts of the world, possibly due to factors such as changes in land use, climate, and human behavior. Increased awareness and improved diagnostic methods may also contribute to the rise in reported cases.

Reservoir:

Certain ixodid ticks through transstadial transmission. Wild rodents, especially *Peromyscus* spp. in the nertheastern and midwestern USA and *Neotoma* spp. in the western USA maintains the enzootic transmission cycle. Deer serves as important mammalian maintenance hosts for vector tick species. The majority of Lyme disease cases result from bites by infected nymphs.

Mode of transmission:

Hard ticks of the genus *Ixodes* are the primary vectors of Lyme disease. The majority of infections are caused by ticks in the nymph stage, as adult ticks are more easily detected and removed as a consequence of their relatively large size. In experimental animals, transmission by *Ixodes scapularis* and *Ixodes pacificus* usually dose not occur until the tick has been attached for 24 hours or more; this may also be true in humans.

In Europe, the commonly known sheep tick, castor bean tick, or European castor bean tick (*Ixodes ricinus*) is the transmitter. In North America, the black-legged tick or deer tick (*Ixodes scapularis*) has been identified as the key to the disease's spread on the east coast. Tick bites often go unnoticed due to the small size of the tick in its nymphal stage, as well as tick secretions that prevent the host from feeling any itch or pain from the bite.

On the west coast, the primary vector is the western black-legged tick (*Ixodes pacificus*). The preponderance of this tick species to feed on host species that are resistant to Borrelia infection appears to diminish transmission of Lyme disease in the West. While Lyme spirochetes have been found in insects other than ticks, reports of actual infectious transmission appear to be rare. Sexual transmission has been anecdotally reported; Lyme spirochetes have been found in semen and breast milk, however transmission of the spirochete by these routes is not known to occur.

Incubation period:

For erythema chronicum migrans (ECM or EM), 3 to 32 days after tick exposure, range is 7 to 10 days.

Period of communicability:

No evidence of natural person to person transmission.

Susceptibility and resistance:

Susceptibility is general. Re-infection has occurred in those treated with antibiotics for early disease.

Methods of control:

Attached ticks should be removed promptly. Protective clothing includes a hat and long-sleeved shirts and long pants that are tucked into socks or boots. Also, light-colored clothing makes the tick more easily visible before it attaches itself. A more effective, community wide method of preventing

Lyme disease is to reduce the numbers of primary hosts on which the deer tick depends such as rodents, other small mammals, and deer. By reducing the deer population back to healthy levels of 8 to 10 per square mile (from the current levels of 60 or more deer per square mile in the areas of the country with the highest Lyme disease rates) the tick numbers can be brought down to very low levels, too few to spread Lyme and other tick-borne diseases.

Antibiotics are the primary treatment for Lyme disease, but the most appropriate antibiotic treatment varies from patient to patient and with the stage of the disease. The antibiotics of choice are doxycycline (in adults), amoxicillin (in children) and ceftriaxone. Alternative choices are cefuroxime and cefotaxime. Macrolide antibiotics have limited efficacy when used alone. Many physicians who treat chronic Lyme disease have noted that combining a macrolide antibiotic such as clarithromycin (biaxin) with hydroxychloroquine (plaquenil) is especially effective in treatment of chronic Lyme disease. New vaccines are being researched using outer surface protein C (OspC) and glycolipoprotein as methods of immunization.

General review

1. Lyme disease, or borreliosis, is an emerging infectious disease caused by at least three species of bacteria from the genus *Borrelia*.

2. Lyme disease is a tick-borne, spirochaetal, zoonotic disease.

3. *Borrelia burgdorferi* is the predominant cause of Lyme disease in the U.S.

4. The acute phase of Lyme disease infection is a characteristic reddish "bull's-eye" rash, with accompanying fever, malaise, and arthralgia or myalgia.

5. Lyme disease is the most common tick-borne disease in North America, Europe and U.S.

6. Deer serve as important mammalian maintenance hosts for vector tick species. The majority of Lyme disease cases result from bites by infected nymphs.

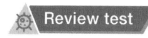 Review test

SCAN ME

Check Your Answers

I. Multiple-choice questions (Four selected one):

1. (   ) What is the predominant cause of Lyme disease in the United States? (A) *Borrelia afzelii*, (B) *Borrelia burgdorferi*, (C) *Borrelia garinii*, (D) *Ixodes scapularis*

2. (   ) Which of the following symptoms is NOT commonly associated with the initial stage of Lyme disease? (A) Rash, (B) Flu-like symptoms, (C) Joint pain, (D) Neurological manifestations

3. (   ) In Taiwan, Lyme disease is categorized as: (A) Category 1, (B) Category 2, (C) Category 3, (D) Category 4

4. (   ) What is the characteristic skin lesion associated with the acute phase of Lyme disease? (A) Maculopapular rash, (B) Vesicular rash, (C) Eczematous rash, (D) "Bull's-eye" rash (erythema migrans)

5. (   ) Late symptoms of Lyme disease, which can appear months or years after initial infection, often progress in a cumulative fashion and may include: (A) Respiratory symptoms, (B) Gastrointestinal symptoms, (C) Neuropsychiatric symptoms, (D) Dermatological symptoms

6. (   ) Chronic Lyme disease can manifest as various neurological disorders, including: (A) Hypertension, (B) Gait disturbances, (C) Visual disturbances, (D) All of the above

7. (   ) Which Borrelia species is predominant in North America and Europe, causing Lyme disease? (A) *Borrelia afzelii*, (B) *Borrelia garinii*, (C) *Borrelia burgdorferi* (*sensu stricto*), (D) *Borrelia hermsii*

8. (   ) What is the primary vector of Lyme disease in the northeastern U.S.? (A) *Ixodes pacificus*, (B) *Ixodes scapularis*, (C) *Amblyomma americanum*, (D) *Dermacentor variabilis*

9. (   ) In what season does the initial infection of Lyme disease primarily occur, with a peak? (A) Fall, (B) Winter, (C) Spring, (D) Summer

10. (   ) Why are nymph stage ticks considered the primary vectors for Lyme disease? (A) They are more resistant to Borrelia infection, (B) They are more easily detected and removed, (C) They have a larger size, (D) They do not secrete substances preventing the host from feeling the bite.

11. (   ) What is a recommended method for preventing Lyme disease through clothing? (A) Wear dark-colored clothing, (B) Wear short-sleeved shirts and shorts, (C) Wear light-colored clothing, (D) Wear heavy jackets

12. (   ) What is a community-wide method mentioned to reduce the incidence of Lyme disease? (A) Increase the deer population, (B) Reduce the number of rodents, (C) Encourage tick habitats, (D) Promote tick attachment

II. Simple answer:

1. What are the potential consequences of late or inadequate treatment of Lyme disease?

2. What is the characteristic appearance of the rash in early-stage Lyme disease, and what does it signify?

3. What is the collective term for the Borrelia species known to cause Lyme disease, and how many genospecies were initially thought to cause Lyme disease?

4. What are some recommended protective measures for avoiding tick bites, especially in tick-prone areas?

7-8 Japanese Encephalitis
(ICD-9 062; ICD-10 A83.0)

😳 Highlight

1. Japanese encephalitis
2. This disease is most prevalent in Southeast Asia and the Far East
3. Domestic pigs and wild birds are reservoirs of the virus
4. *Culex tritaeniorhynchus*
5. The case fatality rates are from 0.3% to 60%
6. Swine; amplifying host and has very important role in epidemiology of the disease
7. Infection with JEV confers life-long immunity
8. All current vaccines are based on the genotype III virus.
9. A formalin-inactivated mouse-brain derived vaccine was first produced in Japan in the 1930s and was validated for use in Taiwan in the 1960s.

Japanese encephalitis is transmitted to humans via the bite of infected mosquitoes. Japanese encephalitis virus (JEV) is a flaviviral (single-stranded RNA) neurologic infection closely related to St. Louis encephalitis and West Nile virus. The disease is spread throughout mostly rural areas of Asia by culicine mosquitoes. It is the most common form of viral encephalitis in Asia. Approximately 3 billion people currently live in areas endemic for Japanese encephalitis; these areas extend from Pakistan to maritime Siberia and Japan.

Japanese encephalitis (JE) previously known as Japanese B encephalitis to distinguish it from von Economo's A encephalitis, which is a disease caused by the mosquito-borne Japanese encephalitis virus. The Japanese encephalitis virus is a virus from the family Flaviviridae. Domestic pigs and wild birds are reservoirs of the virus; transmission to humans may cause severe symptoms. One of the most important vectors of this disease is the mosquito *Culex tritaeniorhynchus*. This disease is most prevalent in Southeast Asia and the Far East.

▣ Identification to the Japanese encephalitis:

The vast majority of Japanese encephalitis infections are asymptomatic: only 1 in 250 infections develop into encephalitis. Severe rigors mark the onset of this disease in humans. Fever, headache and malaise are other non-specific symptoms of this disease which may last for a period of between 1 and 6 days. Signs which develop during the acute encephalitic stage include neck rigidity, cachexia, hemiparesis, convulsions and a raised body temperature between 38-41°C. Mental retardation developed from this disease usually leads to coma. Mortality of this disease varies but is generally much higher in children. Transplacental spread has been noted. Life-long neurological defects such as deafness, emotional lability and hemiparesis may occur in those who have had central nervous system involvement. In known cases some effects also include, nausea, headache, fever,vomiting and sometimes swelling of the testicles.

The case fatality rates of Japanese encephalitis are from 0.3% to 60%. Neurological sequelae occur with variable frequency depending on age and infecting agent; they tend to be most severe in infants infected with JE.

Infectious agent:

The causative agent Japanese encephalitis virus is an enveloped virus of the genus flavivirus; it is closely related to the West Nile virus and St. Louis encephalitis virus. Positive sense single stranded RNA genome is packaged in the capsid, formed by the capsid protein.

Occurrence:

Japanese encephalitis is the leading cause of viral encephalitis in Asia, with 30,000–50,000 cases reported annually. Case-fatality rates range from 0.3% to 60% and depends on the population and on age. Rare outbreaks in U.S. territories in Western Pacific have occurred. Residents of rural areas in endemic locations are at highest risk; Japanese encephalitis does not usually occur in urban areas. Countries which have had major epidemics in the past, but which have controlled the disease primarily by vaccination, include China, Korea, Japan, Taiwan and Thailand. It is most common in rural and agricultural areas where rice paddies provide a suitable environment for the mosquito vectors. Since the national vaccination program was implementing in 1968, there are now around 20 to 30 sporadic JE cases annually in Taiwan (Fig. 7-6).

Other countries that still have periodic epidemics include Vietnam, Cambodia, Myanmar, India, Nepal, and Malaysia. Japanese encephalitis has been reported on the Torres Strait Islands and two fatal cases were reported in mainland northern Australia in 1998. The spread of the virus in Australia is of particular concern to Australian health officials due to the unplanned introduction of *Culex gelidus*, a potential vector of the virus, from Asia.

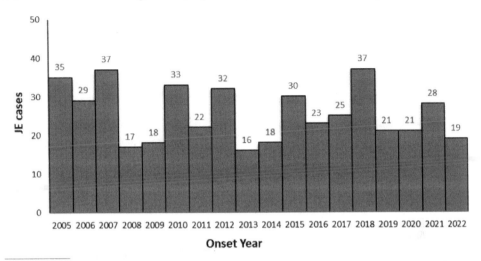

Figure 7-6   Japanese Encephalitis cases in Taiwan, 2005-2022 (CDC, Taiwan, 2023).
(https://www.cdc.gov.tw/En/Category/ListContent/bg0g_VU_
Ysrgkes_KRUDgQ?uaid=FCBms2B8k0PJx4io35AsOw)

🐷 Reservoir:

Swine play as amplifying host and has very important role in epidemiology of the disease. Infection in swine is asymptomatic, except in pregnant sows, when abortion and fetal abnormalities are common sequelae.

The most important vector is *C. tritaeniorhynchus*, which feeds on cattle in preference to humans; it has been proposed that moving swine away from human habitation can divert the mosquito away from humans and swine. The natural host of the Japanese encephalitis virus is bird, not human, and the virus will therefore never be completely eliminated.

Mode of transmission:

The virus is transmitted through the bite of infected mosquitoes, with pigs and birds serving as amplifying hosts. Humans are incidental hosts and do not play a significant role in the transmission cycle. Bite of infective mosquitoes; *Culex tritaeniorhynchus*, *C. vishnui* complex and in the tropics, *C. gelidus*.

Incubation period:

Incubation period is usually 5-15 days.

Period of communicability:

No evidence of natural person to person transmission. Virus is not usually demonstrable in human blood after onset of disease. Mosquitoes remain infective for life. Swine acts as amplifying host and has very important role in epidemiology of the disease. Viraemia in birds usually lasts 2-5 days but may be prolonged in bats, reptiles and amphibia, particulary if interrupted by hiberation.

Susceptibility and resistance:

Susceptibility to clinical disease is usually highest in infancy and old age; inapparent or undiagnosed infection is more common at other ages. Infection results in homologous immunity.

Infection with JEV confers life-long immunity. All current vaccines are based on the genotype III virus. A formalin-inactivated mouse-brain derived vaccine was first produced in Japan in the 1930s and was validated for use in Taiwan in the 1960s and in Thailand in the 1980s. The widespread use of vaccine and urbanisation has led to control of the disease in Japan, Korea, Taiwan and Singapore. The high cost of the vaccine, which is grown in live mice, means that poorer countries have not been able to afford to give it as part of a routine immunisation programme. Vaccination is the most effective way to prevent Japanese encephalitis. The vaccine is recommended for travelers to areas where the disease is endemic and for individuals living in or visiting areas with a high risk of transmission.

Methods of control:

Controlling Japanese encephalitis involves a combination of vaccination, mosquito control measures, and public health strategies. Here are some key control methods:

1. **Routine Vaccination**: Implementing routine vaccination programs in areas where Japanese encephalitis is endemic is a primary control measure. Vaccination is particularly important for individuals at high risk of exposure, such as those living in or traveling to affected regions.

2. **Livestock Vaccination**: Since pigs can serve as amplifying hosts for the virus, vaccinating pigs in areas with a high risk of Japanese encephalitis transmission can help reduce the reservoir of the virus.

3. **Mosquito Control:**

   - Vector Surveillance: Monitoring and studying the mosquito population, especially the Culex species that transmit the virus, can help assess the risk of Japanese encephalitis transmission in a given area.

   - Insecticide Use: Application of insecticides to kill mosquito larvae in breeding sites, such as rice paddies and other standing water sources, can be an effective method of controlling mosquito populations.

   - Bed Nets and Protective Clothing: Encouraging the use of bed nets treated with insecticides and the wearing of long-sleeved clothing can help prevent mosquito bites.

⚗ General review

1. Japanese encephalitis (JE) is a disease caused by the mosquito-borne Japanese encephalitis virus.

2. Domestic pigs and wild birds are reservoirs of the virus; transmission to humans may cause severe symptoms.

3. Swine play as amplifying host and has very important role in epidemiology of the disease.

4. The case fatality rates of Japanese encephalitis are from 0.3% to 60%.

5. Japanese encephalitis is transmitted by infected mosquitoes (*Culex tritaeniorhynchus, Culex vishnui* complex and in the tropics, *Culex gelidus*) bites.

6. Japanese encephalitis vaccine: Live attenuated vaccine (SA 14-14-2 strain). In Taiwan, toddlers reaching 15 months of age should receive the first dose of Japanese encephalitis vaccine and the second dose should be taken after 12 months additionally.

7. Inactivated, Vero cell-derived, alum-adjuvanted vaccine (SA 14- 14-2 strain). Primary immunization consists of two intramuscular doses, 4 weeks apart. A booster is recommended after 1 year.

SCAN ME

Check Your Answers

⚙ Review test

I. Multiple-choice questions (Four selected one):

1. (   ) What is the primary mode of transmission of Japanese encephalitis to humans? (A) Direct contact with infected individuals, (B) Consumption of contaminated food and water, (C) Infected mosquitoes' bites, (D) Airborne droplets from coughing and sneezing

2. ( ) Which family does the Japanese encephalitis virus (JEV) belong to? (A) Retroviridae, (B) Flaviviridae, (C) Orthomyxoviridae, (D) Paramyxoviridae

3. ( ) What is a common early symptom marking the onset of Japanese encephalitis in humans? (A) Skin rash, (B) Severe rigors, (C) Joint pain, (D) Respiratory distress

4. ( ) Which demographic group tends to have a higher mortality rate from Japanese encephalitis? (A) Adults, (B) Elderly individuals, (C) Adolescents, (D) Children

5. ( ) What is the primary vector of the Japanese encephalitis virus? (A) *Aedes aegypti*, (B) Anopheles mosquito, (C) *Culex tritaeniorhynchus*, (D) Simulium blackfly

6. ( ) Which of the following countries has controlled Japanese encephalitis primarily by vaccination? (A) Indonesia, (B) Australia, (C) Thailand, (D) Philippines

7. ( ) What is the primary role of swine in the epidemiology of Japanese encephalitis? (A) Primary reservoir of the virus, (B) Incidental hosts like humans, (C) Important vector for transmission, (D) Amplifying hosts contributing to the spread

8. ( ) Which mosquito species is considered the most important vector for Japanese encephalitis transmission? (A) *Aedes aegypti*, (B) *Culex vishnui* complex, (C) Anopheles mosquito, (D) Simulium blackfly

9. ( ) What is the primary host serving as an amplifying host in the epidemiology of Japanese encephalitis? (A) Humans, (B) Birds, (C) Bats, (D) Swine

10. (　) Which age groups typically exhibit the highest susceptibility to clinical disease from Japanese encephalitis? (A) Adolescents, (B) Infants and the elderly, (C) Young adults, (D) Middle-aged individuals

11. (　) What is the most effective way to prevent Japanese encephalitis? (A) Antibiotic treatment, (B) Mosquito nets, (C) Vaccination, (D) Quarantine measures

II. Simple answer:

1. Please identify one of the important vectors responsible for transmitting Japanese encephalitis.

2. Why is it proposed to move swine away from human habitation as a control measure for Japanese encephalitis?

3. What is the duration of viraemia in birds infected with Japanese encephalitis virus?

4. Which genotype of the virus are all current vaccines based on?

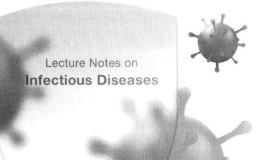

8

CHAPTER

Acute Viral Hepatitis

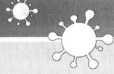

Hepatitis (plural hepatitides) implies injury to liver characterized by presence of inflammatory cells in the liver tissue. Etymologically from ancient Greek *hepar* (ηπαρ) or *hepato-* (ηπατο-), meaning "liver," and suffix *-itis,* denoting inflammation. The condition can be self limiting, healing on its own, or can progress to scarring of the liver. Hepatitis is acute when it lasts less than 6 months and chronic when it persists longer. A group of viruses known as the hepatitis viruses cause most cases of liver damage worldwide. Hepatitis can also be due to toxins (notably alcohol), other infections or from autoimmune process. It may run a subclinical course when the affected person may not feel ill. The patient becomes unwell and symptomatic when the disease impairs liver functions that include, among other things, screening of harmful substances, regulation of blood composition, and production of bile to help digestion.

Acute hepatitis:

Clinically, the course of acute hepatitis varies widely from mild symptoms requiring no treatment to fulminant hepatic failure needing liver transplantation. Acute viral hepatitis is more likely to be asymptomatic in younger people. Symptomatic individuals may present after convalescent stage of 7 to 10 days, with the total illness lasting 2 to 6 weeks.

Initial features are of nonspecific flu-like symptoms, common to almost all acute viral infections and may include malaise, muscle and joint aches, fever, nausea or vomiting, diarrhea, and headache.

More specific symptoms, which can be present in acute hepatitis from any cause, are profound loss of appetite, aversion to smoking among smokers, dark urine, yellowing of the eyes and skin (i.e., jaundice) and abdominal discomfort. Physical findings are usually minimal, apart from jaundice (33%) and tender hepatomegaly (10%). There can be occasional lymphadenopathy (5%) or splenomegaly (5%).

Acute viral hepatitis refers to inflammation of the liver caused by a viral infection. The proportion of acute hepatitis cases are hepatitis A (39.2%), hepatitis B (36.3%), hepatitis C (22.1%), hepatitis D (0.6%), and hepatitis E (1.8%) (Fig. 8-1).

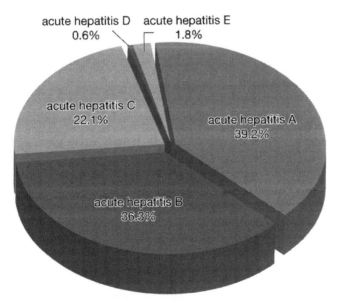

Figure 8-1   Proportion of Acute Hepatitis Cases in Taiwan, 2001-2016 (CDC, Taiwan, 2017)
(https://www.cdc.gov.tw/En/Category/ListContent/bg0g_VU_Ysrgkes_KRUDgQ?uaid=gvF-US_HVAZXQLg1VUXkTw)

Each of these viruses is transmitted differently and has distinct characteristics:

1. **Hepatitis A (HAV):**

   - Transmission: Usually spread through contaminated food or water, or through close contact with an infected person.

   - Acute Symptoms: Fatigue, nausea, abdominal pain, loss of appetite, jaundice (yellowing of the skin and eyes).

   - Vaccine: Available and is effective in preventing infection.

2. **Hepatitis B (HBV):**

   - Transmission: Spread through contact with the blood or other body fluids of an infected person, such as through sexual contact or sharing of needles.

   - Acute Symptoms: Similar to hepatitis A; may also include joint pain.

   - Vaccine: Highly effective and a part of routine childhood immunizations.

3. **Hepatitis C (HCV):**

   - Transmission: Primarily through direct contact with infected blood, often due to sharing needles or other drug paraphernalia.

   - Acute Symptoms: Often mild or asymptomatic; may lead to chronic infection.

   - Treatment: Antiviral medications are available for chronic cases.

4. **Hepatitis D (HDV):**

   - Transmission: Can only infect individuals already infected with hepatitis B.

   - Acute Symptoms: Similar to hepatitis B; can lead to more severe liver disease.

   - Prevention: Hepatitis B vaccination helps prevent hepatitis D.

5. **Hepatitis E (HEV):**

   - Transmission: Usually through the consumption of contaminated water or food.

   - Acute Symptoms: Similar to hepatitis A.

   - Generally, a self-limiting disease, but can be more severe in pregnant women.

Common features of acute viral hepatitis include liver inflammation, elevated liver enzymes, and symptoms like fatigue, jaundice, and abdominal pain. The severity and duration of symptoms can vary among individuals. It's important to note that while acute viral hepatitis can resolve on its own, some individuals may develop chronic hepatitis, which can lead to long-term liver damage. Early diagnosis and appropriate medical care are crucial for managing and treating acute viral hepatitis.

8-1 Viral Hepatitis A (ICD-9 070.1; ICD-10 B15)

Highlight

1. Viral hepatitis A ; infectious hepatitis, epidemic hepatitis, epidemic jaundice, catarrhal jaundice, type A hepatitis, HA
2. HAV infection may be asymptomatic
3. Hepatitis A typical symptoms: fever, malaise, anorexia, nausea, abdominal discomfort, dark urine, and jaundice
4. Hepatitis A virus spreads by the fecal-oral route
5. Approximately 40% of all acute viral hepatitis is caused by HAV
6. The case-fatality rate is 0.3%
7. Hepatitis A vaccines contain a killed or inactivated virus

Viral hepatitis A is also known as infectiuos hepatitis, epidemic hepatitis, epidemic jaundice, catarrhal jaundice, type A hepatitis, and HA. Hepatitis A is the most common vaccine-preventable infection acquired during travel. The risk for acquiring HAV infection for U.S. residents travelling abroad varies with living conditions, length of stay, and the incidence of HAV infection in the area visited. Travellers to North America (except Mexico), Japan, Australia, New Zealand, and developed countries in Europe are at no greater risk for infection than in the United States. For travellers to other countries, risk for infection increases with duration of travel and is highest for those who live in or visit rural areas, trek in back-country areas, or frequently eat or drink in settings of poor sanitation. Nevertheless, many cases of travel-related hepatitis A occur in travellers to developing countries with standard tourist itineraries, accommodations, and food consumption behaviours.

🔹 Identification to the viral hepatitis A:

HAV infection may be asymptomatic or its clinical manifestations may range in severity from a mild illness lasting 1-2 weeks to a severely disabling disease lasting several months. Clinical manifestations of hepatitis A often include fever, malaise, anorexia, nausea, and abdominal discomfort, followed within a few days by jaundice.

Hepatitis A typically has an abrupt onset of symptoms that can include fever, malaise, anorexia, nausea, abdominal discomfort, dark urine, and jaundice. The likelihood of having symptoms with HAV infection is related to the infected person's age. In children <6 years old, most (70%) infections are asymptomatic; if illness does occur its duration is usually <2 months. No chronic or long-term infection is associated with hepatitis A, but 10% of infected persons will have prolonged or relapsing symptoms over a 6- to 9-month period. The overall case-fatality rate among cases reported to CDC is 0.3%; however, the rate is 1.8% among adults >50 years of age.

Hepatitis A does not have a chronic stage and does not cause permanent liver damage. Following infection, the immune system makes antibodies against the hepatitis A virus that confer immunity against future infection. The disease can be prevented by vaccination and hepatitis A vaccine has been proved effective in controlling outbreaks worldwide.

🔹 Infectious agent:

Hepatitis A virus (HAV), a 27 nm picornavirus (positive-strand RNA virus). It has been classified as a member of the family Picornaviridae.

🔹 Occurrence:

Worldwide, geographic areas can be characterized by high, intermediate, or low levels of endemicity. Levels of endemicity are related to hygienic and sanitary conditions of geographic areas.

In developing countries, and in regions with poor hygiene standards, the incidence of infection with this virus approaches 100% and the illness is usually contracted in early childhood. Hepatitis A infection causes no clinical signs and symptoms in over 90% of these children and since the infection confers lifelong immunity, the disease is of no special significance to the indigenous population. In Europe, the United States and other industrialised countries, on the other hand, the infection is contracted primarily by susceptible young adults, most of whom are infected with the virus during trips to countries with a high incidence of the disease.

Hepatitis A occurrence in Taiwan:

1. 1980 survey; there were 43-83% of aged 12-13 year-old pupil infected hepatitis A in Taipei metropolitan.

2. 1989 survey; the hepatitis A infected population were decreased to less than 5% of aged 12-13 year-old pupil infected hepatitis A in Taipei metropolitan.

3. 1991 survey; there were more than 80% of aboriginal of aged 12-13 year-old pupil infected hepatitis A.

4. 1995; Executive Yuan D.O.H. provided vaccine inoculation for prevented hepatitis A infection in aboriginal children.

5. In 2016, Taiwan experienced one of the most severe hepatitis A outbreaks in history.

6. There have been few recent cases of hepatitis A in Taiwan (Fig. 8-2). Almost everyone can fully recover from hepatitis A and have lifelong immunity.

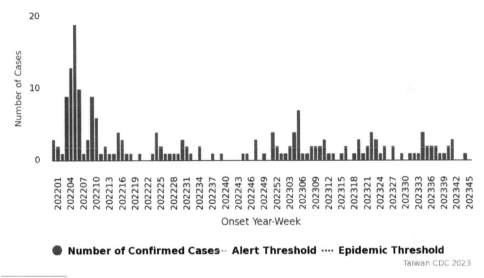

Acute Hepatitis A, Nationwide, Indigenous and Imported, Week 1/2022 - Week 46/2023
[Date of Onset 2022/01/02-2023/11/18]

● **Number of Confirmed Cases** ·· **Alert Threshold** ···· **Epidemic Threshold**

Taiwan CDC 2023

Figure 8-2   Acute hepatitis A, nationwide, indigenous and imported, week1/2022-week/2023 (CDC, Taiwan, 2023) (https://nidss.cdc.gov.tw/en/nndss/disease?id=0701)

🔖 Reservoir:

Man, rarely chimpanzees and other primates.

🔖 Mode of transmission:

The virus spreads by the fecal-oral route and infections often occur in conditions of poor sanitation and overcrowding. Hepatitis A can be transmitted by the parenteral route but very rarely by blood and blood products. Food-borne outbreaks are not uncommon, and ingestion of shellfish cultivated in polluted water is associated with a high risk of infection. Approximately 40% of all acute viral hepatitis is caused by HAV. Infected individuals are infectious prior to onset of symptoms, roughly 10 days following infection.

🔴 Incubation period:

Incubation period is average 28-30 days; range 15-50 days.

🔴 Period of communicability:

Communicability occurs during the latter half of incubation and continues for a few days after onset of jaundice. Most cases are probably non-infectious after the first week of jaundice, although prolonged viral excretion has been documented in infants and children.

🔴 Susceptibility and resistance:

Susceptibility is general. Low incidence of manifest disease in infants and preschool children suggests that mild and anicteric infections are common. Homologous immunity after infection probably lasts for life.

🔴 Methods of control:

HAV can be inactivated by: chlorine treatment (drinking water), formalin (0.35%, 37°C, 72 hours), peracetic acid (2%, 4 hours), beta-propiolactone (0.25%, 1 hour), and UV radiation (2 μW/cm^2/min).

Intervention measures include early detection of infected individuals, interruption of transmission, and protection of the susceptible population. The most important prevention measure is interrupting HAV fecal-oral transmission by promoting good personal hygiene, proper food handling practices, and provision of clean drinking water and effective sanitary facilities. Other prevention measures include active immunization with hepatitis A vaccines and passive immunization with immune globulin.

Hepatitis A vaccines contain a killed or inactivated virus. The immunologic response takes about 4 weeks to become established, and antibodies persist for at least 1 year after the first dose. Booster doses, given at 6 months or later, confer long-term immunity. Studies to date indicate that antibodies are sustained for at least 3 years after vaccination. Patients with suppressed immune systems may require more doses of the vaccine than a person with a healthy immune system in order to develop an immunological response.

 ## General review

1. Hepatitis A virus spreads by the fecal-oral route and infections often occur in conditions of poor sanitation and overcrowding

2. Control methods: active immunization with hepatitis A vaccines and passive immunization with immune globulin

3. 1995; Executive Yuan D.O.H. provided vaccine inoculation for prevented hepatitis A infection in aboriginal children

 ## Review test

SCAN ME

Check Your Answers

I. Multiple-choice questions (Four selected one):

1. ( ) What is another name for viral hepatitis A? (A) Serum Hepatitis, (B) Catarrhal jaundice, (C) Food Hepatitis, (D) Jaundice A

2. ( ) Which of the following regions poses the highest risk for acquiring HAV infection during travel? (A) North America (except Mexico), (B) Europe, (C) Australia, (D) Developing countries with standard tourist itineraries

3. ( ) What is the typical duration of illness in children under 6 years old who develop symptoms of hepatitis A? (A) 1-2 weeks, (B) 2-3 months, (C) Less than 2 months, (D) More than 6 months

4. ( ) What percentage of infected persons may experience prolonged or relapsing symptoms over a 6- to 9-month period? (A) 5%, (B) 10%, (C) 15%, (D) 20%

5. ( ) What is the primary age group affected by hepatitis A in industrialized countries like Europe and the United States? (A) Infants, (B) Children under 6 years old, (C) Susceptible young adults, (D) Elderly individuals

6. ( ) In regions with poor hygiene standards and high levels of endemicity, when is hepatitis A infection typically contracted? (A) Adolescence, (B) Early childhood, (C) Young adulthood, (D) Elderly age

7. ( ) What percentage of children in regions with poor hygiene standards may experience no clinical signs and symptoms following hepatitis A infection? (A) 50%, (B) 70%, (C) Over 90%, (D) 100%

8. ( ) What is the primary mode of transmission for the hepatitis A virus? (A) Respiratory droplets, (B) Sexual contact, (C) Fecal-oral route, (D) Blood transfusions

9. ( ) Ingestion of shellfish cultivated in polluted water is associated with a high risk of hepatitis A infection. What type of outbreak is commonly linked to this mode of transmission? (A) Airborne outbreaks, (B) Waterborne outbreaks, (C) Vector-borne outbreaks, (D) Person-to-person outbreaks

10.( ) What is the primary mode of inactivating the hepatitis A virus in drinking water? (A) UV radiation, (B) Formalin, (C) Peracetic acid, (D) Chlorine treatment

11.( ) How long does the immunologic response typically take to become established after receiving a hepatitis A vaccine? (A) 2 weeks, (B) 4 weeks, (C) 6 weeks, (D) 8 weeks

II. Simple answer:

1. What are some factors that increase the risk of acquiring HAV infection during travel to other countries, according to the provided information?

2. Does hepatitis A have a chronic stage, and what is the overall case-fatality rate reported among cases to the CDC?

3. According to information provided by the Taiwan Centers for Disease Control and Prevention, what measures were mentioned in 1995 to prevent aboriginal children from being infected with hepatitis A?

4. When are infected individuals most infectious, according to the provided information, and for how long does communicability typically continue after the onset of jaundice?

5. What are the key prevention measures mentioned in the provided information for interrupting HAV fecal-oral transmission?

8-2 — Viral Hepatitis B (ICD-9 070.3; ICD-10 B16)

Highlight

1. Hepatitis B; type B hepatitis, serum hepatitis, homologous serum jaundice, Australia antigen hepatitis, HB

2. Symptoms of acute hepatitis B: liver inflammation, vomiting, jaundice, and rarely, death

3. Chronic hepatitis B: liver cirrhosis and liver cancer, a fatal disease

4. HBV transmission: Blood transfusion; Body fluids transmission; Vertical transmission

5. HBsAg is a protein antigen produced by HBV.

6. HBsAg is the earliest indicator of acute hepatitis B.

7. HBsAg disappears from the blood during the recovery period.

8. Anti-HBs presence indicates previous exposure to HBV

9. HBeAg is a viral protein associated with HBV infections

10. Anti-HBe; successful treatment; eliminate HBeAg from the blood

11. Anti-HBc; who have cleared the virus, and usually persists for life

Hepatitis B is also known as type B hepatitis, serum hepatitis, homologous serum jaundice, Australia antigen hepatitis, and HB. Hepatitis B virus infects the liver of hominoidae, including humans, and causes an inflammation called hepatitis. Hepatitis B is a viral infection that attacks the liver and can cause both acute and chronic diseases. The virus is transmitted through contact with the blood or other body fluids of an infected person. It is a DNA virus and one of many unrelated viruses that cause viral hepatitis. The disease was originally known as serum hepatitis and has caused epidemics in parts of Asia and Africa. Hepatitis B is endemic in China and various other parts of Asia. The proportion of the world's population currently infected with the virus is estimated at 3 to 6%, but up to a third have been exposed. Symptoms of the acute illness caused by the virus include liver inflammation, vomiting, jaundice, and rarely, death. Chronic hepatitis B may eventually cause liver cirrhosis and liver cancer, a fatal disease with very poor response to current chemotherapy. The infection is preventable by vaccination.

Identification to the hepatitis B:

Hepatitis B virus infection may either be acute (self-limiting) or chronic (long-standing). Persons with self-limiting infection clear the infection spontaneously within weeks to months. Children are less likely than adults to clear the infection. More than 95% of people who become infected as adults or older children will stage a full recovery and develop protective immunity to the virus. However, only 5% of newborns that acquire the infection from their mother at birth will clear the infection. Of those infected between the age of one to six, 70% will clear the infection.

Acute infection with hepatitis B virus is associated with acute viral hepatitis - an illness that begins with general ill-health, loss of appetite, nausea, vomiting, body aches, mild fever, dark urine, and then progresses to development of jaundice. It has been noted that itchy skin has been an indication as a possible symptom of all hepatitis virus types. The illness lasts for a few weeks and then gradually improves in most affected people. A few patients may have more severe liver disease (fulminant hepatic failure), and may die as a result of it. The infection may be entirely asymptomatic and may go unrecognized.

Hepatitis B surface antigen (HBsAg) is a protein antigen produced by HBV. This antigen is the earliest indicator of acute hepatitis B and frequently identifies infected people before symptoms appear. HBsAg disappears from the blood during the recovery period. In some people, chronic infection with HBV may occur and HBsAg remains positive. The hepatitis B surface antibody (anti-HBs) is the most common test. Its presence indicates previous exposure to HBV, but the virus is no longer present and the person cannot pass on the virus to others. The antibody also protects the body from future HBV infection. In addition to exposure to HBV, the antibodies can also be acquired from successful vaccination. This test is done to determine the need for vaccination (if anti-HBs is absent), or following the completion of vaccination against the disease, or following an active infection.

Hepatitis B e-antigen (HBeAg) is a viral protein associated with HBV infections. Unlike the surface antigen, the e-antigen is found in the blood only when there are viruses also present. When the virus goes into "hiding," the e-antigen will no longer be present in the blood. HBeAg is often used as a marker of ability to spread the virus to other people (infectivity). Measurement of e-antigen may also be used to monitor the effectiveness of HBV treatment; successful treatment will usually eliminate HBeAg from the blood and lead to development of antibodies against e-antigen (anti-HBe). There are some types (strains) of HBV that do not make e-antigen; these are especially common in the Middle East and Asia. In areas where these strains of HBV are common, testing for HBeAg is not very useful. Anti-HBe is an antibody produced in response to the Hepatitis B e antigen. In those who have recovered from acute hepatitis B infection, anti-HBe will be present along with anti-HBc and anti-HBs. In those with chronic hepatitis B, usually anti-HBe becomes positive when the virus goes into hiding or is eliminated from the body. In strains that do not make HBe antigen, anti-HBe is also positive.

Anti-hepatitis B core antigen (anti-HBc) is an antibody to the hepatitis B core antigen. The core antigen is found on virus particles but disappears early in the course of infection. This antibody is produced during and after an acute HBV infection and is usually found in chronic HBV carriers as well as those who have cleared the virus, and usually persists for life. Anti-HBc testing is either specific for the IgM antibody, anti-HBc, IgM, which indicates acute infection, or measures total antibody, anti-HBC, which indicates past infection, either acute or chronic.

Infectious agent:

Hepatitis B is a large (42 nm) enveloped DNA virus, which contains 27 nm core (HBcAg) and the particle coated with lipoprotein envelop (HBsAg) (Fig. 8-3). The major antigenic determinant of HBsAg is the "a" antigen; antibodies to this antigen confer protection after infection or vaccination. HBV giving four phenotypes, adw, adr, ayw and ayr. The frequency of these phenotypes varies in different parts of the world. In Taiwan, HBV phenotypes are almost adw type.

Occurrence:

Occurrence is worldwide. Hepatitis B is a major global health problem and the most serious type of viral hepatitis. According to the World Health Organization (WHO), an estimated 257 million people are living with hepatitis B virus infection (WHO, 2023). The incidence of acute disease and prevalence of carriage varies considerably from country to country. In south-east Asia, 10-20% of the population may be carriers. In Taiwan, among pregnant female approximately 7.8% are "e" antigen positive, therefore, the newborn is 6-8% were carrier per year.

Hepatitis B Virus
Baltimore Group VII (dsDNA-RT)

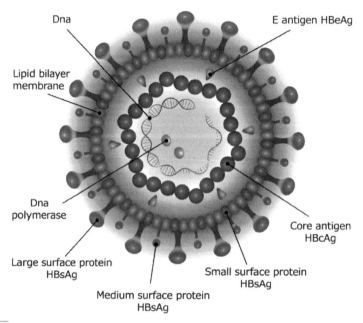

Figure 8-3   Diagram of Hepatitis B virus Particle structure

In the past, recipients of blood products were at high risk. In countries where pretransfusion screening of blood for HBsAg is required, and where pooled blood clotting factors are processed to destroy the virus, this risk has been virtually eliminated; however, it is still present in many developing countries. Contaminated and inadequately sterilized syringes and needles have resulted in outbreaks of hepatitis B among patients; this has been a major mode of transmission worldwide. Outbreaks have been reported among patients in dialysis centers in many countries through failure to adhere to recommended infection control practices against transmission of HBV and other blood-borne pathogens in these settings.

🔹 Reservoir:

Man and chimpanzee are susceptible.

🔹 Mode of transmission:

Body substances capable of transmitting HBV include: Blood transfusion; Body fluids transmission (semen, vaginal discharges); Vertical transmission.

Possible forms of transmission include unprotected sexual contact, blood transfusions, re-use of contaminated needles and syringes, and vertical transmission from mother to child during childbirth. Without intervention, a mother who is positive for the hepatitis B surface antigen confers a 20% risk of passing the infection to her offspring at the time of birth. This risk is as high as 90% if the mother is also positive for the hepatitis B e antigen. HBV can be transmitted between family members within households, possibly by contact of nonintact skin or mucous membrane with secretions or saliva containing HBV.

The risk groups for hepatitis B in developed countries include: Intravenous drug abusers, homosexual men, sexual contacts of antigen-positive persons, residents in long-stay homes for mentally handicapped people, renal dialysis patients, recipients of multiple blood products, surgeons, dentists and morticians, and infants of e antigen positive mothers.

🔹 Incubation period:

Usually 45-180 days, averages are 60-90 days. Incubation period is dependent on virus volume, transmission way and host immunity.

🔋 Period of communicability:

The acute stage and chronic carrier patients are infective. The asymptomatic infection induces chronic carrier, who was been infected in infant stage. e antigen-positive carriers are high communicability.

🔋 Susceptibility and resistance:

Susceptibility is general. Usually, the disease is milder and often anicteric (non-jaundice publication) in children. In infants it is predominatly asymptomatic. Solid immunity follows infection if antibody to HBsAg (anti-HBs) develops and HBsAg is negative.

🔋 Methods of control:

1. Pre-exposure prophylaxis with non-replicating vaccine.
2. Post-exposure prophylaxis with specific immunoglobulin and vaccine.
3. Universal antenatal screening.
4. Universal testing of donated blood products.
5. Use of condoms.
6. Use of clean needles and other skin-piercing equipment.
7. Safe disposal of hospital sharps.
8. Use of disposable hemodialysis equipment.

The hepatitis B vaccine is an effective way to prevent infection. It is usually given as a series of three shots. Several vaccines have been developed for the prevention of hepatitis B virus infection. These rely on the use of one of the viral envelope proteins (hepatitis B surface antigen or HBsAg). The vaccine was originally prepared from plasma obtained from patients who had long-standing hepatitis B virus infection. However, currently, these are more often made using recombinant DNA technology, though plasma-derived vaccines continue to be used; the two types of vaccines are equally effective and safe. Following vaccination hepatitis B surface antigen may be detected in serum for several days; this is known as vaccine antigenaemia.

General review

1. Hepatitis B virus infection may either be acute (self-limiting) or chronic (long-standing)

2. HBeAg is often used as a marker of ability to spread the virus to other people (infectivity)

3. Measurement of e-antigen may also be used to monitor the effectiveness of HBV treatment

4. Anti-HBe; successful treatment will usually eliminate HBeAg from the blood and lead to development of antibodies against e-antigen

5. Anti-HBc produced during and after an acute HBV infection and is usually found in chronic HBV carriers, who have cleared the virus, and usually persists for life

6. Anti-HBc testing is either specific for the IgM antibody, anti-HBc, IgM, which indicates acute infection

7. In Taiwan, among pregnant female approximately 7.8% are "e" antigen positive, therefore, the newborn is 6-8% were carrier per year

8. HBV transmission: Blood transfusion; Body fluids transmission (semen, vaginal discharges); Vertical transmission

Review test

I.   Multiple-choice questions (Four selected one):

1. (   ) What is another name for Hepatitis B? (A) Type A Hepatitis, (B) Serum Hepatitis, (C) Influenza Hepatitis, (D) Gastrointestinal Hepatitis

2. (   ) What is the estimated proportion of the world's population currently infected with Hepatitis B? (A) 1 to 2%, (B) 3 to 6%, (C) 7 to 10%, (D) 11 to 15%

3. (   ) What is the primary indicator of acute hepatitis B and often identifies infected individuals before symptoms appear? (A) Hepatitis B e-antigen (HBeAg), (B) Anti-hepatitis B core antigen (anti-HBc), (C) Hepatitis B surface antibody (anti-HBs), (D) Hepatitis B surface antigen (HBsAg)

4. (   ) What percentage of newborns infected with hepatitis B from their mothers at birth are likely to clear the infection? (A) 5%, (B) 20%, (C) 50%, (D) 95%

5. (   ) Which antibody indicates previous exposure to HBV, but the virus is no longer present, and the person cannot pass on the virus to others? (A) Anti-hepatitis B core antigen (anti-HBc), (B) Hepatitis B surface antibody (anti-HBs), (C) Anti-HBe, (D) Hepatitis B e-antigen (HBeAg)

6. (   ) What symptom is commonly associated with acute viral hepatitis, including hepatitis B? (A) Cough, (B) Itchy skin, (C) Headache, (D) Muscle pain

7. ( ) When is Hepatitis B e-antigen (HBeAg) present in the blood? (A) Only during acute infection, (B) Only when the virus goes into "hiding", (C) Throughout the recovery period, (D) Only in chronic carriers

8. ( ) Which of the following is NOT mentioned as a possible form of hepatitis B transmission? (A) Blood transfusions, (B) Vertical transmission, (C) Airborne transmission, (D) Unprotected sexual contact

9. ( ) What is the risk of a mother passing hepatitis B to her offspring at the time of birth if she is positive for the hepatitis B surface antigen, and this risk increases if she is also positive for the hepatitis B e antigen? (A) 5%, (B) 20%, (C) 50%, (D) 90%

10. ( ) How is the hepatitis B vaccine typically administered to individuals for prevention? (A) Intravenous injection, (B) Single shot, (C) Series of two shots, (D) Series of three shots

11. ( ) What technology is commonly used to produce hepatitis B vaccines, although plasma-derived vaccines are still in use? (A) Live attenuated virus, (B) Inactivated virus, (C) Recombinant DNA technology, (D) Conventional chemical synthesis

II. Simple answer:

1. What are some symptoms of the acute illness caused by Hepatitis B?

2. What does the presence of Anti-hepatitis B core antigen (anti-HBc) indicate, and what are the two types of anti-HBc testing mentioned?

3. What is the term for the detection of hepatitis B surface antigen in serum for several days after vaccination, and how is this phenomenon known?

8-3 · Viral Hepatitis C (ICD-9 070.5; ICD-10 B17.1)

Highlight

1. Hepatitis C; non-A non-B hepatitis; HCV infection
2. HCV is spread by blood-to-blood contact.
3. HCV transmission: Blood transfusion; body fluids transmission; HCV is primarily transmitted parenterally
4. No vaccine against hepatitis C is available

Hepatitis C is also known as parenterally transmitted non-A non-B hepatitis, non-B transfusion associated hepatitis, posttransfusion non-A non-B hepatitis, and HCV infection. Hepatitis C is a blood-borne infectious disease that is caused by hepatitis C virus (HCV), infecting the liver. The infection can cause liver inflammation (hepatitis) that is often asymptomatic, but ensuing chronic hepatitis can result later in cirrhosis (fibrotic scarring of the liver) and liver cancer. HCV is spread by blood-to-blood contact. No vaccine against hepatitis C is available. The symptoms of infection can be medically managed, and a proportion of patients can be cleared of the virus by a long course of anti-viral medicines. Although early medical intervention is helpful, people with HCV infection often experience mild symptoms, and consequently do not seek treatment. Hepatitis C is a major global health problem and the most serious type of viral hepatitis. An estimated 150-200 million people worldwide are infected with hepatitis C.

Identification to the hepatitis C:

Hepatitis C is a common cause of blood-borne hepatitis, when blood transfusion infected hepatitis C, which will going to be chronic infection (70%). Approximately 40% may have persisting hepatitis with the risk of late cirrhosis or hepatocellular carcinoma. The onset of hepatitis C is usually insidious with anorexia, vague abdominal discomfort, nausea, vomiting, dark urine, and joint pain, progressing to jaundice less frequently than hepatitis B.

Acute Hepatitis C refers to the first 6 months after infection. It can range in severity from a mild illness with few or no symptoms to a serious condition requiring hospitalization. Chronic Hepatitis C is a long-term infection that can last a lifetime. Over time, it can lead to serious liver problems, including cirrhosis, liver failure, or liver cancer.

Infectious agent:

Hepatitis C virus (HCV) is an RNA virus related to the flaviviruses and animal pestiviruses. Hepatitis C is a small (30-50 nm) lipo-enveloped ssRNA virus, with a 9.4-kb positive-sense genome, encoding a single polypeptide.

Occurrence:

Worldwide distribution, HCV prevalence is directly related to the prevalence of persons who routinely share injection equipment and to the prevalence of poor parenteral practices in health care settings.

In Taiwan, the prevalence of transfusion-transmitted hepatitis C is 69 %. Since 1992; provided hepatitis C testing of donated blood products, and then the disease was decreased. So far, HCV infection remains a public health issue with an estimated prevalence of 3.3% (1.8-5.5%) in the general population and there are several regional disparities in terms of prevalence of hepatitis C in Taiwan (CDC, Taiwan, 2021).

🔋 Reservoir:

Man and chimpanzee are susceptible.

🔋 Mode of transmission:

Blood transfusion; body fluids transmission (semen, vaginal discharges); HCV is primarily transmitted parenterally. Sexual and mother-to-child have been documented but appears far less efficient or frequent than the parenteral route.

🔋 Incubation period:

Ranges from 2 weeks to 6 months, usually 6-9 weeks.

🔋 Period of communicability:

From one or more weeks before onset of first symptoms through the acute clinical course of the disease and chronic carrier stages all are communicable.

🔋 Susceptibility and resistance:

Susceptibility is general. Repeated bouts of acute hepatitis C have been reported but it is not known whether these represent infection by different agents or recrudescence of the original infection.

🔋 Methods of control:

1. Avoiding High-Risk Behaviors: Hepatitis C is commonly transmitted through the sharing of needles and other equipment for injecting drugs. Avoiding intravenous drug use or ensuring the use of clean, sterile equipment can help prevent the spread of the virus.

2. Practicing Safe Sex: While the risk of sexual transmission of Hepatitis C is considered to be low, it's still a good practice to use barrier methods, such as condoms, especially if you have multiple sexual partners or engage in high-risk sexual behaviors.

3. Screening: Identifying individuals with Hepatitis C through screening is crucial, especially among high-risk groups such as intravenous drug users, individuals with a history of blood transfusions or organ transplants before widespread screening, and those born to mothers with Hepatitis C.

4. General measures for the prevention of hepatitis B apply also to hepatitis C.

5. Needle exchange schemes help to reduce new cases among intravenous drug users.

6. Currently, there is no vaccine for Hepatitis C. However, vaccination against Hepatitis B can prevent co-infection with both viruses, which can lead to more severe liver disease.

General review

1. HCV infection can cause liver inflammation (hepatitis) that is often asymptomatic, but ensuing chronic hepatitis can result later in cirrhosis (fibrotic scarring of the liver) and liver cancer

2. HCV transmission: Blood transfusion; body fluids transmission (semen, vaginal discharges); HCV is primarily transmitted parenterally

SCAN ME

Check Your Answers

Review test

I. Multiple-choice questions (Four selected one):

1. ( ) How is Hepatitis C primarily spread? (A) Airborne droplets, (B) Fecal-oral route, (C) Blood-to-blood contact, (D) Casual contact

2. ( ) What percentage of individuals infected with hepatitis C through blood transfusion may develop chronic infection? (A) 30%, (B) 40%, (C) 50%, (D) 70%

3. ( ) Which of the following symptoms is less frequently associated with the onset of Hepatitis C compared to Hepatitis B? (A) Jaundice, (B) Vague abdominal discomfort, (C) Dark urine, (D) Joint pain

4. ( ) What is the key factor directly related to the prevalence of Hepatitis C worldwide? (A) Water contamination, (B) Airborne transmission, (C) Sharing injection equipment, (D) Foodborne transmission

5. ( ) What was the prevalence of transfusion-transmitted hepatitis C in Taiwan before the implementation of hepatitis C testing of donated blood products? (A) 30%, (B) 49%, (C) 69%, (D) 80%

6. ( ) Which high-risk group is crucial to target for screening to identify individuals with Hepatitis C? (A) Individuals with a history of organ transplants, (B) Individuals born to mothers with Hepatitis C, (C) Individuals with a history of blood transfusions, (D) All of the above

7. ( ) What is a general preventive measure applicable to both Hepatitis B and Hepatitis C? (A) Needle exchange schemes, (B) Safe sex practices, (C) Blood transfusion, (D) Vaccination

II. Simple answer:

1. How many people worldwide are estimated to be infected with hepatitis C?

2. Please define Acute Hepatitis C and its duration. What are the potential outcomes of Chronic Hepatitis C?

3. Please describe the impact of hepatitis C testing on donated blood products in Taiwan since 1992. What is the current estimated prevalence of HCV infection in the general population, and are there regional disparities in Taiwan?

4. Please list three modes of transmission for Hepatitis C, and briefly discuss which one is considered less efficient or frequent.

8-4 Viral Hepatitis D (ICD-9 070.5; ICD-10 B17.0)

 Highlight

1. Hepatitis D is also known as delta hepatitis, hepatitis delta virus, delta agent hepatitis, delta associated hepatitis

2. HDV is considered to be a subviral satellite

3. HDV can propagate only in the presence of another virus, the hepatitis B virus (HBV)

4. Transmission of HDV can occur either via simultaneous infection with HBV (coinfection or superinfection)

5. Both superinfection and coinfection with HDV results in more severe

6. In combination with hepatitis B virus, hepatitis D has the highest mortality rate of 20%

7. Hepatitis D may be self-limiting or it may progress to chronic hepatitis

Hepatitis D is also known as delta hepatitis, hepatitis delta virus, delta agent hepatitis, delta associated hepatitis. Hepatitis D is a disease caused by a small circular RNA virus (hepatitis delta virus or hepatitis D virus, HDV). HDV is considered to be a subviral satellite because it can propagate only in the presence of another virus, the hepatitis B virus (HBV). Transmission of HDV can occur either via simultaneous infection with HBV (coinfection) or via infection of an individual previously infected with HBV (superinfection). Both superinfection and coinfection with HDV results in more severe complications compared to infection with HBV alone. These complications include a greater likelihood of experiencing liver failure in acute infections and a greater likelihood of developing liver cancer in chronic infections. In combination with hepatitis B virus, hepatitis D has the highest mortality rate of all the hepatitis infections of 20%.

Identification to the hepatitis D:

The onset of hepatitis D is usually abrupt, with signs and symptoms resembling those of hepatitis B. Hepatitis D may be severe and is always associated with a coexistent hepatitis B virus infection. Hepatitis D may be self-limiting, or it may progress to chronic hepatitis. The symptoms of hepatitis D are similar to those of hepatitis B and can include fatigue, jaundice (yellowing of the skin and eyes), abdominal pain, nausea, and vomiting.

Infectious agent:

The hepatitis D agent is a 35-37 nm virus-like particle consisting of a coat of hepatitis B surface antigen and a unique internal antigen, δ antigen. Encapsulated with the δ antigen is a linear ss RNA that is thought to be the genome of the δ antigen.

Occurrence:

Worldwide, prevalence is varies and widely. Attack rate are highest in young adults, often with male predominance. In Taiwan, the high risk populations are; intravenous drug users, prostitutions, and hepatitis B carriers, their infection rate are 40-80%.

Reservoir:

Man; possibly transmissible to marmosets and chimpanzees.

Mode of transmission:

The transmission mode is thought to be similar to that of hepatitis B virus, including blood and serous body fluids, contaminated needles and syringes, plasma derivatives such as anti-hemophilic factor and mother-to-

infant transmission. In Taiwan, prostitution is a high risk behavior of transmission.

Incubation period:

Approximately 2-8 weeks.

Period of communicability:

Blood is potentially infectious during all phase of active δ infection. Peak infectivity probably occurs just prior to onset of illness, when particles containing the δ antigen are readily detected in the blood.

Susceptibility and resistance:

All persons susceptible to hepatitis B or who are HBV carriers can be infected with δ. Severe disease can occur even in children. In Taiwan; the hepatitis D infection rate among children are rare.

✏ Methods of control:

1. Prevention of hepatitis B virus infection will prevent infection with hepatitis D.

2. Needle exchange schemes help to reduce new cases among intravenous drug users.

3. Condom use.

4. HBIG, IG or HBV vaccine is useful in protecting HBV carriers after exposure to δ agent.

🔥 General review

1. In Taiwan, the high risk populations are; intravenous drug users, prostitutions, and hepatitis B carriers, their infection rate are 40–80%

2. In Taiwan, prostitution is a high risk behavior of HDV transmission

3. All persons susceptible to hepatitis B or who are HBV carriers can be infected with δ

4. HBIG, IG or HBV vaccine is useful in protecting HBV carriers after exposure to δ agent

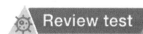

SCAN ME

Check Your Answers

I.   Multiple-choice questions (Four selected one):

1. (   ) What is another name for Hepatitis D? (A) Gamma hepatitis, (B) Delta hepatitis, (C) Alpha hepatitis, (D) Omega hepatitis

2. (   ) How does Hepatitis D propagate, and what is its relationship with another virus? (A) Propagates independently; no relationship with other viruses, (B) Propagates in the presence

of the common cold virus, (C) Propagates only in the presence of Hepatitis C virus, (D) Propagates only in the presence of Hepatitis B virus

3. (　) What is the unique internal antigen associated with the hepatitis D virus? (A) Gamma antigen, (B) Alpha antigen, (C) Delta antigen, (D) Omega antigen

4. (　) How does the onset of hepatitis D typically manifest, and what is it always associated with? (A) Gradual onset; always associated with hepatitis A, (B) Abrupt onset; always associated with a coexistent hepatitis C virus infection, (C) Abrupt onset; always associated with a coexistent hepatitis B virus infection, (D) Gradual onset; always associated with hepatitis E.

5. (　) Which of the following populations in Taiwan is identified as a high-risk group for Hepatitis D transmission with an infection rate ranging from 40-80%? (A) Elderly individuals, (B) University students, (C) Intravenous drug users, prostitutes, and hepatitis B carriers, (D) Outdoor enthusiasts

6. (　) What is a significant high-risk behavior for Hepatitis D transmission in Taiwan, according to the information provided? (A) Consuming contaminated water, (B) Smoking, (C) Prostitution, (D) Excessive alcohol consumption

7. (　) Who is susceptible to hepatitis D infection according to the information provided? (A) Only adults, (B) Only children, (C) Only HBV carriers, (D) All persons susceptible to hepatitis B or who are HBV carriers

8. ( ) What is mentioned as a method to reduce new cases of hepatitis D among intravenous drug users? (A) Increased alcohol consumption, (B) Needle exchange schemes, (C) Avoiding vaccination, (D) Condom use

9. ( ) According to the information, what is a recommended control method for preventing hepatitis D infection? (A) Eating a balanced diet, (B) Avoiding outdoor activities, (C) Regular exercise, (D) Prevention of hepatitis B virus infection

10.( ) What is identified as useful in protecting HBV carriers after exposure to the hepatitis D agent? (A) Antibiotics, (B) Condom use, (C) Needle exchange schemes, (D) HBIG, IG, or HBV vaccine

II. Simple answer:

1. What are the complications associated with both superinfection and coinfection with Hepatitis D?

2. Please describe the structure of the hepatitis D agent.

3. Please describe the worldwide occurrence and prevalence of Hepatitis D, highlighting the demographics most affected.

8-5 **Viral Hepatitis E** (ICD-9 070.5; ICD-10 B17.2)

Highlight

1. Hepatitis E: Enterically transmitted non-A non-B hepatitis, epidemic non-A non-B hepatitis, and fecal-oral non-A non-B hepatitis

2. Hepatitis E is behaving rather like hepatitis A and circulates by fecal-oral route

3. Hepatitis E is severe in pregnancy

4. The incidence of hepatitis E is highest in adults between the ages of 15 and 40

5. Hepatitis E is a "self-limiting" disease

6. Man is the natural host of HEV

7. Domestic animals have been reported as a reservoir for the hepatitis E virus

8. No vaccine or immunoglobulin is available for HEV

Hepatitis E is also known as enterically transmitted non-A non-B hepatitis, epidemic non-A non-B hepatitis, and fecal-oral non-A non-B hepatitis. Hepatitis E is a viral hepatitis caused by infection with a virus called hepatitis E virus (HEV). Infection with this virus was first documented in 1955 during an outbreak in New Delhi, India. Hepatitis E is endemic in various parts of Asia, Africa, and Central America. Outbreaks are more common in regions with poor sanitation and hygiene practices, especially after heavy rainfall or flooding, which can contaminate water sources. Immunocompromised individuals may also experience more severe cases.

🔋 Identification to the hepatitis E:

Hepatitis E is behaving rather like hepatitis A and circulates by fecal-oral route. It is unaccountably severe in pregnancy, causing a mortality of 20 %, compared with less than 1% in non-pregnant patients. Jaundice is often prolonged, lasting 4 or 5 weeks. The symptoms of Hepatitis E can range from mild to severe and may include fever, fatigue, loss of appetite, nausea, vomiting, abdominal pain, and jaundice. In general, Hepatitis E is a self-limiting disease, and most people recover fully within a few weeks. However, it can be more severe in pregnant women, especially in the third trimester, leading to a higher risk of complications.

🔋 Infectious agent:

Hepatitis E is a small (32-24 nm) non-enveloped RNA virus. In acute stage, could found 32 nm virus-like particles in stool from infected patient. There are different genotypes of HEV. Genotypes 1 and 2 are typically associated with waterborne transmission in developing countries, while genotypes 3 and 4 are associated with zoonotic transmission and are found in developed countries.

🔋 Occurrence:

Epidemics have been identified in several countries, particularly in South-east Asia and China. In these outbreaks, young adults, especially males, are predominantly affected. Travelers to regions with high Hepatitis E prevalence may be at risk of contracting the virus through contaminated food and water.

The incidence of hepatitis E is highest in adults between the ages of 15 and 40. Though children often contract this infection as well, they less frequently become symptomatic. Mortality rates are generally low, for hepatitis E is a "self-limiting" disease, in that it usually goes away by itself and the patient recovers. However, during the duration of the infection (usually several weeks), the disease severely impairs a person's ability to work, care for family members, and obtain food. Hepatitis E occasionally develops into an acute severe liver disease and is fatal in about 2% of all cases.

Reservoir:

Man is the natural host of HEV; some non-human primates, e.g. chimpanzees, monkeys, tamarins are reported as susceptible to natural infection with human strains of HEV. Domestic animals have been reported as a reservoir for the hepatitis E virus, with some surveys showing infection rates exceeding 95% among domestic pigs.

Mode of transmission:

The source of infection is usually contaminated water; person-to-person spread by the fecal-oral route also occurs.

Incubation period:

The range is 15-64 days, average are 26-42 days.

Period of communicability:

The communicable period is uncertain, but probably coincides with the phase of increasing transaminase (AST, ALT/serum).

Susceptibility and resistance:

Uncertain; over 50% of HEV infections may be anicteric; the expression of icterus appears to increase with increasing age.

⭑ Methods of control:

General sanitary measures and personal hygiene are effective in limiting spread. Improving sanitation is the most important measure, which consists in proper treatment and disposal of human waste, higher standards for public water supplies, improved personal hygiene procedures and sanitary food preparation. Thus, prevention strategies of this disease are similar to those of many others that plague developing nations, and they require large scale international financing of water supply and water treatment projects. No vaccine or immunoglobulin is available. Here are some key control methods for Hepatitis E:

1. **Improving Sanitation**: Implementation of proper sewage disposal systems and promoting safe drinking water practices can help reduce the risk of contamination.

2. **Hygiene Promotion**: Public health campaigns that emphasize good hygiene practices, including regular handwashing with soap and water, can help prevent the spread of the virus.

3. **Monitoring and Surveillance**: Establishing robust monitoring and surveillance systems is essential to track the incidence and prevalence of Hepatitis E.

4. **Outbreak Response**: In areas prone to outbreaks, having a rapid response plan in place is crucial. This may involve providing medical care, clean water, and implementing sanitation measures promptly.

5. **Pregnancy Management**: Early detection and appropriate management of pregnant women with Hepatitis E can reduce the risk of complications.

6. **International Collaboration**: Due to the global nature of Hepatitis E, international collaboration is essential. Sharing information, resources, and best practices can contribute to more effective control efforts.

⚫ General review

1. HEV infection was first documented in 1955 during an outbreak in New Delhi, India.

2. Hepatitis E is unaccountably severe in pregnancy, causing a mortality of 20 %

3. Hepatitis E occasionally develops into an acute severe liver disease, and is fatal in about 2% of all cases.

4. Domestic pigs are reservoir for the hepatitis E virus, infection rates is exceeding 95%

5. The source of HEV infection: contaminated water; person-to-person spread by the fecal-oral route

6. No vaccine or immunoglobulin is available for HEV

SCAN ME

Check Your Answers

⚫ Review test

I. Multiple-choice questions (Four selected one):

1. ( ) What is another name for Hepatitis E? (A) Enterically transmitted non-A non-B hepatitis, (B) Epidemic non-A non-B hepatitis, (C) Fecal-oral non-A non-B hepatitis, (D) All of the above

2. ( ) When was the first documented outbreak of Hepatitis E reported? (A) 1955, (B) 1960, (C) 1975, (D) 1982

3. ( ) Which regions are mentioned as endemic for Hepatitis E in the provided information? (A) North America and Europe, (B) Asia, Africa, and Central America, (C) Australia and South America, (D) Middle East and Oceania

4. (   ) What is the size of the Hepatitis E virus (HEV) in the acute stage? (A) 15-20 nm, (B) 24-32 nm, (C) 40-50 nm, (D) 60-70 nm

5. (   ) Which genotypes of HEV are associated with waterborne transmission in developing countries? (A) Genotypes 3 and 4, (B) Genotypes 1 and 2, (C) Genotypes 2 and 3, (D) Genotypes 1 and 3

6. (   ) In which regions have epidemics of Hepatitis E been identified, with young adults, especially males, predominantly affected? (A) North America and Europe, (B) South-east Asia and China, (C) Australia and Africa, (D) Middle East and Oceania

7. (   ) What age group experiences the highest incidence of Hepatitis E? (A) Children under 5, (B) Adults between 40-60, (C) Adults between 15-40, (D) Elderly above 65

8. (   ) Which of the following non-human primates is reported as susceptible to natural infection with human strains of Hepatitis E virus (HEV)? (A) Gorillas, (B) Baboons, (C) Chimpanzees, (D) Lemurs

9. (   ) Among domestic animals, which species is commonly reported as a reservoir for the Hepatitis E virus, with infection rates sometimes exceeding 95%? (A) Cattle, (B) Sheep, (C) Domestic Pigs, (D) Chickens

10. (   ) What is a key component of outbreak response in areas prone to Hepatitis E outbreaks? (A) Providing medical care, (B) Pregnancy management, (C) Monitoring and surveillance, (D) Hygiene promotion

II. Simple answer:

1. What is the mortality rate for pregnant women with severe Hepatitis E, and how does it compare to non-pregnant patients?

2. What is the mortality rate for Hepatitis E, and how does the disease impact a person's daily life during the infection?

3. What are the primary sources of infection for Hepatitis E, and how is person-to-person spread typically facilitated?

4. Why is international collaboration considered essential in the control efforts of Hepatitis E?

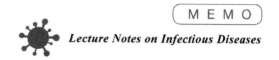

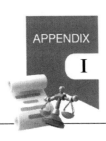

Laws and Regulations on Communicable Diseases Control in Taiwan
傳染病防治法施行細則

中華民國七十四年九月九日行政院衛生署(74)衛署防字第 548919 號令訂定發布全文 12 條

中華民國一百零五年七月六日衛生福利部部授疾字第 1050100789 號令修正發布第 10、13、16 條文

第 1 條　本細則依傳染病防治法（以下簡稱本法）第七十六條規定訂定之。

第 2 條　本法所稱預防接種，指為達預防疾病發生或減輕病情之目的，將疫苗施於人體之措施。

　　　　本法所稱疫苗，指配合預防接種或防疫需要之主動及被動免疫製劑。

第 3 條　本法所定調查，其具體措施如下：

　　　　一、疫情調查：為瞭解經通報之傳染病個案之感染地、接觸史、旅遊史及有無疑似病例所為之各種措施。

　　　　二、流行病學調查：為瞭解傳染病發生之原因、流行狀況及傳染模式所為之各種措施。

　　　　三、病媒調查：為瞭解地區病媒之種類、密度及其消長等所為之各種措施。

　　　　四、其他調查：前三款調查以外，為瞭解傳染病發生之狀況及原因，所為之各種措施。

第 4 條　本法所稱檢驗，指為確定診斷或研判疫情，由實驗室就相關檢體進行化驗、鑑定或其他必要之檢查等行為。

第 5 條　本法所稱疫區，指有傳染病流行或有疫情通報，經中央或地方主管機關依本法第八條第一項規定發布之國際疫區或國內疫區。

第 5-1 條　本法第九條所定傳播媒體之範圍，包括平面或電子新聞媒體、網際網路，及以有線、無線、衛星或其他電子傳輸設施傳送聲音、影像、文字或數據者。

本法第九條所定錯誤或不實訊息之發表人，包括自然人及法人在內。

第 6 條　本法第二十三條所稱各種已經證實媒介傳染病之飲食物品、動物或動物屍體，指經主管機關調查或檢驗其可致傳染於人者。

第 7 條　地方主管機關依本法第二十五條第二項規定所為之通知，應以書面為之。但情況急迫者，不在此限。

第 8 條　地方主管機關依本法第三十八條規定所為之通知，得以書面、言詞或電子資料傳輸等方式為之。

第 9 條　未經指定為隔離治療機構之醫療機構，發現各類應隔離治療之傳染病病人，應配合各級主管機關依本法第四十四條第一項規定所為處置，依醫療法等相關法令規定進行轉診事宜。

第 10 條　本法第四十四條第一項第二款所稱必要時，指該傳染病病人有傳染他人之虞時。

本法第四十四條第三項所定由中央主管機關支應之各類傳染病病人施行隔離治療之費用，指比照全民健康保險醫療服務給付項目及支付標準核付之醫療費用及隔離治療機構之膳食費。

負擔家計之傳染病病人，因隔離治療致影響其家計者，主管機關得依社會救助法等相關法令予以救助。

第 11 條　主管機關依本法第四十八條第一項規定為留驗、檢查或施行預防接種等必要處置時，應注意當事人之身體及名譽，並不得逾必要之程度。

第 12 條　醫事機構或該管主管機關依本法第四十九條規定施行必要之消毒或其他適當之處置時，應依傳染病種類及其傳染特性，於傳染病病人原居留之病房或住（居）所內外，對可能受到體液、分泌物與排泄物污染之場所及物品，或潛在可能具有傳染性之病媒，執行清潔、消毒、殺菌、滅蟲及進行具感染性廢棄物之清理等相關措施。

第 13 條　醫事機構依本法第五十條第一項規定施行消毒及其他必要處置時，應依感染管制相關規定，對因傳染病或疑似傳染病致死之屍體，施予終末消毒；相關人員於執行臨終護理、終末消毒、屍體運送、病理解剖及入殮過程中，應著個人防護衣具，以防範感染；主管機關處置社區內因傳染病或疑似傳染病致死之屍體時，亦同。

前項屍體，如係因疑似第一類傳染病或第五類傳染病所致者，應先以具防護功能之屍袋包覆，留置適當場所妥善冰存，並儘速處理。

第 14 條　本法第五十條第四項所定二十四小時之起算時點如下：

一、屍體經中央主管機關依本法第五十條第二項規定施行病理解剖者，自解剖完成時起算。

二、無前款情形者，自醫師開具死亡證明書或檢察機關開具相驗屍體證明書時起算。

本法第五十條第四項所稱依規定深埋，指深埋之棺面應深入地面一公尺二十公分以下。

第 15 條　中央主管機關依第五十條第二項、第三項規定施行病理解剖檢驗前，應會同地方主管機關確實與死者家屬充分溝通，始得作成傳染病或疑似傳染病屍體病理解剖檢驗通知書，或疑似預防接種致死屍體病理解剖檢驗通知書，送達死者家屬。

第 16 條　中央主管機關為因應傳染病防治需要，得委任所屬疾病管制署辦理下列事項：

一、依本法第三十四條規定之感染性生物材料與實驗室生物安全管理事項。

二、依本法第三十九條第四項規定要求醫事機構、醫師或法醫師限期提供傳染病病人或疑似疫苗接種後產生不良反應個案之相關資料。

三、本法第四十六條第一項第一款傳染病檢體採檢及第二款檢驗機構管理之相關規定。

四、本法第五十條第二項、第三項規定之傳染病或疑似傳染病,或疑似預防接種致死屍體之病理解剖檢驗相關事項。

五、本法第五十八條至第六十條規定之國際及指定特殊港埠檢疫相關事項。

第 17 條　本細則自發布日施行。

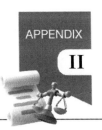

Tetanus (Lockjaw; Neonatal Tetanus)
(ICD-10 A33)

The word tetanus comes from the Ancient Greek: τέτανος, romanized: tetanos, means 'to stretch'. Tetanus, also known as lockjaw, is a bacterial infection caused by *Clostridium tetani* and characterized by muscle spasms. In the most common type, the spasms begin in the jaw, and then progress to the rest of the body. Each spasm usually lasts for a few minutes. Spasms occur frequently for three to four weeks. Some spasms may be severe enough to fracture bones. Other symptoms of tetanus may include fever, sweating, headache, trouble swallowing, high blood pressure, and a fast heart rate. Onset of symptoms is typically 3 to 21 days following infection. Recovery may take months, but about 10% of cases prove to be fatal.

🔸 Identification to the Tetanus:

Tetanus often begins with mild spasms in the jaw muscles—also known as lockjaw. Similar spasms can also be a feature of trismus. The spasms can also affect the facial muscles, resulting in an appearance called risus sardonicus (is a highly characteristic, abnormal, sustained spasm of the facial muscles that appears to produce grinning). Chest, neck, back, abdominal muscles, and buttocks may be affected. Back muscle spasms often cause arching, called opisthotonus. Sometimes, the spasms affect muscles utilized during inhalation and exhalation, which can lead to breathing problems.

Prolonged muscular action causes sudden, powerful, and painful contractions of muscle groups, called tetany. These episodes can cause fractures and muscle tears. Other symptoms include fever, headache, restlessness, irritability, feeding difficulties, breathing problems, burning sensation during urination, urinary retention, and loss of stool control. Even with treatment, about 10% of people who contract tetanus die. The mortality rate is higher in unvaccinated individuals, and in people over 60 years of age.

Infectious agent:

Clostridium tetani. A rod-shaped, Gram-positive bacterium, typically up to 0.5 μm wide and 2.5 μm long. It is motile by way of various flagellums that surround its body. Spores of tetanus bacteria are everywhere in the environment, including soil, dust, and manure. The spores develop into bacteria when they enter the body. *C. tetani* cannot grow in the presence of oxygen. It grows best at temperatures ranging from 33 - 37 °C. Unlike other vaccine-preventable diseases, tetanus is not spread from person to person.

Occurrence:

Tetanus occurs in all parts of the world but is most frequent in hot and wet climates where the soil has a high organic content. In 2015, there were about 209,000 infections and about 59,000 deaths globally. This is down from 356,000 deaths in 1990. In the US, there are about 30 cases per year, almost all of which were in people who had not been vaccinated. An early description of the disease was made by Hippocrates in the 5th century BC. The cause of the disease was determined in 1884 by Antonio Carle and Giorgio Rattone at the University of Turin, and a vaccine was developed in 1924.

The disease occurs almost exclusively in people who are inadequately immunized. It is more common in hot, damp climates with soil rich in organic matter. Manure-treated soils may contain spores, as they are widely distributed in the intestines and feces of many animals, such as horses, sheep, cattle, dogs, cats, rats, guinea pigs, and chickens. In agricultural areas, a significant number of human adults may harbor the organism.

Reservoir:

Soil is the main reservoir of *C. tetani* but many animals, both herbivores and omnivores, carry the bacilli in their intestines and excrete the spores in their faeces. The spores can also be found on skin surfaces and in sewage water. Rarely, tetanus can be contracted through surgical procedures, intramuscular injections, compound fractures, and dental infections. Animal bites can transmit tetanus.

Mode of transmission:

Tetanus is different from other vaccine-preventable diseases because it does not spread from person to person. Tetanus is spread by the direct transfer of *C. tetani* spores from soil and excreta of animals and humans to wounds and cuts. It is not transmitted from person to person.

Incubation period:

Incubation period is varying from 3-21 days, with an average of 8 days. In neonatal tetanus, symptoms usually appear from 4 - 14 days after birth, averaging about 7 days.

Period of communicability:

Tetanus is not contagious from person to person. It is the only vaccine-preventable disease that is infectious, but not contagious.

Susceptibility and resistance:

The risk of death from tetanus is highest among people 60 years of age or older. Diabetes, a history of immunosuppression, and intravenous drug use may be risk factors for tetanus. People cannot naturally acquire immunity to tetanus, the best way to prevent tetanus is to vaccinate your patients. CDC recommends tetanus vaccines for all infants and children, preteens and adolescents, and adults. A complete vaccine series has a clinical efficacy of virtually 100% for tetanus.

Methods of control:

Tetanus can be prevented by vaccination with tetanus toxoid. In children under the age of 2 months, the tetanus vaccine is often administered as a combined vaccine, DPT/DTaP vaccine, which also includes vaccines against diphtheria and pertussis. For adults and children over seven, the Td vaccine (tetanus and diphtheria) or Tdap (tetanus, diphtheria, and acellular pertussis) is commonly used.

1. Post-exposure prophylaxis:

Tetanus toxoid can be given in case of suspected exposure to tetanus. In such cases, it can be given with or without tetanus immunoglobulin (also called tetanus antibodies or tetanus antitoxin). It can be given as intravenous therapy or by intramuscular injection.

2. Mild cases of tetanus can be treated with:

Tetanus immunoglobulin (TIG), also called tetanus antibodies or tetanus antitoxin. It can be given as intravenous therapy or by intramuscular injection. Antibiotic therapy to reduce toxin production. Metronidazole intravenous (IV) injection is a preferred treatment. Benzodiazepines can be used to control muscle spasms. Options include diazepam and lorazepam, oral or IV.

3. Severe cases will require admission to intensive care.

Table Principles of tetanus prevention and treatment measures for wounds after injury

Type of wound / Treatment measure / Tetanus immunity situation	Clean, minor wounds		All other wounds	
	Tdap or Td* (or Toxoid)	TIG	Tdap or Td* (or Toxoid)	TIG
Unknown or less than 3 doses of tetanus toxoid containing vaccine	Recommend catch-up vaccination	No indication	Recommend catch-up vaccination	Recommend catch-up vaccination
3 or more doses of tetanus toxoid containing vaccine	No indication (But the last dose has passed Those with 10 years need to booster)	No indication	No indication (But the last dose has passed Those with 5 years need to booster)	No indication

(CDC, Taiwan, 2023)

Note:
1. Active immunity vaccine:
   (1) Tdap: Tetanus toxoid and diphtheria with acellular pertussis vaccine
   (2) Td: Tetanus toxoid with diphtheria vaccine
   (3) Toxoid: Tetanus toxoid
2. Passive immunity vaccine:
   (1) TIG: Tetanus immunoglobulin

RRFERENCES

Adak T, Sharma V, Orlov V (1998). "Studies on the Plasmodium vivax relapse pattern in Delhi, India.". *Am J Trop Med Hyg* **59** (1): 175-9.

Adams S, Brown H, Turner G (2002). "Breaking down the blood-brain barrier: signaling a path to cerebral malaria?". *Trends Parasitol* **18** (8): 360-6.

Alan G. Barbour and Wolfram R. Zückert (1997). Genome sequencing: New tricks of tick-borne pathogen. *Nature* **390**, 553-554 (11 December 1997), doi: 10.1038/37475.

Arevalo J, Ramirez L, Adaui V, *et al.* (2007). "Influence of Leishmania (Viannia) species on the response to antimonial treatment in patients with American tegumentary leishmaniasis". *J Infect Dis* **195**: 1846–51.

Aylward R (2006). Eradicating polio: today's challenges and tomorrow's legacy. *Ann Trop Med Parasitol* **100** (5–6): 401–13.

Badaro R, Lobo I, Munõs A, *et al.* (2006). "Immunotherapy for drug-refractory mucosal leishmaniasis". *J Infect Dis* **194**: 1151–59.Baillie, Mike (1997). *A Slice Through Time*, p124.

Baker JP, Katz SL (2004). "Childhood vaccine development: an overview". *Pediatr. Res.* **55** (2): 347-56.

Balentine J and Kessler D (March 7, 2006). "Scarlet Fever". *eMedicine.* emerg/518.

Bannister B.A., Begg N.T. and Gillespie S.H. (2000). Infectious disease. 2nd Ed. Blackwell Science Ltd.

Barnett, ED (March 2007). "Yellow fever: epidemiology and prevention.". *Clin Infect Dis* **44** (6): 850-6.

Bastida G, Nos P, Aguas M, Beltrán B, Rubín A, Dasí F, Ponce J (2005). "Incidence, risk factors and clinical course of thiopurine-induced liver injury in patients with inflammatory bowel disease.". *Aliment Pharmacol Ther* **22** (9): 775-82.

Bell C, Devarajan S, Gersbach H (2003). "*The long-run economic costs of AIDS: theory and an application to South Africa*" (PDF). World Bank Policy Research Working Paper No. 3152. Retrieved on 2008-04-28.

Bonah C (2005). "The 'experimental stable' of the BCG vaccine: safety, efficacy, proof, and standards, 1921–1933". *Stud Hist Philos Biol Biomed Sci* **36** (4): 696–721.

Bruce AJ, Rogers RS (2004). "Oral manifestations of sexually transmitted diseases". *Clin. Dermatol.* **22** (6): 520–7.

Call S, Vollenweider M, Hornung C, Simel D, McKinney W (2005). "Does this patient have influenza?". *JAMA* **293** (8): 987-97.

Carter JA, Ross AJ, Neville BG, Obiero E, Katana K, Mung'ala-Odera V, Lees JA, Newton CR (2005). "Developmental impairments following severe falciparum malaria in children". *Trop Med Int Health* **10**: 3-10.

CDC (2005-07-06). Lyme Disease Erythema Migrans.

Centers for Disease Control (2003). SARS local transmission in Taiwan (CDC/DOH, Taiwan).

Centers for Disease Control (2007). Alert level of meningococcal meningitis in Taiwan, 2006-2007 (CDC/DOH, Taiwan).

Centers for Disease Control, USA (2012). Levels of endemicity for hepatitis E virus (www.cdc.gov/hepatitis/HEV/HEV fag.htm).

Chabria SB, Lawrason J (2007). "Altered mental status, an unusual manifestation of early disseminated Lyme disease: A case report" *J. Med. Case Reports.* **1** (1): 62.

Chaves SS, Gargiullo P, Zhang JX, *et al.* (2007). "Loss of vaccine-induced immunity to varicella over time". *N Engl J Med* **356** (11): 1121–9.

Chen Q, Schlichtherle M, Wahlgren M (2000). "Molecular aspects of severe malaria.". *Clin Microbiol Rev* **13** (3): 439-50.

Cohen JI (2004). Chapter 175: Enteroviruses and Reoviruses, in Kasper DL, Braunwald E, Fauci AS, *et al* (eds.): Harrison's Principles of Internal Medicine, 16th ed., McGraw-Hill Professional, 1144.

Cooke FJ, Wain J, Threlfall EJ (2006). "Fluoroquinolone resistance in *Salmonella* Typhi (letter)". *Brit Med J* **333** (7563): 353–4.

Cox F (2002). "History of human parasitology.". *Clin Microbiol Rev* **15** (4): 595-612.

Cox FE (2002). "History of human parasitology". *Clin. Microbiol. Rev.* **15** (4): 595-612.

Dayan GH, Castillo-Solórzano C, Nava M, *et al* (2006). "Efforts at rubella elimination in the United States: the impact of hemispheric rubella control". *Clin. Infect. Dis.* **43 Suppl 3**: S158–63.

Dengue Fever – Information Sheet. World Health Organization, October 9, 2006. Retrieved on 2007-11-30.

Digestive System Diagram (2005).Los Altos Feeding Clinic, 2235 Grant Rd. Ste 2Los Altos, CA 94024.

Donta ST (2002). "Late and chronic Lyme disease". *Med Clin North Am* **86** (2): 341-9.

Dyne P and McCartan K (October 19, 2005). "Pediatrics, Scarlet Fever". *eMedicine.* emerg/402.

Edlich RF, Winters KL, Long WB, Gubler KD (2005). "Rubella and congenital rubella (German measles)". *J Long Term Eff Med Implants* **15** (3): 319–28.

Eichelberger, L. (2007) SARS and New York's Chinatown: The politics of risk and blame during an epidemic of fear. *Social Science and Medicine* **65**(6):1284-95.

Elbers A, Koch G, Bouma A (2005). "Performance of clinical signs in poultry for the detection of outbreaks during the avian influenza A (H7N7) epidemic in The Netherlands in 2003.". *Avian Pathol* **34** (3): 181-7.

Epidemic and Pandemic Alert and Response (EPR), World Health Organization (WHO)

Escalante A, Freeland D, Collins W, Lal A (1998). "The evolution of primate malaria parasites based on the gene encoding cytochrome b from the linear mitochondrial genome.". *Proc Natl Acad Sci U S A* **95** (14): 8124-9.

Fact sheets: Pharyngitis. www.bupa.co.uk/individuals/health-information/directory/p/pharyngitis

Fatahzadeh M, Schwartz RA (2007). "Human herpes simplex virus infections: epidemiology, pathogenesis, symptomatology, diagnosis, and management". *J. Am. Acad. Dermatol.* **57** (5): 737–63; quiz 764–6.

Feldman C (2005). "Pneumonia associated with HIV infection". *Curr. Opin. Infect. Dis.* **18** (2): 165–170.

Fidel PL (2002). "Immunity to Candida". *Oral Dis.* **8**: 69-75.

Fine P, Floyd S, Stanford J, Nkhosa P, Kasunga A, Chaguluka S, Warndorff D, Jenkins P, Yates M, Ponnighaus J (2001). "Environmental mycobacteria in northern Malawi: implications for the epidemiology of tuberculosis and leprosy". *Epidemiol Infect* **126** (3): 379-87.

Fouchier, RAM, Kuiken, T, Schutten, M et al (2003). Aetiology: Koch's postulates fulfilled for SARS virus. *Nature* **423**:240.

Gambel JM, DeFraites R, Hoke C, *et al.* (1995). "Japanese encephalitis vaccine: persistence of antibody up to 3 years after a three-dose primary series (letter)". *J Infect Dis* **171**: 1074.

Gao F, Bailes E, Robertson DL, et al (1999). "Origin of HIV-1 in the Chimpanzee Pan troglodytes troglodytes". *Nature* **397** (6718): 436–441.

Gottfried, Robert S. (1983). The Black Death. New York: The Free Press.

Gubler DJ (1998). "Dengue and dengue hemorrhagic fever". *Clin. Microbiol. Rev.* **11** (3): 480–96.

Gupta R, Warren T, Wald A (2007). "Genital herpes". *Lancet* **370** (9605): 2127–37.

Guss DA (1994). "The acquired immune deficiency syndrome: an overview for the emergency physician, Part 1". *J. Emerg. Med.* **12** (3): 375–384.

Guss DA (1994). "The acquired immune deficiency syndrome: an overview for the emergency physician, Part 2". *J. Emerg. Med.* **12** (4): 491–497.

Harris J, Khan A, LaRocque R, Dorer D, Chowdhury F, Faruque A, Sack D, Ryan E, Qadri F, Calderwood S (2005). "Blood group, immunity, and risk of infection with *Vibrio cholerae* in an area of endemicity". *Infect Immun* **73** (11): 7422-7.

Hayashi T, Hayashi K, Maeda M, Kojima I (1996). "Calcium spirulan, an inhibitor of enveloped virus replication, from a blue-green alga Spirulina platensis". *J Nat Prod* **59** (1): 83-7.

Health Protection Agency. The gonococcal resistance to antimicrobials surveillance programme: Annual report 2005. Retrieved on 2006-10-28.

Henneberg M, Henneberg RJ (2002). "Reconstructing Medical Knowledge in Ancient Pompeii from the Hard Evidence of Bones and Teeth", in J Renn, G Castagnetti (eds): *Homo Faber: Studies on Nature. Technology and*

Science at the Time of Pompeii,. Rome: "L'ERMA" di Bretschneider, pp.169-187.

Hepatitis C: Global Prevalence: Update 2003(World Health Organisation (1999). Wkly Epid Rec. 1997; 74: 425-427; Farci P. et al. (2000). Semin Liver Dis. 2000; 20: 103-126; Wasley A et al. Semin Liver Dis. 2000; 20: 1-16).

Heuner K, Swanson M (editors). (2008). *Legionella: Molecular Microbiology.* Caister Academic Press.

Heymann D.L. (2004). "Control of communicable diseases manual" 18th Ed. WHO. APHA.

Hviid A, Rubin S, Mühlemann K (2008). "Mumps". *Lancet* **371** (9616): 932–44.

Iademarco MF, Castro KG (2003). "Epidemiology of tuberculosis". *Seminars in respiratory infections* **18** (4): 225-40.

Influenza: Viral Infections: Merck Manual Home Edition. Retrieved on 2008-03-15, from http://www.merck.com.

Joy D, Feng X, Mu J, *et al* (2003). "Early origin and recent expansion of Plasmodium falciparum.". *Science* **300** (5617): 318-21.

Judith M. Bennett and C. Warren Hollister, *Medieval Europe: A Short History* (New York: McGraw-Hill, 2006), 372.

Kanra G, Isik P, Kara A, Cengiz AB, Secmeer G, Ceyhan M (2004). "Complementary findings in clinical and epidemiologic features of mumps and mumps meningoencephalitis in children without mumps vaccination". *Pediatr Int* **46** (6): 663-8.

Karch H, Tarr P, Bielaszewska M (2005). "Enterohaemorrhagic *Escherichia coli* in human medicine.". *Int J Med Microbiol* **295** (6-7): 405–18.

Kasper DL, Braunwald E, Fauci AS, Hauser SL, Longo DL, Jameson JL, Isselbacher KJ, Eds. (2004). *Harrison's Principles of Internal Medicine*, 16th, McGraw-Hill Professional.

Ken K.S. wang. 2002. Environmental Hygienic Vector Control. New Wun Ching Developmental Publishing Co., Ltd. 86pp

Kerr AA, McQuillin J, Downham MA, Gardner PS (1975). "Gastric 'flu influenza B causing abdominal symptons in children". *Lancet* **1** (7902): 291–5.

Khandekar R, Sudhan A, Jain BK, Shrivastav K, Sachan R (2007). "Pediatric cataract and surgery outcomes in Central India: a hospital based study.". *Indian J Med Sci* **61** (1): 15–22.

Koelle DM, Corey L (2008). "Herpes Simplex: Insights on Pathogenesis and Possible Vaccines". *Annu Rev Med* **59**: 381–395.

Kurane I, Takashi T (2000). "Immunogenicity and protective efficacy of the current inactivated Japanese encephalitis vaccine against different Japanese encephalitis virus strains". *Vaccine* **18 Suppl**: 33–5.

Lau, SKP, Woo, PCY, Li, KSM et al. (2005). Severe acute respiratory syndrome coronavirus-like virus in Chinese horseshoe bats. *Proceedings of the National Academy of Sciences* **102**(29):14040–14045.

Lee JY, Bowden DS (2000). "Rubella virus replication and links to teratogenicity". *Clin. Microbiol. Rev.* **13** (4): 571-87.

Leone P (2005). "Reducing the risk of transmitting genital herpes: advances in understanding and therapy". *Curr Med Res Opin* **21** (10): 1577–82.

Li, W, Shi, A, Yu, M et al (2005) Bats are natural reservoirs of SARS-like coronaviruses. *Science* **310**(5748):676–679.

Lowen AC, Mubareka S, Steel J, Palese P (2007). "Influenza virus transmission is dependent on relative humidity and temperature". *PLoS Pathog.* **3** (10): 1470–6.

Magnarelli L, Anderson J (1988). "Ticks and biting insects infected with the etiologic agent of Lyme disease, *Borrelia burgdorferi.*" (PDF). *J Clin Microbiol* **26** (8): 1482-6.

Mattoo S, Cherry JD (2005). "Molecular pathogenesis, epidemiology, and clinical manifestations of respiratory infections due to *Bordetella pertussis* and other *Bordetella* subspecies". *Clin Microbiol Rev* **18** (2): 326-82.

McCormick, M (2003). "Rats, Communications, and Plague: Toward an Ecological History," *Journal of Interdisciplinary History* **34**: 25.

McLeod K (2000). "Our sense of Snow: John Snow in medical geography". *Soc Sci Med* **50** (7-8): 923-35.

McPherson RA, Pincus MR(2007) *Henry's Clinical Diagnosis and Management by Laboratory Methods* (21st ed). Chapter 54. W.B. Saanders Company.

Medical Health Infromation (2014).Diarrhea related to pathogenic germs. www.Hostgator.com/1penny.

Mendis K, Sina B, Marchesini P Carter R (2001). "The neglected burden of Plasmodium vivax malaria.". *Am J Trop Med Hyg* **64** (1-2 Suppl): 97-106.

MMWR, Weekly Special issue of Epidemiologic Notes and Reports Follow-up on Respiratory Illness –Philadelphia (reprinted January 24, 1997, Vol **46**(03); 50-56)

MMWR. Weekly March 21. 2008/55(53); 1-94, from http://www.cdc.gov/mmwr/preview/mmwrhtml/mm5553a1.htm

Mondal D, Petri Jr WA, Sack RB, *et al.* (2006). "*Entamoeba histolytica*-associated diarreal illness is negatively associated with the growth of preschool shildren: evidence from a prospective study". *Trans R Soc Trop Med H* **100** (11): 1032–38.

Moosa MY, Sobel JD, Elhalis H, Du W, Akins RA (2004). "Fungicidal activity of fluconazole against Candida albicans in a synthetic vagina-simulative medium". *Antimicrob. Agents Chemother.* **48** (1): 161–7.

Murin S, Bilello K (2005). "Respiratory tract infections: another reason not to smoke.". *Cleve Clin J Med* **72** (10): 916-20.

Nadir A, Reddy D, Van Thiel DH (2000). "Cascara sagrada-induced intrahepatic cholestasis causing portal hypertension: case report and review of herbal hepatotoxicity". *Am. J. Gastroenterol.* **95** (12): 3634-7.

nu107018 www.fotosearch.com

Odds FC (1987). "Candida infections: an overview". *Crit. Rev. Microbiol.* **15** (1): 1–5.

Palefsky J (2007). "Human papillomavirus infection in HIV-infected persons". *Top HIV Med* **15** (4): 130–3.

Palella FJ Jr, Delaney KM, Moorman AC, et al (1998). "Declining morbidity and mortality among patients with advanced human immunodeficiency virus infection. HIV Outpatient Study Investigators". *N. Engl. J. Med* **338** (13): 853–860.

Pappas PG (2006). "Invasive candidiasis". *Infect. Dis. Clin. North Am.* **20** (3): 485–506.

Parker A, Staggs W, Dayan G *et al.* (2006). "Implications of a 2005 measles outbreak in Indiana for sustained elimination of measles in the United States". *N Engl J Med* **355** (5): 447–55.

Peltola H, Kulkarni PS, Kapre SV, Paunio M, Jadhav SS, Dhere RM (2007). "Mumps outbreaks in Canada and the United States: Time for new thinking on mumps vaccines". *Clin Infect Dis* **45**: 459–66.

Petersen LR, Marfin AA (2005). "Shifting epidemiology of Flaviviridae". *J Travel Med* **12 Suppl 1**: S3-11.

Raviglione MC, O'Brien RJ (2004). "Tuberculosis", in Kasper DL, Braunwald E, Fauci AS, Hauser SL, Longo DL, Jameson JL, Isselbacher KJ, eds.: *Harrison's Principles of Internal Medicine*, 16th ed., McGraw-Hill Professional, 953–66.

Reid AH, Fanning TG, Hultin JV, Taubenberger JK (1999). "Origin and evolution of the 1918 "Spanish" influenza virus hemagglutinin gene". *Proc. Natl. Acad. Sci. U.S.A.* **96** (4): 1651-6.

Restrepo BI (2007). "Convergence of the tuberculosis and diabetes epidemics: renewal of old acquaintances". *Clin Infect Dis* **45**: 436–8.

Rhinehart E. and McGoldrick M. (2006). "Infection control in home care and hospital". 2nd Ed. Jones, Bartlett publishers Sudburry Massachusetts. pp. 7-14.

Richard B. Jamess, MD, PhD (2006). "Syphilis- Sexually Transmitted Infections, 2006.". *Sexually transmitted diseases treatment guidelines*. Retrieved from http://www.health.am/sex/syphilis/.

Richardson M, Elliman D, Maguire H, Simpson J, Nicoll A (2001). "Evidence base of incubation periods, periods of infectiousness and exclusion policies for the control of communicable diseases in schools and preschools". *Pediatr. Infect. Dis. J.* **20** (4): 380–91.

Rima BK, Earle JA, Yeo RP, Herlihy L, Baczko K, ter Muelen V, Carabana J, Caballero M, Celma ML, Fernandez-Munoz R (1995). Temporal and geographical distribution of measles virus genotypes. *J Gen Virol* **76**:1173–1180.

Rothman AL (2004). "Dengue: defining protective versus pathologic immunity". *J. Clin. Invest.* **113** (7): 946–51.

Rothschild B, Martin L, Lev G, Bercovier H, Bar-Gal G, Greenblatt C, Donoghue H, Spigelman M, Brittain D (2001). "Mycobacterium tuberculosis complex DNA from an extinct bison dated 17,000 years before the present". *Clin Infect Dis* **33** (3): 305-11.

Ryan KJ, Ray CG (editors) (2004). *Sherris Medical Microbiology*, 4th ed., McGraw Hill, 299–302.

Ryan KJ, Ray CG (editors) (2004). *Sherris Medical Microbiology*, 4th ed., McGraw Hill, 434–7.

Ryder S, Beckingham I (2001). "ABC of diseases of liver, pancreas, and biliary system: Acute hepatitis". *BMJ* **322** (7279): 151-153.

SARS in China square 3 (2002). Canadian Environmental Health Atlas. www.ehatlas.ca

Scheinfeld N, Lehman DS (2006). An evidence-based review of medical and surgical treatments of genital warts. *Dermatol Online J* **12** (3): 5.

Shafer MA, Moscicki AB (2006). "Sexually Transmitted Infections, 2006." *Sexually Transmitted Infections*: 1-8. Retrieved Apr. 04, from http://www.health.am.

Shukla N, Poles M (2004). "Hepatitis B virus infection: co-infection with hepatitis C virus, hepatitis D virus, and human immunodeficiency virus.". *Clin Liver Dis* **8** (2): 445-60.

Skoulidis F, Morgan MS, MacLeod KM (2004). "Penicillium marneffei: a pathogen on our doorstep?". *J. R. Soc. Med.* **97** (2): 394–396.

Snow RW, Guerra CA, Noor AM, Myint HY, Hay SI (2005). "The global distribution of clinical episodes of Plasmodium falciparum malaria". *Nature* **434** (7030): 214-7.

Sobero R, Peabody J (2006). "Tuberculosis control in Bolivia, Chile, Colombia and Peru: why does incidence vary so much between neighbors?". *Int J Tuberc Lung Dis* **10** (11): 1292–5.

Soto J, Toledo JT (2007). "Oral miltefosine to treat new world cutaneous leishmaniasis". *Lancet Infect Dis* **7** (1): 7.

Steere AC, Sikand VK, Schoen RT, Nowakowski J (2003). "Asymptomatic infection with *Borrelia burgdorferi*". *Clin. Infect. Dis.* **37** (4): 528-32.

Stegmann BJ, Carey JC (2002). "TORCH Infections. Toxoplasmosis, Other (syphilis, varicella-zoster, parvovirus B19), Rubella, Cytomegalovirus (CMV), and Herpes infections". *Curr Womens Health Rep* **2** (4): 253–8.

Suarez, D; Spackman E, Senne D, Bulaga L, Welsch A, Froberg K (2003). "The effect of various disinfectants on detection of avian influenza virus by real time RT-PCR". *Avian Dis* **47** (3 Suppl): 1091–5.

Sundar S, Chakravarty J, Rai VK, *et al.* (2007). "Amphotericin B Treatment for Indian Visceral Leishmaniasis: Response to 15 Daily versus Alternate-Day Infusions". *Clin Infect Dis* **45**: 556–561.

Takhampunya R, Ubol S, Houng HS, Cameron CE, Padmanabhan R (2006). "Inhibition of dengue virus replication by mycophenolic acid and ribavirin". *J. Gen. Virol.* **87** (Pt 7): 1947–52.

Tang J, Kaslow RA (2003). "The impact of host genetics on HIV infection and disease progression in the era of highly active antiretroviral therapy". *AIDS* **17** (Suppl 4): S51–S60.

Tebruegge M, Kuruvilla M, Margarson I (2006). "Does the use of calamine or antihistamine provide symptomatic relief from pruritus in children with varicella zoster infection?". *Arch. Dis. Child.* **91** (12): 1035-6.

Tom Solomon (2006). "Control of Japanese Encephalitis—within our grasp?" **355** (9): 869-871.

Trichomoniasis at EMedicine. Aug. 10, 2005. Retrieved Mar. 11, 2008, from http://www.emedicinehealth.com/trichomoniasis/page3_em.htm

Typhoid Mary: An Urban Historical publisher=Anthony Bourdain Hardcover. New York. 2001:148. ISBN 1582341338

US Centers for Disease Control and Prevention. Varicella Treatment Questions & Answers. *CDC Guidelines*. CDC. Retrieved on 2007-08-23.

Vaginitis/Trichomoniasis:Treatment for trichomoniasis, American Social Heath Association. Retrieved March 12, 2008.

Versteegh FGA, Schellekens JFP, Fleer A, Roord JJ. (2005). "Pertussis: a concise historical review including diagnosis, incidence, clinical manifestations and the role of treatment and vaccination in management.". *Rev Med Microbiol* **16** (3): 79–89.

Walter T, Lebouche B, Miailhes P, *et al.* (2006). "Symptomatic relapse of neurologic syphilis after benzathine penicillin G therapy for primary or secondary syphilis in HIV-infected patients". *Clin Infect Dis* **43** (6): 787-90.

Webber D, Kremer M (2001). Stimulating Industrial R&D for Neglected Infectious Diseases: Economic Perspectives (PDF). *Bulletin of the World Health Organization* **79**(8): 693–801.

WHO Confirmed Human Cases of H5N1 Data published by WHO Epidemic and Pandemic Alert and Response (EPR). Accessed 24 Oct. 2006.

WHO. Summary of probable SARS cases with onset of illness from 1 November 2002 to 31 July 2003.

Workowski K, Berman S (2006). "Sexually transmitted diseases treatment guidelines, 2006.". *MMWR Recomm Rep* **55** (RR-11): 1-94.

World Health Organisation (2007). Current WHO phases of pandemic alert.

World Health Organisation (2007). Diphtheria global annual reported incidence and DTP3 coverage, 1980-2006. WHO/IVB database.

World Health Organisation (2007). Individual infection progress. *Weekly epidemiological record.*

World Health Organisation (2007). Poliomyelitis global annual reported incidence and vaccine IPV (Pol 3) coverage, 1980-2006. WHO/IVB database.

World Health Organisation (2007). The trend of global disease. *Weekly epidemiological record.*

World Health Organisation (2008). "Typhoid vaccines: WHO position paper". *Weekly epidemiological record* **83** (6): 49–60.

Wu J, Chen C, Sheen I, Lee S, Tzeng H, Choo K (1995). "Evidence of transmission of hepatitis D virus to spouses from sequence analysis of the viral genome.". *Hepatology* **22** (6): 1656-60.

www.doctortipster.com

www.eastmed.co.nz/meningitis-children-adults-symptoms-signs-vaccination-vaccine.php

www.healthylive world.com

www.jica.jp/english/publications/report/network/archive_2004/vol_24_3.html

www.life in the fastlane.com

www.nidss.cdc.gov.tw/en/NIDSS_diagram Figure 5-2.aspx?dt

www.pathmicro.med.sc.edu/virol/picorna.htm

www.patient.co.uk

www.som.flinders.edu.au/Fuswikis/dsrswikiol/doku.php?id

www.who.int.immunization/monitoring_surveillance/burden/vpd/surveill
ance_type/passive/pertussis/en/

www.who.int/immunization/monitoring_surveillance/burden/diphtheria/e
n/ index.html

www.who.int/immunization_monitoring/diseases/poliomyetis/en/index.ht
ml

Yellow fever fact sheet. *WHO—Yellow fever*. Retrieved on 2006-04-18.

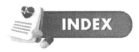

F

I

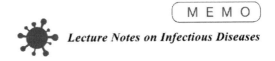

MEMO

Lecture Notes on Infectious Diseases

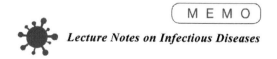

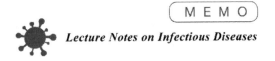

MEMO

Lecture Notes on Infectious Diseases

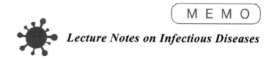

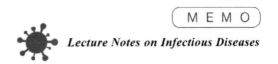

MEMO

Lecture Notes on Infectious Diseases

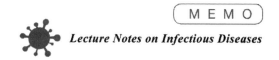

Lecture Notes on Infectious Diseases, 4th Edition

Author: Ken K. S. Wang

Publisher: New Wun Ching Developmental Publishing Co., Ltd.
   9F, No. 362, Sec. 2, Zhongshan Rd., Zhonghe Dist., New Taipei City 235026, Taiwan
   +886-2-2244 8188
Publication date: July 15th,2024
Suggested retail price: New Taiwan dollar (NT$) 580

ISBN 978-626-392-026-2

To customers outside Taiwan (R.O.C.):
You can view the introduction of this book on:
https://www.wun-ching.com.tw/book_detail.asp?seq=13344
If you want to buy this book, please write an email to inform us the quantity you want to purchase and the address you can receive the books, then we will tell you how to completed the purchasing.
Our email address for overseas customers: crm@wun-ching.com.tw